PLE

MCQs IN MEDICINE FOR THE FRCA

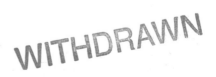

QBASE ANAESTHESIA: 3

MCQs IN MEDICINE FOR THE FRCA

Edited by

Edward J Hammond MA BM BCh MRCP FRCA
Specialist Registrar
Shackleton Department of Anaesthetics
Southampton University Hospital NHS Trust

Andrew K McIndoe MB ChB FRCA
Consultant Anaesthetist
Sir Humphry Davy Department of Anaesthesia
Bristol Royal Infirmary

Contributors
Punit Ramrakha
Emert White
Tom Peck
Justine Nanson
Andrew Padkin
Richard Protheroe
David Jones

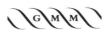

Greenwich Medical Media Ltd
219 The Linen Hall
162-168 Regent Street
London
W1R 5TB

ISBN: 1 900 151 588

First Published 1999

Distributed worldwide by
Oxford University Press

Designed and Produced by
Diane Parker, Saldatore Limited

Printed in Great Britain by
Ashford Colour Press

CONTENTS

FOREWORD

Multiple Choice Examinations (MCQ's) form part of the assessment process in many postgraduate examinations. The MCQ paper is perceived as a threatening test of breadth of knowledge. It is said that the use of negative marking discourages guessing and that candidates fail by answering too many questions. Whilst not a substitute for knowledge and adequate preparation, the assessment of an individuals exam technique can provide valuable feedback that may lead to improved performance. Candidates should remember that knowledge and technique act synergistically to improve scores.

Our experience in teaching MCQ technique to candidates suggests that the advice "do not guess" is not correct. Candidates are consistently surprised at the positive benefits of their educated and wild guesses. From a statistical viewpoint, for true random guesses, the negative marking system employed by the Royal College of Anaesthetists tends to produce a null score rather than a negative score. However, with proper preparation, a candidate's acquisition of knowledge and insight can skew the distribution towards a positive score. This may significantly improve an individual's performance in the MCQ section of the examination. The QBase CD-ROM has been designed to allow candidates to analyse how their guessing strategy affects their performance at MCQ's examinations.

QBase 3: MCQ's in Medicine for the FRCA has been developed in response to comments from candidates sitting the Final FRCA Examination. Many have found revising for the General Medicine component of the examination difficult. This book contains 555 MCQ's in Medicine that complement those in QBase 2. The questions are provided with comprehensive explanations and references for further reading. They broadly cover the subject of General Medicine with a bias towards areas particularly relevant to anaesthesia. Some questions are more difficult than others. Do not be disheartened. They are aimed at the level of knowledge an SHO might be expected to achieve after completing six months of general medicine. The questions have designed to assist your revision of this vast topic rather than just test your knowledge. Candidates specialising in intensive care medicine may find these questions a useful refresher for their general medical knowledge.

The accompanying CD-ROM contains the latest version of the QBase Interactive MCQ Examination software. It allows the candidate to generate customised exams for revision or assessment purposes. Furthermore the system provides detailed structured analysis of performance and exam technique using the unique "Confidence Option" facility. This CD will update previous versions of QBase. It should be used repeatedly to improve exam technique.

We hope that candidates will find this book and CD-ROM a useful adjunct to their revision for the Final FRCA Examination.

Edward Hammond
Andrew McIndoe
QBase Series Developers/Editors
September 1998

NOTES FOR USERS OF QBASE ON CD-ROM

Since we released the first version of QBase, we have tried to respond to the requests and suggestions of trainees on how we can improve it. This latest version of the program contains improvements in the exam analysis functions. These allow you to review your performance based on all the questions in the exam or by subject allowing you to identify areas that need further revision. This also allows you to see whether your technique varies with the subject of the question.

The QBase program resides on your hard disk and reads the data from whatever QBase CD is in your CD drive. If you reinstall QBase from this CD (see back of book for instructions) it will update previous version of the program. Owners of previous QBase titles will then have all the new functions available to them. All QBase CDs will work with the new program. To check for successful installation of the new program, look at the Quick Start Menu screen. It should have 6 exam buttons. Exam 6 will be used by QBase titles containing the appropriate predefined examination.

Many of you have requested shorter examinations. The exams directory on this CD contains a large number of predefined examinations. To access these exams, go to the Main Menu screen and select the 'Resit exam' option. From the dialogue box that appears, select the exam directory on your CD drive and then the exam you wish to attempt. The table that follows gives details of the exams available. You can save the exam to your hard disk as normal. To further enhance your revision, instead of selecting the 'Resit exam' button, we suggest you select the 'Resit shuffled exam' button. The leaves within each question will be randomly shuffled removing your ability to remember the pattern of the answers rather than the facts. The questions in these exams follow the order in the book.

The Autoset an exam option on this CD selects questions from only some of the subjects. You will be presented with exams containing 25 questions made up as follows; Cardiology 6, Respiratory 3, Gastro/Hepatobiliary 2, Renal 2, Neurology 2, Endocrine 2, Haematology 2, Inf Disease 1, Psychiatry 1, Paeds 1, Med Biochem 2, and Pharmacology 1. These shorter exams focus more closely on questions that may appear in the actual Final FRCA paper. The 6 predefined exams on this CD are constructed in this way. You can generate your own customised exams using the "Create your own exam" option. We have provided the revision exams details below to allow you to do all the questions in the book without repetition.

We hope that you will find these notes, suggestions and improvements in the program useful in your preparation for the exam. Don't be discouraged if you only achieve a low overall score at first. The standard of the questions probably exceeds that required of the average anaesthetic trainee sitting the Final FRCA. However the material covered is highly relevant and should also assist your clinical practice.

Edward Hammond
Andrew McIndoe
QBase Series Developers/Editors
September 1998

Exams included in the exams directory of QBase 3

Exam name	No of Questions	Subjects	Type	Time Allowed
Cardio1	20	Cardiology	Revision	40 mins
Cardio2	20	Cardiology	Revision	40 mins
Cardio3	20	Cardiology	Revision	40 mins
Cardio4	20	Cardiology	Revision	40 mins
Cardio5	20	Cardiology	Revision	40 mins
Resp1	20	Respiratory	Revision	40 mins
Resp2	20	Respiratory	Revision	40 mins
Resp3	10	Respiratory	Revision	20 mins
Gastro	25	Gastroenterology	Revision	50 mins
Hepato	25	Hepatobiliary	Revision	50 mins
Renal1	20	Renal	Revision	40 mins
Renal2	10	Renal	Revision	20 mins
Neuro1	20	Neurology	Revision	40 mins
Neuro2	20	Neurology	Revision	40 mins
Neuro3	25	Neurology	Revision	50 mins
Endo1	20	Endocrine	Revision	40 mins
Endo2	15	Endocrine	Revision	30 mins
Metab	10	Metabolism	Revision	20 mins
Haem1	20	Haematology	Revision	40 mins
Haem2	15	Haematology	Revision	30 mins
InfDis1	20	Infectious Dis	Revision	40 mins
InfDis2	10	Infectious Dis	Revision	20 mins
Psych	25	Psychiatry	Revision	50 mins
Subst	10	Substance abuse	Revision	20 mins
Immun	10	Immunology	Revision	20 mins
Paeds	20	Paediatrics	Revision	40 mins
MedBio1	20	Medical Biochem	Revision	40 mins
MedBio2	15	Medical Biochem	Revision	30 mins
Pharm	25	Pharmacology	Revision	50 mins
Rheum	15	Rheumatology	Revision	30 mins
Exam1	25	Mixed	Mock	50 mins
Exam2	25	Mixed	Mock	50 mins
Exam3	25	Mixed	Mock	50 mins
Exam4	25	Mixed	Mock	50 mins
Exam5	25	Mixed	Mock	50 mins
Exam6	25	Mixed	Mock	50 mins

QUESTIONS

CARDIOLOGY

QUESTION 1

The following features are characteristic of Fallot's tetralogy

A. A loud pan-systolic murmur
B. A loud first heart sound
C. Fixed splitting of the second heart sound
D. Atrial fibrillation in 75% of cases
E. Increasing incidence with increasing maternal age

QUESTION 2

Recognised causes of secondary hypertension include

A. Acromegaly
B. Thyrotoxicosis
C. Pregnancy
D. Persistent ductus arteriosus
E. Primary hyperaldosteronism

QUESTION 3

The following drugs are known to cause a prolonged QT interval

A. Amitryptilline
B. Chlorpropramide
C. Sotalol
D. Disopyramide
E. Digoxin

QUESTION 4

Regarding aortic stenosis

A. An ejection click is common in calcific aortic stenosis
B. Subvalvular stenosis is not associated with aortic regurgitation
C. In supravalvular stenosis, the facies may be characteristic
D. May be a cause of unequal upper limb pulses
E. Normal coronary arteries should prompt a search for a non-cardiac cause for chest pain

QUESTION 5

When a patent ductus arteriosus is diagnosed following delivery

A. An ejection systolic murmur is heard
B. Blood flow is usually left to right
C. Closure is encouraged by an increase in the PaO_2
D. Indomethacin may be used to help close the duct
E. Prostacyclin keeps the duct open

QUESTION 6

Pulmonary hypertension is associated with

A. An increased frequency in men if the aetiology is unknown
B. Left atrial myxoma
C. A loud second heart sound
D. Sickle cell disease
E. The Graham-Steele murmur

QUESTION 7

Recognised causes of a sinus tachycardia include

A. Anaemia
B. Thyrotoxicosis
C. Mitral stenosis
D. Hypoglycaemia
E. Malignant hyperthermia

QUESTION 8

Procedural antibiotic prophylaxis is required in patients with

A. Aortic valve replacement
B. Mitral valve prolapse
C. Previous history of infective endocarditis
D. Ostium secundum ASD
E. Mitral stenosis

QUESTION 9

Bicuspid aortic valves

A. Are associated with coarctation of the aorta
B. Calcification is uncommon
C. Incompetence is more common than stenosis
D. Are associated with Turner's syndrome
E. Are a feature of Marfan's syndrome

QUESTION 10

Features of acute cardiac tamponade include

A. Ascites
B. Hypotension
C. Pulsus paradoxus
D. Loud heart sounds
E. Distended pulmonary veins

QUESTION 11

In constrictive pericarditis

A. Ascites is often out of proportion to the degree of dependent oedema
B. Pedal oedema is a prominent feature
C. Atrial fibrillation is a common finding
D. A pansystolic murmur which increases on inspiration is characteristic
E. Prominent 'v' waves are present in the neck

QUESTION 12

With reference to congenital heart lesions

A. ASD is the most common lesion
B. VSD's account for 10% of congenital lesions
C. Patent ductus arteriosus is more common in females
D. Patent ductus arteriosus accounts for 10% of all lesions
E. Fallot's has a higher than normal incidence in first degree relatives

QUESTION 13

In the sick sinus syndrome

A. Atrial fibrillation is rare
B. A pacemaker is seldom required
C. Acute MI is the commonest cause of death
D. Syncopal attacks are the commonest presentation
E. There is a recognised association with AV nodal disease

QUESTION 14

P waves are absent in

A. Atrial flutter
B. Atrial fibrillation
C. Nodal tachycardia
D. Ventricular tachycardia
E. Hypokalaemia

QUESTION 15

In infective endocarditis

A. Bacteria are commonly found in the kidney
B. Renal lesions are due to glomerulonephritis
C. Frank haematuria suggests an unrelated cause
D. Renal involvement is associated with a poor prognosis
E. Persistent hypocomplementaemia is the rule

QUESTION 16

Pulmonary hypertension

A. Causes wide splitting of S2
B. Is a cause of the Graham-Steele murmur
C. Can cause peripheral cyanosis
D. Is a cause of atrial fibrillation
E. Causes giant a waves in the JVP

QUESTION 17

Recognised associations with coarctation of the aorta include

A. Cerebral aneurysms
B. Bicuspid pulmonary valve
C. VSD
D. Patent ductus arteriosus
E. Marfan's syndrome

QUESTION 18

Concerning the Tetralogy of Fallot

A. Clubbing is apparent from birth
B. It is the commonest form of cyanotic congenital heart disease
C. Squatting reduces the cyanosis
D. It characteristically has a stenotic overriding aorta
E. Beta-blockers have a useful therapeutic role

QUESTION 19

The following are associated with aortic regurgitation

A. Coarctation of the aorta
B. Syphilis
C. Hypertension
D. Ankylosing spondylitis
E. Marfan's syndrome

QUESTION   20

Mid-systolic murmurs are features of

A. Coarctation of the aorta
B. Hypertrophic Cardiomyopathy
C. VSD
D. Patent ductus arteriosus
E. ASD

QUESTION   21

With reference to congenital heart disease

A. Congenital cardiac malformations occur in about 3% of live births
B. There is an overall female preponderance
C. Patent ductus arteriosus is more common in males
D. Clubbing commonly occurs
E. Down's syndrome is associated with endomyocardial cushion defects

QUESTION   22

Recognised causes of a pericardial effusion include

A. Coxsackie B virus infection
B. Thyrotoxicosis
C. SLE
D. Hodgkin's disease
E. Chronic renal failure

QUESTION   23

The following are recognised features of an uncomplicated patent ductus arteriosus

A. Cyanosis
B. Wide pulse pressure
C. Clubbing
D. Soft heart sound in the pulmonary area
E. Apical late diastolic murmur

QUESTION   24

The severity of mitral stenosis can be judged by

A. Degree of left ventricular enlargement
B. Length of the diastolic murmur
C. Proximity of opening snap to the second heart sound
D. Patient symptoms
E. Echocardiographic Doppler studies

QUESTION 25

The following are recognised causes of inverted P waves in lead I

A. Dextrocardia
B. Ventricular tachycardia
C. Nodal rhythm
D. Reversed limb lead
E. HOCM

QUESTION 26

The following are true regarding AV block

A. Diphtheria can produce a narrow complex complete heart block
B. A permanent pacemaker should always be used in asymptomatic broad complex complete heart block
C. Decreasing PR interval suggests Wenckebach's phenomenon
D. Irregular cannon waves suggest complete heart block
E. Patients with second degree block are usually asymptomatic

QUESTION 27

The following suggest predominant incompetence in mixed mitral valve disease

A. Displaced, thrusting apex beat
B. Loud first heart sound
C. Presence of a third heart sound
D. Atrial fibrillation
E. Left parasternal heave

QUESTION 28

The following signs are characteristic of a pulmonary embolus (PE)

A. Dyspnoea
B. Large 'a' wave in the JVP trace
C. Raised systolic blood pressure
D. Cyanosis
E. Gallop rhythm

QUESTION 29

In a patient with ischaemic heart disease

A. Dyspnoea following prolonged angina suggests severe left ventricular disease
B. An atrial sound may be audible only during an attack of angina
C. A fall in BP on exercise suggests severe coronary artery disease
D. Tachycardia induced by pacing is more likely to produce pain than exercise
E. Pain at rest without a rise in serum enzymes may be due to coronary artery spasm

QUESTION 30

In endocarditis

A. Enterococci are highly sensitive to penicillins
B. *Streptococcus bovis* is frequently associated with lesions in the bowel
C. Indolent infection late after cardiac surgery is often due to infection with Staphylococcus aureus
D. Anticoagulation is indicated to reduce the risk of emboli when large vegetations are present
E. Mycotic aneurysms may rupture after complete eradication of infection

QUESTION 31

The prolonged repolarisation syndrome may be associated with the following

A. Erythromycin therapy
B. Terfenadine
C. Astemizole
D. Hypermagnesaemia
E. Bradycardia

QUESTION 32

Recognised complications of mitral valve prolapse include

A. Exercise-induced ventricular arrhythmias
B. Infective endocarditis
C. Supraventricular ectopics
D. Atypical chest pains
E. Pericarditis

QUESTION 33

Digoxin

A. Has been proven to prolong survival in patients with chronic heart failure
B. May be used for the control of fetal arrhythmias in pregnancy
C. Is not known to be teratogenic
D. Digoxin-like substances secreted by the placenta may interfere with digoxin assays during pregnancy
E. Provides effective control of heart rate in patients with AF at rest and during exercise

QUESTION 34

The long QT syndrome is associated with

A. Hypercalcaemia
B. Hypokalaemia
C. Aminophylline
D. Sotalol
E. Chlorpromazine

QUESTION 35

The following factors predispose to the development of dissecting aortic aneurysm

A. Hypertension
B. Marfan's syndrome
C. Hypercholesterolaemia
D. Bicuspid aortic valve
E. Pregnancy

QUESTION 36

Metabolic predispositions to digoxin toxicity include

A. Hypokalaemia
B. Hypermagnesaemia
C. Hypocalaemia
D. Hypothyroidism
E. Hypoxia

QUESTION 37

The presence of prominent T waves in the ECG indicates

A. Hypothermia
B. Hypokalaemia
C. Hypocalcaemia
D. Hyperkalaemia
E. Hypomagnesaemia

QUESTION 38

Findings in a patient with emphysema and cor pulmonale include

A. Hypoxia
B. Left axis deviation of the ECG
C. Tricuspid regurgitation
D. Large 'a' wave in the JVP
E. Parasternal heave

QUESTION 39

On auscultation of the heart, an opening snap

A. Is a low pitched sound best heard with the bell of the stethoscope
B. Occurs at a variable distance from the second heart sound
C. Represents the sudden opening of the mitral valve
D. Varies in position with respiration
E. Occurs earlier in diastole the more severe the degree of stenosis

QUESTION 40

Nicorandil

A. Is a potassium channel inhibitor
B. Reduces preload and afterload
C. Is absolutely contraindicated in the presence of beta-blockers
D. Is used in the treatment of angina
E. Headaches may occur when treatment is started

QUESTION 41

Hypertrophic cardiomyopathy

A. Is a recognised cause of sudden death
B. May be associated with thiamine deficiency
C. Is commonly associated with mitral regurgitation
D. Has a recognised association with ACE gene polymorphism
E. Is familial in 50% of cases

QUESTION 42

Losartan

A. Is an Angiotensin II receptor antagonist
B. Produces reduced renin activity
C. Causes a dry cough similar to captopril
D. Is safe in patients taking amiloride
E. Has no active metabolites

QUESTION 43

The first heart sound

A. Is best heard at the left sternal edge
B. Is due to the closure of the mitral tricuspid valves
C. Is usually split
D. Is loud in patients with thyrotoxicosis
E. Is quiet in patients with mitral stenosis

QUESTION 44

The QRS complex on the ECG

A. Is caused by ventricular myocardial repolarisation
B. Will normally contain a Q-wave up to half the height of the R-wave
C. Corresponds with the phase of isovolumetric contraction
D. Is shortened in tricyclic poisoning
E. May be used to assess rotation of the heart along its longitudinal axis

QUESTION 45

The third heart sound

A. Is due to rapid ventricular filling
B. Is a normal finding in children and young adults
C. Is referred to as the sound of cardiac distress
D. Occurs immediately following mitral and tricuspid valve opening
E. Occurs in mitral incompetence

QUESTION 46

Coarctation of the aorta

A. Is twice as common in men as in women
B. May be associated with webbing of the neck
C. Is associated with a pansystolic murmur
D. Is preductal in origin in 20% of cases
E. Is associated with a patent ductus arteriosus

QUESTION 47

Concerning the JVP

A. It is usually measured from the sternal notch
B. The normal value is usually less than 3 cm of water
C. Steep x descent is associated with constrictive pericarditis
D. Steep y descent is associated with tricuspid regurgitation
E. The level rises in expiration in cardiac tamponade

QUESTION 48

The following statements are true of the normal ECG

A. It represents the vector sum of the depolarization potentials of all myocardial cells
B. At the body surface, the potential difference generated is about 10mV
C. Two perpendicular axes are required to represent the spatial vector
D. The diastolic potential difference is maintained by a high intracellular potassium concentration
E. The resting intracellular voltage of the myocardium is -70mV

QUESTION   49

The following are true of the T wave on the ECG

A. It represents ventricular repolarisation
B. It is normally less than 1mV in the standard leads
C. Digoxin toxicity is associated with increased T wave amplitude
D. 50% of people have an inverted T wave in V2
E. T wave inversion in V4 may be a normal finding

QUESTION   50

Characteristic features of the ECG in hypothermia include

A. J waves
B. Long PR interval
C. Wide QRS complex
D. Nodal bradycardia
E. Long QT interval

QUESTION   51

In a patient with a broad complex tachycardia, the following would favour a diagnosis of SVT rather than VT

A. Left axis deviation
B. P waves
C. Capture beats
D. QRS < 0.14 seconds
E. Classical RBBB morphology

QUESTION   52

Reversed splitting of the second heart sound occurs in

A. Left bundle branch block
B. Right bundle branch block
C. Severe aortic stenosis
D. Large patent ductus arteriosus
E. Pulmonary stenosis

QUESTION   53

Right bundle branch block

A. May be a normal finding
B. Is associated with atrial septal defects
C. Is associated with ventricular septal defects
D. Results in a QRS duration of at least 100 msec
E. Occurs in hyperkalaemia

QUESTION 54

The third heart sound

A. May be a normal finding in a person over 40
B. Is present in right ventricular failure
C. Occurs in mitral stenosis
D. Occurs in constrictive pericarditis
E. Is a mid–systolic sound

QUESTION 55

A prolonged QT interval in the ECG

A. May be associated with congenital deafness
B. May occur in patients on chlorpromazine
C. Is associated with an abnormal pathway between atria and ventricles
D. Is associated with Torsades de Pointes tachycardia
E. Is a recognised consequence of hypomagnesaemia

QUESTION 56

A fourth heart sound

A. May be physiological
B. Occurs late in diastole
C. Occurs in acute mitral regurgitation
D. May indicate ventricular volume overload
E. Occurs in pulmonary stenosis

QUESTION 57

Mid–diastolic murmurs occur in

A. Mitral stenosis
B. Atrial myxoma
C. Hypertrophic cardiomyopathy
D. Rheumatic fever
E. Aortic regurgitation

QUESTION 58

The following are likely to cause serious complications during pregnancy

A. Mitral stenosis
B. Secundum atrial septal defect
C. Ventricular septal defect with normal pulmonary artery pressure
D. Isolated aortic regurgitation
E. Primary pulmonary hypertension

QUESTION   59

The following are accentuated in the strain phase of the Valsalva manoeuvre

A. Murmur of Hypertrophic Cardiomyopathy
B. Length of the murmur of mitral valve prolapse
C. Murmur of aortic stenosis
D. Murmur of mitral regurgitation
E. Fourth heart sound

QUESTION 60

Mortality in myocardial infarction is reduced by

A. Nifedipine
B. Beta-blockers
C. ACE inhibitors
D. Intravenous magnesium
E. Intravenous nitrates

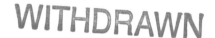

QUESTION   61

Lown-Ganong Levine syndrome is associated with

A. Normal P wave
B. Short PR interval
C. Broad QRS complex
D. Accessory pathway between the atria and ventricles
E. Positive delta wave in V1

QUESTION   62

Ventricular septal defect (VSD)

A. Occurring at approximately 1 in 500 live births is the commonest congenital cardiac defect
B. Is uncommon in Down's syndrome
C. When large, should not be surgically corrected below 3 years of age
D. Makes the shunt right to left, resulting in central cyanosis
E. Produces a loud diastolic murmur

QUESTION   63

A fourth heart sound

A. Occurs in aortic incompetence
B. Occurs late in systole
C. May be a normal finding in elderly patients
D. May be palpated
E. Occurs in hypertension

QUESTION 64

In rheumatic fever

A. Patients may develop a fleeting polyarthritis affecting the small joints
B. Affecting the heart, 40% of patients have both mitral and aortic valve disease
C. The causative bacterium is a group B Streptococcus
D. Only the pericardium is involved
E. Mitral valvulitis leads to a transient diastolic mitral (Carey-Coombs) murmur

QUESTION 65

Complications of mitral valve prolapse include

A. Pericarditis
B. Chest pain
C. Ventricular dysrhythmias
D. Infective endocarditis
E. Cerebral embolism in young adults

QUESTION 66

Constrictive pericarditis is associated with

A. Peripheral oedema
B. A raised jugular venous pressure (JVP)
C. Pulsus paradoxus
D. A steep 'y' descent on JVP trace
E. Tuberculosis

QUESTION 67

Concerning the second heart sounds

A. Physiological splitting is associated with greater separation of the sounds during expiration
B. Atrial septal defects are associated with a widely split second heart sound
C. Reversed splitting occurs in right bundle branch block
D. Left ventricular failure may be associated with reversed splitting
E. Coarcation of the aorta may be associated with greater splitting of the sounds in expiration

QUESTION 68

The following are normal findings on the ECG

A. PR interval of 0.22 s
B. Mean frontal QRS axis of –40
C. R wave in aVL of 12 mm
D. Right bundle branch block
E. Q wave in lead III

QUESTION   69

In a patient with broad complex tachycardia

A. Presence of any Q wave in V6 in LBBB pattern tachycardia is strongly suggestive of ventricular tachycardia
B. P-waves just after every QRS complex are diagnostic of ventricular tachycardia
C. Variation of the tachycardia cycle length by >10 ms between adjacent beats usually excludes ventricular tachycardia
D. In a RBBB pattern tachycardia, if the R' is taller than the R wave it is likely to be supraventricular
E. If no pre-excitation is seen on ECG during sinus rhythm, then it is not an atrioventricular re-entrant tachycardia

QUESTION   70

Digoxin toxicity may cause

A. Prolongation of the PR interval
B. Prolongation of the QT interval
C. Diarrhoea
D. Photophobia
E. Blurred vision

QUESTION   71

Digoxin in therapeutic doses has the following effects on the normal ECG

A. Prolongation of the R-R interval
B. Shortening of the corrected QT interval
C. T wave flattening
D. U waves
E. First degree heart block

QUESTION   72

Coronary artery stents

A. Reduce the need for emergency CABG after failed angioplasty
B. Are most effective in small <3 mm arteries
C. Require life-long anticoagulation
D. Preclude the use of nuclear magnetic resonance imaging
E. Can easily be seen on a lateral chest film

QUESTION 73

In coarctation of the aorta

A. Renal hypoperfusion activates the renin-angiotensin system resulting in hypertension
B. There is a tendency to intracranial haemorrhage
C. It is important to maintain a normal to high mean arterial pressure following surgical correction
D. More than 50% are associated with a bicuspid aortic valve
E. The constriction is usually proximal to the origin of the left subclavian artery

QUESTION 74

In a 65 year old patient with mitral stenosis

A. Rheumatic fever is the most likely cause
B. Atrial flutter is a contraindication to valvotomy
C. Pulmonary oedema may develop if the mitral valve orifice area is 1 cm²
D. Right ventricular failure may develop
E. Pulmonary artery wedge pressure reflects left ventricular end diastolic pressure

QUESTION 75

Paradoxical splitting of the second heart sound is caused by

A. Right bundle branch block
B. Subaortic stenosis
C. Valvular aortic stenosis
D. Hypertensive heart disease with LVF
E. Atrial septal defect

QUESTION 76

Tall R waves in lead V1 on the ECG are seen in

A. Right bundle branch block
B. Ebstein's anomaly
C. Wolff-Parkinson-White syndrome
D. Acute pulmonary embolism
E. Dextrocardia

QUESTION 77

Regarding vagotonic manoeuvres in the presence of supraventricular arrhythmias

A. Right sided carotid sinus massage generally impairs AV nodal conduction
B. Left sided carotid sinus massage generally slows the sinus rate
C. Arrhythmias involving circus movement may convert to sinus rhythm
D. Ocular pressure is effective
E. The Valsalva manoeuvre is the most effective

QUESTION 78

The following findings are consistent with an atrial septal defect

A. Right ventricular heave
B. Loud second heart sound
C. Fixed splitting of the first heart sound
D. Mid-systolic ejection murmur in the pulmonary area
E. Pulmonary venous plethora on the chest X-ray

QUESTION 79

Dilated cardiomyopathy

A. Secondary to alcohol abuse presents predominantly with right heart failure
B. Occurring peripartum is associated with a high risk of recurrence in subsequent pregnancy
C. Is associated with anthracycline therapy
D. Is associated with selenium deficiency
E. With a LVED dimension of >7cm is an indication for cardiac transplantation

QUESTION 80

Wide splitting of the second heart sound is a characteristic feature of

A. Severe aortic stenosis
B. Right bundle branch block
C. Atrial septal defect
D. Ventricular septal defect
E. Tetralogy of Fallot

QUESTION 81

Wolff-Parkinson-White syndrome is associated with

A. Short PR interval
B. Increase in the QT interval
C. A positive QRS complex in V1 if the accessory bundle is on the left side
D. Atrioventricular re-entrant tachycardia treated effectively with digoxin
E. Characteristic delta wave during tachydysrhythmias

QUESTION 82

The normal right coronary artery

A. Supplies the inferior aspect of the left ventricle
B. Supplies the AV node
C. Divides into the circumflex and marginal arteries
D. Supplies the right ventricle and part of the septum
E. Arises from the posterior aortic sinus

QUESTION 83

The following are recognised features in patients presenting with a left atrial myxoma

A. Syncope
B. Atrial fibrillation
C. Apical systolic murmur
D. Systemic emboli
E. Raised serum immunoglobulins

QUESTION 84

Hypertrophic obstructive cardiomyopathy is associated with

A. Systolic anterior motion of the posterior leaflet of the mitral valve
B. Slow rising pulse
C. Palpable fourth heart sound
D. Double apical impulse
E. Long PR interval

QUESTION 85

The following features distinguish an ostium primum from a secundum atrial septal defect

A. Systolic ejection murmur at the upper left sternal border
B. Fixed split second heart sound
C. Right atrial enlargement on chest X-ray
D. Left axis deviation on the ECG
E. Parasternal heave on palpation of the precordium

QUESTION 86

The following statements concerning the jugular venous pulse are correct

A. The a wave coincides with the fourth heart sound
B. The c wave coincides with tricuspid valve closure
C. Cannon waves are seen in tricuspid incompetence
D. The x descent is slowed in tricuspid stenosis
E. The v wave represents ventricular filling

QUESTION 87

In atrial flutter

A. The atrial rate is commonly 230 bpm
B. Digoxin often converts the rhythm to atrial fibrillation
C. The heart is usually otherwise normal
D. Carotid sinus massage usually slows the AV conduction
E. The radial pulse is usually regular or regularly irregular

QUESTION 88

In atrial fibrillation

A. The femoral pulse is irregularly irregular
B. The ECG shows 'f' waves
C. Patients are usually symptomatic
D. Chronic alcohol abuse is a recognised cause
E. The atrial rate is about 400

QUESTION 89

In hypertrophic cardiomyopathy

A. The genetic defect is a point mutation at a single locus on chromosome 14
B. Dual chamber pacing can reduce the outflow tract gradient and improve symptoms
C. Non-sustained ventricular tachycardia is a marker for sudden death risk
D. Patients with recurrent VF may require implantation of a cardioverter defibrillator
E. Squatting makes the systolic murmur louder

QUESTION 90

On the ECG

A. The P wave denotes sino-atrial activity
B. The initial deflection in V1 is negative
C. The T wave is negative in aVr
D. There is usually a Q wave in V6
E. The R wave is bigger than the S wave in V1

QUESTION 91

Concerning the ECG

A. The PR interval represents the time for the impulse to pass from the sinus node to the AV node
B. Atrial repolarization is represented by a biphasic P wave in V1
C. The normal QRS axis lies between –30 and +90
D. An axis of +120 is consistent with right posterior hemiblock
E. The S wave is greater than the R wave in III in Left axis deviation

QUESTION 92

With regard to the Wolff-Parkinson-White syndrome

A. The ventricular rate is usually slow if the patient is in AF
B. Digoxin is the treatment of choice
C. Ventricular and supraventricular tachydysrhythmias are equally common
D. Defects in the cardiac septa are common
E. The accessory pathway always links the right atrium and ventricle

QUESTION 93

Regarding the jugular venous pressure

A. The x descent is rapid in cardiac tamponade
B. Regular cannon waves are seen in nodal tachycardia
C. Inspection of the normal adult usually reveals a, c and v waves
D. The physiological third heart sound is synchronous with the x descent
E. Fixed elevation is seen with IVC obstruction

QUESTION 94

In atrial septal defect (ASD)

A. There is a male preponderance
B. Splitting of the second heart sound increases in expiration
C. The shunt is left to right
D. If left uncorrected, pulmonary hypertension may develop
E. The ECG usually shows left bundle branch block and left axis deviation

QUESTION 95

In Wolff-Parkinson-White syndrome

A. There is often a history of rheumatic fever
B. Type B is associated with deep Q and S waves in V1
C. Sudden death is a recognised complication
D. Ebstein's anomaly may be an associated condition
E. Antidromic tachycardia is more common than orthodromic

QUESTION 96

Cyanosis may be present in

A. Tricuspid atresia
B. Patent Ductus Arteriosus
C. Eisenmenger's syndrome
D. Ostium primum ASD
E. Fallot's tetralogy

QUESTION 97

Causes of a dominant a wave in the JVP include

A. Tricuspid stenosis
B. Pulmonary stenosis
C. Complete heart block
D. Pulmonary hypertension
E. Atrial septal defect

QUESTION 98

The following ECG changes are associated with the correct cause

A. U waves – Hypothermia
B. T wave flattening – Hypothyroidism
C. Short QT Interval – Hypercalcaemia
D. Biphasic P wave in V1 – Mitral stenosis
E. T wave inversion – Hypokalaemia

QUESTION 99

The following findings are associated with an ostium primum ASD

A. Wide splitting of the second heart sound
B. Right axis deviation
C. Mid-diastolic murmur
D. Pulmonary systolic murmur
E. Mitral incompetence

QUESTION 100

Features of digoxin toxicity include

A. Xanthopsia
B. Gynaecomastia
C. Hypokalaemia
D. T wave inversion
E. Headaches

RESPIRATORY

QUESTION 101

The following are true

A. The trachea starts at the level of C6 and ends at T4
B. The left main bronchus passes under the aortic arch and is approximately 5 cm long
C. Pores of Kohn allow communication between alveoli of adjoining lobules
D. There are 18 divisions between the trachea and the alveolus
E. Type I pneumocytes secrete surfactant

QUESTION 102

The right lung

A. Has one fissure
B. Has no Sibson's fascia
C. Has two pulmonary veins
D. Is related to the azygous vein
E. Has 7 bronchopulmonary segments

QUESTION 103

Regarding normal Pulmonary Function Tests (PFTs)

A. The FEV1 is greater than 70% of the FVC
B. The FRC can be measured by spirometry
C. The peak flow rate is a measure of intrinsic airway disease
D. Compliance must be measured dynamically
E. Peak expiratory flow rate is correlated to age, sex, height and race

QUESTION 104

A trachea deviated to the right on palpation may be caused by

A. A nodular goitre
B. A right sided pneumothorax
C. Collapse of the left lung
D. A massive left sided empyema
E. Asthma

QUESTION   105

In consolidated lobar pneumonia there is

A. Reduced chest wall movement ipsilaterally
B. A dull percussion note
C. Bronchial breathing
D. Reduced vocal resonance
E. Expiratory polyphonic wheeze

QUESTION   106

Tension pneumothorax is characterised by

A. Mediastinal deviation to the opposite side
B. Cyanosis
C. Hypertension
D. Dullness to percussion
E. Decreased air entry

QUESTION   107

Good indicators of life threatening asthma include

A. A pulse rate greater than 120 bpm
B. A low $PaCO_2$
C. Pulsus paradoxus greater than 20 mmHg
D. Widespread polyphonic wheeze
E. Peak expiratory flow rate of 350 l/min

QUESTION   108

Characteristics of finger clubbing include

A. Increased nail bed curvature in all directions
B. Nail base fluctuation
C. Finger pulp swelling
D. Nail base skin oedema
E. Nail base telangiectasia

QUESTION   109

Causes of finger clubbing include

A. Chronic bronchitis
B. Cystic fibrosis
C. Inflammatory bowel disease
D. Mesothelioma
E. Acute bacterial endocarditis

QUESTION 110

Central cyanosis is an expected feature in

A. Fibrosing alveolitis
B. SVC obstruction
C. Polycythaemia
D. Hypothermia
E. Ankylosing spondylitis

QUESTION 111

Typical findings in right lower lobe collapse include

A. Decreased chest expansion
B. Stony dull percussion
C. Bronchial breath sounds
D. Decreased vocal resonance
E. Crepitations

QUESTION 112

Typical features of Staphylococcal pneumonia include

A. Multiple lung abscesses which persist as thin walled cysts
B. A recognised association with influenza viral infection
C. Close contact with birds
D. Pneumothorax
E. Hyponatraemia, diarrhoea and a prodromal viral illness

QUESTION 113

In cystic fibrosis

A. The lungs are structurally normal at birth
B. Older children develop nasal polyps
C. The mode of inheritance is autosomal dominant with poor penetration
D. There is generalised endocrine dysfunction
E. The vas deferens and epididymis are absent

QUESTION 114

Features of primary tuberculosis include

A. Swinging pyrexia
B. Erythema nodusum
C. Bilateral hilar lymphadenopathy
D. Caseation within the regional lymph nodes
E. Predilection for the upper lung zones

QUESTION   115

Miliary tuberculosis

A. Is a benign form of tuberculosis seen in older people
B. Is diagnosed from typical CXR appearances
C. May have CXR appearances in common with sarcoidosis
D. May be associated with a negative Mantoux test
E. Can produce chest lesions up to 10mm diameter

QUESTION   116

Honeycomb lung occurs

A. After treatment with bleomycin
B. In sarcoidosis
C. In rheumatoid arthritis
D. In smokers
E. In ankylosing spondylitis

QUESTION   117

Extrapulmonary manifestations of bronchial carcinoma include

A. Weight loss
B. Hypocalcaemia
C. Myasthenic syndrome
D. Acanthosis nigricans
E. Gynaecomastia

QUESTION   118

In Legionnaires' disease

A. Malaise, myalgia, headache and a pyrexia up to 40°C are common features
B. Hypernatraemia is a recognised finding
C. Lymphopenia is a recognised finding
D. The presenting cough is often dry
E. Lung cavitation commonly occurs

QUESTION   119

In Pickwickian syndrome (obstructive sleep apnoea)

A. The main symptoms are hypersommnolence, snoring and restless sleep
B. Abnormal daytime PaO_2 and $PaCO_2$ may occur
C. Nocturnal positive nasal airway pressure devices is a recognised and effective treatment
D. Is commoner in women
E. May result in sudden death

QUESTION 120

In Sarcoidosis

A. There is multi-system granulomatous disease
B. Bilateral hilar lymphadenopathy is rare
C. Pulmonary function tests reveal an obstructive pattern
D. Erythema nodosum is rare
E. Hypocalcaemia is found in 10% of cases

QUESTION 121

Regarding arterial blood gases

A. Normal H^+ concentration is 40 mmol/L
B. Bicarbonate values are calculated not measured
C. Standard bicarbonate requires a normal $PaCO_2$
D. A low $PaCO_2$ is a feature of aspirin overdose
E. A low PaO_2 prevents apnoea in some patients

QUESTION 122

Patients with adult respiratory distress syndrome (ARDS)

A. Have a low pulmonary vascular resistance
B. Have a lower mortality if treated early with nitric oxide
C. Have a high thoracic compliance
D. Due to a fat embolus have a survival rate of about 90%
E. By definition must be ventilated

QUESTION 123

Asbestosis

A. Typically produces upper lobe fibrosis
B. Characteristically produces calcification on the diaphragmatic pleural surface
C. Produces a restrictive lung disease
D. Causes sputum eosinophilia
E. Is associated with an increased incidence of mesothelioma

QUESTION 124

The following statements about whooping cough are true

A. It rarely occurs before six months of age
B. Is infective only in the paroxysmal phase
C. Lymphocytosis is characteristic
D. May rarely occur in immunised children
E. May cause rectal prolapse

QUESTION 125

Children with acute laryngotracheobronchitis

A. Are usually apyrexial
B. Are best treated with humidified oxygen and steroids
C. May have inspiratory stridor
D. Usually have a bacterial cause
E. Usually drool

QUESTION 126

Recognised lung complications of rheumatic disease include

A. Pleural effusion
B. Fibrosing alveolitis
C. Pulmonary eosinophilia
D. Bronchogenic carcinoma
E. Stridor

QUESTION 127

The following may contribute to the pathology of bronchiectasis

A. Cystic fibrosis
B. Coarctation
C. Measles
D. Bordetella pertussis
E. Achalasia

QUESTION 128

Recognised complications of Mycoplasma pneumonia include

A. Leucocytosis
B. Pericarditis
C. Thrombocytopenia
D. Diarrhoea and vomiting
E. Subphrenic abscess

QUESTION 129

The following are true regarding spontaneous pneumothorax

A. Breathlessness and pleuritic chest pain are usually present
B. Bronchial breathing is heard over the affected hemithorax
C. Is 5 times more common in women when not associated with serious lung pathology
D. Pleuradesis should be considered for recurrent pneumothoraces
E. The lower lobes are the first to collapse (when the patient is erect)

QUESTION 130

The following may result in shadowing on the CXR in patients with AIDS

A. Pneumocystis carinii
B. Cytomegalovirus
C. Kaposi's sarcoma
D. Mycobacterium avium intracellulare
E. Cryptococcus

QUESTION 131

The following are true

A. Altitude sickness may be prevented by breathing oxygen
B. Drowning is likely to occur more rapidly in sea water than in fresh water
C. 'Bends' are caused by bubbles of CO_2 forming and causing emboli
D. A diver suffering from the bends requires rapid decompression
E. Pre-treatment with acetazolamide is of value in preventing the bends

QUESTION 132

The following are recognised non-metastatic presenting features of carcinoma of the lung

A. Painful hands and wrists
B. Tetany
C. Polyuria
D. Hyperpigmentation
E. Ataxia

QUESTION 133

Regarding carcinoma of the lung

A. Radiotherapy is the treatment of choice for adenocarcinomas
B. Exposure to petroleum products increases risk of alveolar cell carcinoma
C. Adenocarcinomas are commonly peripheral in the lung parenchyma
D. Alveolar cell carcinoma may be of multicentric origin
E. Squamous cell tumours metastasise early

QUESTION 134

Cigarette smoking is implicated in the causation of

A. Thyroid cancer
B. Bronchial cancer
C. Cervical cancer
D. Bladder cancer
E. Colon cancer

QUESTION 135

The following statements concerning asbestosis are true

A. Pleural plaques are pre-malignant
B. It produces pulmonary nodules and fibrosis
C. Carcinoma of the bronchus is a recognised complication
D. Is commonly associated with a positive anti-nuclear antibody
E. It produces finger clubbing and fine end inspiratory crepitations in the lung bases

QUESTION 136

In patients with sarcoidosis

A. Heart failure is usually secondary to lung involvement and cor pulmonale
B. Asymptomatic hilar lymphadenopathy is a common presentation
C. Pulmonary involvement is usually seen on transbronchial biopsy even in extra-pulmonary presentations of the disease
D. 50% of patients will have a positive tuberculin test
E. A fall in serum ACE levels with corticosteroid treatment correlates with disease response

QUESTION 137

The following are associated with pulmonary granulomata

A. Sarcoidosis
B. Histoplasmosis
C. Chicken pox pneumonia
D. Berylliosis
E. Farmers' lung

QUESTION 138

The following are associated with calcification on the chest radiograph

A. Varicella zoster
B. Mitral stenosis
C. Farmer's lung
D. Silicosis
E. Asbestos exposure

QUESTION 139

Causes of pulmonary cavitation include

A. Aspiration pneumonia
B. Invasive aspergillosis
C. Septic emboli
D. Pneumocystis carinii pneumonia
E. Churg-Strauss syndrome

QUESTION 140

Differential diagnosis of upper zone infiltrates on CXR includes

A. Asbestosis
B. Pulmonary haemosiderosis
C. Ankylosing spondylitis
D. Histiocytosis X
E. Bronchiectasis

QUESTION 141

Pleural effusions with a protein content of 22 g/l may be found in

A. Nephrotic syndrome
B. 'Wet' beri beri
C. Hypothyroidism
D. Systemic lupus
E. Acute intermittent porphyria

QUESTION 142

Clinical features of carbon dioxide retention include

A. Papilloedema
B. Extensor plantars
C. Miosis
D. Low volume pulse
E. Hypertension

QUESTION 143

An elevated $PaCO_2$ may be found with

A. Severe kyphoscoliosis
B. Mild uncomplicated asthma
C. Barbiturate overdose
D. Raised intracranial pressure
E. Early stages of cryptogenic fibrosing alveolitis

QUESTION 144

Indications for long-term low-flow oxygen therapy include

A. Age less than 70 years
B. PaO_2 <7.3 kPa on air
C. Respiratory muscle weakness
D. Cyanotic congenital heart disease
E. Obstructive sleep apnoea

QUESTION 145

Cystic fibrosis

A. Diagnosis is established with sweat sodium >40 mEq/l
B. Is inherited in an autosomal recessive manner
C. Diabetes occurs in 25%
D. Is the commonest cause of recurrent bronchopulmonary infections in childhood
E. Both males and females are infertile

QUESTION 146

The following are features of Pickwickian syndrome

A. Morbid obesity
B. Nocturnal insomnia
C. Polycythaemia
D. Pulmonary hypertension
E. Reduced libido

QUESTION 147

Respiratory failure

A. $PaCO_2$ is <8.0 kPa by definition
B. Lactic acidosis may occur
C. Is always due to pre-existing lung disease
D. Should always be treated with 100% oxygen
E. Is a recognised complication of diphtheria

QUESTION 148

The following predispose to anaerobic lung infections

A. Diabetes
B. Pulmonary fibrosis
C. Alcoholism
D. Old age
E. Poor dentition

QUESTION 149

Mycoplasma pneumonia
A. Is associated with an autoimmune haemolytic anaemia
B. May be diagnosed by culture from throat swab
C. Is associated with an aseptic meningitis
D. Causes hepatosplenomegaly
E. May be complicated by erythema nodosum

QUESTION 150

Legionella pneumophila

A. Is the causative organism of Pontiac fever
B. Infection is associated with encephalopathy and headache
C. Pneumonia is associated with hyponatraemia and hypophosphataemia
D. Tetracycline is the treatment of choice
E. Infection is associated with lymphocytosis

GASTRO

QUESTION 151

Metabolic consequences of vomiting may include

A. Alkalosis
B. Decreased urinary chloride excretion
C. Increased urinary sodium excretion
D. Decreased intracellular H^+ ions
E. Increased urinary potassium excretion

QUESTION 152

Achalasia

A. Is characterised by failure of the lower oesophageal sphincter to relax on initiation of swallowing
B. Results in complete absence of oesophageal contractility
C. Can present with pneumonia
D. Can respond to treatment with sub-lingual nifedipine
E. Is associated with a 30% risk of carcinoma of the oesophagus

QUESTION 153

Regarding peptic ulcer disease

A. Peptic ulcer disease is associated with hypoparathyroidism
B. Gastric ulcers are two to three times more common than duodenal ulcers
C. Misoprostol aids healing by inhibition of gastrin production
D. Gastric ulcers are most commonly found on the greater curve of the stomach
E. Helicobacter pylori eradication usually cures peptic ulcer disease

QUESTION 154

In Zollinger-Ellison syndrome

A. There is an association with acromegaly
B. There is excessive gastrin secretion in the stomach
C. Diarrhoea is a common feature
D. Treatment is usually medical
E. The tumour is usually benign

QUESTION 155

In Coeliac disease

A. There is an association with haplotype HLA-B8
B. Splenic atrophy may result in the presence of Howell-Jolly bodies in the blood film
C. There is an association with exfoliative dermatitis
D. Serum anti-mitochondrial antibodies are found in the majority of cases
E. A gluten-free diet results in a rapid clinical improvement although abnormal small bowel morphology persists.

QUESTION 156

Regarding carcinoid tumours

A. They may present with acute appendicitis
B. 20% of patients develop carcinoid syndrome
C. There is an association with mitral incompetence
D. Pellegra may be a feature
E. Excessive 5-HT (serotonin) production causes facial flushing in carcinoid syndrome

QUESTION 157

In Crohn's disease

A. The terminal ileum is often affected
B. A 'cobblestone' appearance in affected bowel is characteristic
C. Granulomas are a common feature
D. Mortality in patients with Crohn's disease is twice that of the normal population
E. Cholangiocarcinoma is more common than in the general population

QUESTION 158

Ulcerative colitis may be differentiated from Crohn's disease by the following

A. In ulcerative colitis, extra-gastrointestinal complications are more common
B. Ulcerative colitis occurs more frequently in women
C. Granulomas are commonly seen on histological examination in ulcerative colitis
D. The ileum is not affected in ulcerative colitis
E. Uveitis and episcleritis are a feature of Crohn's disease but not ulcerative colitis

QUESTION 159

Malabsorption

A. Of vitamin B12 occurs in Crohn's disease
B. If due to tropical sprue may be caused by an enterotoxin producing coliform bacteria
C. Can occur due to bacterial overgrowth in structurally normal small intestine
D. May occur following a 30% resection of the gut
E. May be associated with characteristic periodic acid-Schiff (PAS)-positive macrophages on electron microscopy (EM)

QUESTION 160

In intestinal tuberculosis (TB)

A. There is chylous ascitic fluid
B. The duodenum and jejunum are most commonly affected
C. Occurrence is more common in HIV infection than in the general population
D. About 10% of patients show radiological evidence of pulmonary TB
E. Medical treatment should be continued for a minimum of 6 months

QUESTION 161

Concerning oesophageal motility

A. Primary peristalsis is stimulated by a food bolus in the mouth
B. Secondary peristalsis is initiated by the vagus nerve as part of the swallowing reflex
C. Tertiary non-propulsive waves are frequent in young adults
D. Spontaneous contractions show a low amplitude pattern in brain stem death
E. Activity may be increased by sodium nitroprusside (SNP)

QUESTION 162

In radiological investigation of the gastrointestinal tract

A. Carbon dioxide producing granules or tablets can be used to improve contrast, thus accuracy
B. Enteroclysis (small bowel enema) involves introducing large volumes of barium beyond the duodenum
C. Small bowel obstruction results in fluid levels being seen on a supine plain abdominal film
D. Adverse reactions to barium are common
E. Endoscopic ultrasound is used in tumour staging

QUESTION   163

Gastrointestinal problems in Human Immunodeficiency Virus (HIV) positive patients include

A. Dysphagia due to Cytomegalovirus (CMV) or Herpes simplex infection
B. Mycobacterium avium intracellulare infection
C. Bloody diarrhoea due to Shigella infection
D. Increased risk of appendicitis due to CMV infection
E. Weight loss and steatorrhoea due to non-infective enteropathy

QUESTION   164

Acquired Immunodeficiency Syndrome (AIDS) is associated specifically with the following mouth conditions

A. Geographic tongue lesions
B. Kaposi's sarcoma, particularly on the hard palate
C. Stevens-Johnson syndrome
D. Hairy leucoplakia
E. Candidiasis

QUESTION   165

The following are true of gastrointestinal peptides

A. Somatostatin inhibits secretion and action of most other gut hormones
B. Substance P increases small bowel motility
C. Vasoactive intestinal peptide (VIP) causes splanchnic vasoconstriction
D. Gastrin stimulates growth of gut mucosa
E. Neuropeptide Y has a role in regulation of intestinal blood flow

QUESTION   166

Colorectal carcinoma

A. Is rare in Africa but not in Africans living in this country
B. Has a chromosomal link with Familial Adenomatous Polyposis (FAP)
C. Screening with universal colonoscopy has been proved to be of benefit
D. Occurs most commonly in the transverse colon
E. Tumours are not sensitive to chemotherapy

QUESTION 167

In Irritable Bowel Syndrome (IBS)

A. The pain is classically situated in the right iliac fossa
B. Motility abnormalities can be demonstrated
C. Bowel habit may be normal
D. Mebeverine is a useful treatment
E. The presence of diverticulae on barium enema excludes IBS as a cause for pain

QUESTION 168

In patients with an hiatus hernia

A. The hernia may be rolling or sliding
B. They are always clinically significant
C. Surgery is commonly required to alleviate reflux from a rolling para-oesophageal hernia
D. 'Rolling' is the most common type
E. The diagnosis is made when patients present with reflux

QUESTION 169

Constipation is a feature of

A. Hypocalcaemia
B. Spinal injury
C. Post-gastrectomy
D. Myxoedema
E. Tricyclic anti-depressant therapy

QUESTION 170

In a patient who presents with dysphagia

A. Syringomyelia is a possible cause
B. Constant dysphagia and pain suggest oesophagitis is the cause
C. Barrett's oesophagus pre-disposes to development of squamous cell carcinoma of the oesophagus
D. Hyperkeratosis of the palms and soles is a recognised association
E. If the cause is carcinoma, 50% of patients will have widespread distant metastases by the time of presentation

QUESTION   171

The following are significantly associated with oesophageal carcinoma

A. Caustic oesophageal stricture
B. Lead poisoning
C. Achalasia of the cardia
D. Tylosis
E. Chronic iron deficiency

QUESTION   172

The following features may be associated with iron-deficiency

A. A sensitive and painful glossitis
B. Dysphagia
C. Increased liver iron
D. Koilonychia
E. Dermatitis herpetiformis

QUESTION   173

Severe pyloric stenosis is accompanied by the following changes

A. Elevated urea
B. Rise in $PaCO_2$
C. Raised haematocrit
D. Reduced plasma sodium
E. Reduced transferrin

QUESTION   174

The following are associated with Gastro-intestinal bleeding

A. Dermatitis herpetiformis
B. Pseudoxanthoma elasticum
C. Acanthosis nigricans
D. Psoriasis
E. Neurofibromatosis

QUESTION   175

Regarding ulcerative colitis

A. The disease is exacerbated by smoking
B. Sacroilitis responds to treatment of Colitis
C. Is associated with sclerosing cholangitis
D. Crypt abscesses are pathognomonic of Ulcerative Colitis
E. Pseudopolyps are pre-malignant

HEPATOBILIARY

QUESTION   176

Regarding the liver

A. The hepatic artery supplies 50% of the total blood flow and 75% of the oxygen
B. The liver receives 25% of the cardiac output during exercise
C. Riedel's lobe is occasionally palpable in the normal abdomen
D. The epithelial lining of liver sinusoids incorporates phagocytic and fat storage cells
E. The right and left hepatic ducts combine to form the common bile duct

QUESTION   177

The liver is responsible for breakdown of the following

A. Glycogen
B. Urea
C. Bilirubin
D. Vasopressin
E. Very low–density lipo-proteins (VLDLs)

QUESTION   178

The following are true of liver function tests

A. Alkaline phosphatase (ALP) may be raised in the absence of clinical jaundice
B. High levels of aspartate transaminase (AST) are a feature of acute myocardial infarction
C. Hypoglobulinaemia occurs in chronic liver disease
D. Alanine aminotransferase (ALT) is a mitochondrial enzyme which is less specific for the liver than AST
E. Elevation of (gamma–glutamyl transpeptidase (gamma GT) in cholestasis parallels that of AST

QUESTION   179

Gilbert's syndrome

A. Shows an autosomal recessive pattern of inheritance
B. Affects up to 5% of the population
C. When investigated shows only a raised conjugated bilirubin
D. Produces hyperbilirubinaemia which worsens following a large meal
E. Is confirmed by normal histology on liver biopsy

QUESTION 180

The following haematological abnormalities are associated with liver disease

A. Pancytopaenia
B. Hypochromic microcytic anaemia
C. Macrocytic anaemia
D. Target cells
E. Aplastic anaemia

QUESTION 181

Regarding immunological tests in liver disease

A. Antimitochondrial antibody is associated with autoimmune chronic active hepatitis (CAH)
B. Raised alpha-fetoprotein (AFP) is associated with hepatocellular carcinoma
C. A low serum IgM is found in primary biliary cirrhosis (PBC)
D. High titres of kidney microsomal antibodies can be found in the serum of patients with CAH
E. Persistent elevation of Hepatitis B surface antigen (HbsAg) following acute infection correlates with development of chronic liver disease

QUESTION 182

The following are symptoms or signs of acute liver disease

A. Spider naevi
B. Hypothermia
C. Raised intracranial pressure
D. Hyperglycaemia
E. Hyperventilation

QUESTION 183

The following viruses are recognised causes of hepatitis

A. Flavivirus
B. Herpes simplex type 2
C. Human immunodeficiency virus
D. Ebola virus
E. Delta virus

QUESTION 184

Regarding hepatitis viruses

A. Non-A, non-B hepatitis causes 90% of post-transfusion hepatitis
B. Hepatitis E carrier state is common
C. All are RNA viruses
D. Only hepatitis B causes liver cancer
E. Death from fulminant hepatic failure occurs in 20% of pregnant women with hepatitis E

QUESTION 185

Chronic hepatitis can result from

A. Methyldopa
B. Methotrexate
C. Ulcerative colitis
D. Hepatitis C
E. Haemachromatosis

QUESTION 186

Hurler's syndrome

A. Inheritance is X-linked
B. Is a lipid storage disease
C. Causes cirrhosis
D. Commonly causes disturbances in liver function
E. Is associated with corneal clouding

QUESTION 187

The following statements about liver transplantation are true

A. 1 year survival is good but 5 year survival is very poor
B. Operative mortality is high
C. Chronic hepatitis C is an indication for transplantation
D. Portal vein thrombosis is a relative contraindication to transplantation
E. Ductopaenic rejection responds to immunosuppressive therapy

QUESTION 188

In a patient with portal hypertension

A. The circulation is hyperdynamic
B. Vasodilatation occurs due to endotoxaemia
C. Liver function is always deranged
D. Ascitic fluid usually contains more than 11g/litre of protein
E. Portosystemic shunting is the treatment of choice to prevent recurrent variceal bleeding

QUESTION 189

Ascites

A. Results in intravascular volume depletion
B. Is a feature of Meig's syndrome
C. Requires stringent fluid restriction
D. May result in spontaneous bacterial peritonitis
E. If resistant, can be managed with a peritoneo-venous shunt

QUESTION 190

Portosystemic encephalopathy

A. Occurs following portocaval shunt operations
B. May be precipitated by paracentesis
C. Is confirmed by measuring raised blood ammonia
D. Results in a decreased frequency of normal alpha waves (8-13 Hz) to delta waves (1.5-3 Hz) on electroencephalogram (EEG)
E. May be precipitated by constipation

QUESTION 191

Causes of cirrhosis of the liver include

A. Primary biliary cirrhosis
B. Haemachromatosis
C. Use of the oral contraceptive pill
D. Renal tumours
E. Caroli's disease

QUESTION 192

During pregnancy

A. Serum total protein is reduced
B. Hepatic blood flow is increased
C. Hyperemesis gravidarum can cause jaundice
D. Acute fatty liver is associated with cell necrosis and macroscopic fat deposition
E. Viral hepatitis is the cause in 40% of women who become jaundiced

QUESTION 193

Reye's syndrome

A. Is a disease of childhood
B. Usually presents with jaundice
C. Aspirin has been implicated in epidemiological studies
D. Has a 50% mortality
E. Causes macrovesicular fatty infiltration of the liver

QUESTION 194

The following are implicated in development of hepatocellular carcinoma

A. Hepatitis C
B. Hepatitis B
C. Hepatolenticular degeneration
D. Schistosomiasis
E. Danazol therapy

QUESTION 195

Regarding the pancreas

A. The main pancreatic duct joins the cystic duct to enter the duodenum via the ampulla of Vater
B. Endocrine cells form 90% of the pancreas
C. Enzyme secretion by exocytosis utilises membrane phosphoinositides
D. Serum pancreatic polypeptide is elevated in all endocrine tumours
E. Serum amylase is a useful index of pancreatic function in patients with chronic pancreatitis

QUESTION 196

Gallstones

A. Are present in 10-20% of the population world-wide
B. May be the result of diminished bile salt synthesis
C. Are a feature of acromegaly
D. Occur more often following ileal disease or resection
E. Are present in over 90% of patients with acute cholecystitis

QUESTION 197

The following are associated with bilateral parotid enlargement

A. Sarcoidosis
B. Cystic fibrosis
C. Alcoholic liver disease
D. Acromegaly
E. Diabetes mellitus

QUESTION 198

In hepatitis B infection

A. The presence of delta agent is indicative of chronic infection
B. Minimal change glomerulonephritis is a recognised complication
C. Anicteric neonatal infection often results in persistent infection
D. 10% of patients have splenomegaly
E. Anti-HBs antibody implies past infection with hepatitis B

QUESTION   199

Regarding hepatic encephalopathy

A. EEG shows 2 Hz classic spike and wave pattern
B. Blood ammonia levels are found in 90%
C. Bromocriptine may be of benefit
D. Flumazenil is contraindicated
E. Branched chain amino acid preparations are effective

QUESTION   200

Hepatitis A infection may lead to

A. Hepatic encephalopathy
B. Chronic liver disease
C. Gallstones
D. FitzHugh-Curtis syndrome
E. Arthritis

RENAL

QUESTION   201

The following urinary measurements suggest pre-renal as opposed to intrinsic renal failure

A. Urine specific gravity < 1.010
B. Urine osmolality >500 mosmol/l
C. Urine sodium >40 mmol/l
D. Fractional excretion of sodium < 1%
E. Urine protein >150 mg/l

QUESTION   202

The following diseases would account for an enlarged kidney

A. Diabetes mellitus
B. Amyloidosis
C. Renal cell carcinoma
D. Acromegaly
E. Urinary tract obstruction

QUESTION 203

Immune complex mediated glomerulonephritis may be caused by

A. Goodpasture's syndrome
B. Systemic lupus erythematosis
C. Streptococcal infection
D. Epstein–Barr viral infection
E. Aminoglycoside treatment

QUESTION 204

Diabetic nephropathy can cause the following

A. Kimmelstiel–Wilson lesions
B. Microalbuminuria
C. Haematuria
D. Normochromic normocytic anaemia
E. A raised erythrocyte sedimentation ratio (ESR)

QUESTION 205

The following renal complications can occur as a result of diabetes mellitus

A. Hypertension
B. Pyelonephritis
C. Renal papillary necrosis
D. Minimal change glomerulonephritis
E. Nephrotic syndrome

QUESTION 206

Direct renal involvement can occur in

A. Polyarteritis nodosa
B. Schistosoma haematobium infection
C. Tuberculosis
D. Staphlococcal infection
E. Malaria

QUESTION 207

The following therapeutic measures may be used to treat hyperkalaemia in acute renal failure

A. Calcium resonium
B. Dextrose and insulin infusion
C. Nebulised salbutamol
D. Hypoventilation
E. Frusemide

QUESTION 208

The following drugs are nephrotoxic

A. Kanamycin
B. Clarithromycin
C. Frusemide
D. Amphotericin B
E. Cephaloridine

QUESTION 209

A raised urea associated with normal renal function may be found in the following circumstances

A. Acute renal failure
B. Dehydration
C. Corticosteroid therapy
D. Tetracycline treatment
E. Upper gastro-intestinal haemorrhage

QUESTION 210

A raised creatinine associated with normal renal function can occur in the following circumstances

A. Muscle damage
B. High muscle mass
C. Cimetidine therapy
D. Liver failure
E. Red meat ingestion

QUESTION 211

Chronic renal failure may lead to the following complications

A. Pericarditis
B. Peripheral neuropathy
C. Tertiary hyperparathyroidism
D. Pruritus
E. Secondary hyperparathyroidism

QUESTION   212

The following statements about renal replacement therapy are true

A. Haemofiltration may be useful in removing cardiodepressant substances accumulating in septic shock
B. Dialysis is a recognised cause of pancreatitis
C. Dialysis is a recognised cause of peritonitis
D. A transplanted kidney is anastomosed to the renal artery and vein
E. Insulin may be added to the dialysate fluid in order to control blood sugar levels

QUESTION   213

The following statements are true

A. Renal cell carcinoma may be associated with polycythaemia
B. Nephroblastomas may be associated with hemihypertrophy and aniridia
C. Adult Polycystic Kidney Disease (APKD) is associated with liver cysts and Berry aneurysms
D. APKD invariably leads to hypertension
E. APKD is an autosomal recessive disease

QUESTION   214

Hyponatraemia may be found in the following

A. Syndrome of Inappropriate Antidiuretic Hormone
B. Chlorpropamide treatment
C. Adrenocortical insufficiency
D. Excessive use of loop diuretics
E. Heart failure

QUESTION   215

The following may cause hyperkalaemia

A. Amiloride treatment
B. Conn's syndrome
C. Carbenoxolone treatment
D. Addison's disease
E. Acute renal failure

QUESTION 216

In a well-hydrated, normal individual, the following changes are to be expected 1 hour after changing from the supine to the upright position

A. Rise in haematocrit
B. Fall in venous serum colloid osmotic pressure
C. Rise in serum vasopressin concentration
D. Fall in diastolic blood pressure
E. Fall in rate of urine flow

QUESTION 217

The following contribute to hyperkalaemia in patients with mild–moderate renal failure

A. Increased potassium intake
B. Hypoaldosteronism
C. Impaired renal potassium excretion
D. Fall in GFR to < 30% of normal
E. Erythropoietin therapy

QUESTION 218

The urinary bladder

A. Derives sensory supply from both the sympathetic and parasympathetic nervous system
B. Motor supply to the vesical sphincter is parasympathetic
C. Motor supply to the bladder wall is sympathetic
D. Venous drainage is to the inferior mesenteric vein
E. Is supported by ligamentous thickenings of the pelvic fascia

QUESTION 219

Regarding the nephron in the healthy kidney

A. The calculated creatinine clearance by the kidney is greater than the true GFR
B. Carbonic anhydrase in the proximal convoluted tubule is responsible for bicarbonate resorption
C. The ascending loop of Henlé is impermeable to water
D. Aldosterone controls sodium resorption in the distal tubule
E. Water deprivation tests the proximal tubular function

QUESTION 220

Bartter's syndrome is typically

A. X-linked
B. Responsive to indomethacin
C. Associated with hypokalaemia
D. Associated with hypertension
E. Asymptomatic until the third decade

QUESTION 221

The following are true about IgA nephropathy

A. Commonly presents as the nephrotic syndrome
B. Immunofluorescent studies of the renal biopsy establish the diagnosis
C. Haematuria is common
D. Its recurrence in renal allografts usually leads to graft failure
E. Prognosis is favourable in most patients

QUESTION 222

The following are true concerning nephrotic syndrome

A. Plasma volume is increased
B. Is usually associated with renal sodium wasting
C. Occurs with diffuse or focal forms of glomerulonephritis
D. Patients are susceptible to infections
E. Albumin infusions are beneficial

QUESTION 223

The following are recognised complications of chronic renal failure

A. Dementia
B. Hepatitis E
C. Infertility
D. Arthropathy
E. Gout

QUESTION 224

The following are recognised adverse effects of NSAIDs on the kidney

A. Nephrotic syndrome
B. Increased sodium wasting
C. Hyperreninaemic hypertension
D. Papillary necrosis
E. Hypokalaemia

QUESTION 225

The following drugs are associated with acute interstitial nephritis

A. Diclofenac sodium
B. Carbamazepine
C. Erythromycin
D. Losartan
E. Allopurinol

QUESTION 226

Adult polycystic kidney disease

A. Is linked to the short arm of chromosome 16
B. Renal cysts are present from birth
C. Subclinical pancreatic cysts are present in the majority of patients
D. Is associated with mitral valve prolapse
E. Is associated with diverticulosis of the colon

QUESTION 227

The following are features of renal osteodystrophy

A. Hypophosphataemia
B. Hypocalcaemia
C. Hypomagnesaemia
D. Elevated circulating parathormone
E. Periarticular bone cysts

QUESTION 228

The following disorders are associated with bilateral renal enlargement

A. Amyloidosis
B. Renal artery stenosis
C. Acute interstitial nephritis
D. Nephrocalcinosis
E. Radiation nephritis

QUESTION 229

Erythropoietin

A. Is synthesised by cells of the juxtaglomerular apparatus
B. Stimulates maturation of the erythroid line
C. Increases iron absorption from the GI tract
D. Is associated with hyperkalaemia
E. Therapy may be complicated by hypertension

QUESTION 230

The following drugs require dose reduction in renal failure

A. Frusemide
B. Heparin
C. Digoxin
D. Cimetidine
E. Doxazosin

NEUROLOGY

QUESTION 231

Horner's syndrome can result from the following

A. Stellate ganglion blockade
B. Syringobulbia
C. Vitamin B12 deficiency
D. Carcinoma of bronchus
E. Tabes dorsalis

QUESTION 232

The following conditions are associated with miosis

A. Argyll-Robertson pupil
B. Hypothermia
C. Holmes-Adie pupil
D. Diabetes mellitus
E. Posterior communicating artery aneurysm

QUESTION 233

Causes of papilloedema include

A. Cavernous sinus thrombosis
B. Gout
C. Hypertension
D. Hypocalcaemia
E. Leukaemia

QUESTION 234

Structures passing through the cavernous sinus include

A. Optic nerve
B. Oculomotor nerve
C. Ophthalmic division of trigeminal nerve
D. Internal carotid artery
E. Olfactory nerve

QUESTION 235

The following cause facial nerve palsy within the petrous temporal bone

A. Sarcoidosis
B. Acoustic neuroma
C. Mumps
D. Glomus tumour
E. Herpes zoster

QUESTION 236

Lesions of the eighth cranial nerve

A. Inhibit the sensation of taste to the posterior two-thirds of the tongue
B. Are the sole cause of nystagmus
C. Cause nystagmus with fast movement to the opposite side on warm caloric testing
D. Increase bone conduction
E. Are caused by glomus tumours of the jugular foramen

QUESTION 237

The following signs are consistent with the diagnosis of pseudobulbar palsy

A. Fasciculation of the tongue
B. Dysarthria
C. Emotional lability
D. Absent gag reflex
E. Cog wheel rigidity

QUESTION 238

Spastic paraparesis is caused by

A. Subacute combined degeneration of the cord
B. Huntingdon's chorea
C. Motor neurone disease
D. Syringomyelia
E. Syphilis

QUESTION 239

Upper motor neurone lesions are characterised by

A. Preservation of abdominal reflexes
B. Muscle wasting
C. Clonus
D. Immediate increase in tone
E. Fibrillation potentials on EMG

QUESTION 240

The following movement disorders occur in diseases of the extrapyramidal system

A. Dysdiadokinesis
B. Bradykinesis
C. Chorea
D. Cog-wheel rigidity
E. Nystagmus

QUESTION 241

The clinical features of spinal cord compression are

A. Severe pain above the level of the lesion
B. Contralateral pyramidal signs
C. Sphincter disturbance
D. Pain made worse by coughing
E. Contralateral loss of pain and temperature sensation

QUESTION 242

Arterial supply of the brain

A The circle of Willis is supplied by the vertebral arteries
B. The anterior spinal artery is formed from a contributory branch from each vertebral artery
C. The posterior inferior cerebellar artery is a branch of the basilar artery
D. The posterior cerebral artery arises from the circle of Willis
E. The middle cerebral artery is a direct continuation of the common carotid artery

QUESTION 243

The clinical features of transient ischaemic attacks arising from the vertebrobasilar system are

A. Amaurosis fugax
B. Aphasia
C. Hemianopic visual loss
D. Tetraparesis
E. Dysarthria

QUESTION 244

The lateral medullary syndrome is characterised by

A. Thromboembolism of either the vertebral artery or posterior inferior cerebellar artery
B. Contralateral spinothalamic sensory loss
C. Contralateral Horner's syndrome
D. Contralateral facial numbness
E. Ipsilateral ataxia

QUESTION 245

Subarachnoid haemorrhage

A. Arteriovenous malformations are the commonest cause
B. Calcium-channel blocking agents are unhelpful
C. Lumbar puncture should be performed immediately to confirm the diagnosis
D. May present with a third nerve palsy
E. Hydrocephalus is a recognised complication

QUESTION 246

Subdural haemorrhage

A. Is always caused by severe head trauma
B. The latent interval between injury and symptoms may be weeks
C. Is common in the elderly
D. The level of consciousness fluctuates
E. Always requires drainage

QUESTION 247

Risk factors for dural venous thrombosis are

A. Oral contraceptive pill
B. Central venous cannulation
C. Paranasal sinus infection
D. Dehydration
E. Epilepsy

QUESTION 248

The following statements are true of partial seizures

A. May be preceded by an olfactory aura
B. Presents as twitching in a finger which progresses to involve the whole limb
C. 3 Hz spike and wave activity on EEG
D. An initial tonic phase is followed by rhythmic jerking
E. Onset in adult life mandates a cerebral CT scan

QUESTION 249

In cataplexy

A. The EEG findings are a characteristic feature of the condition
B. Attacks are precipitated by sudden surprises
C. There is an association with obstructive sleep apnoea
D. Hypnagogic hallucinations occur on waking
E. Treatment is with methylphenidate

QUESTION 250

Clinical features of Parkinson's disease include

A. Festinant gait
B. Intention tremor
C. Bradykinesia
D. Cogwheel rigidity
E. Extensor planter responses

QUESTION 251

Huntington's chorea

A. Inheritance is autosomal dominant
B. A mutation has been identified on chromosome 4
C. Is characterised by chorea in childhood
D. There is depletion of angiotensin-converting enzyme in the substantia nigra
E. Death occurs rapidly after the onset

QUESTION 252

Features of Gilles de la Tourette syndrome are

A. Inheritance as a sex-linked recessive
B. Coprolalia
C. Echolalia
D. Obsessive-compulsive symptoms
E. Treatment with haloperidol is effective

QUESTION 253

Multiple sclerosis

A. There is a positive association with HLA B 27
B. Visual evoked responses are normal
C. Peripheral nerve studies are normal
D. Oligoclonal IgG is present in the CSF
E. Internuclear ophthalmoplegia occurs

QUESTION 254

Typical changes in the CSF in bacterial meningitis include

A. Less than 5 mononuclear cells per cubic mm
B. 200 polymorphonuclear cells per cubic mm
C. Acid-fast bacilli demonstrated on Ziehl-Nielsen staining
D. Oligigoclonal IgG
E. Gram-positive intracellular diplocci

QUESTION 255

Neurological sequelae following infection with Herpes varicella zoster include

A. Acute disseminated encephalomyelitis
B. Subacute sclerosing panencephalitis
C. Ramsay Hunt syndrome
D. Reye's syndrome
E. Meningosarcoma

QUESTION 256

Features of tertiary syphilis include

A. Dementia
B. Optic atrophy
C. Pupils that respond to light but not to accommodation
D. Ataxia
E. Neuropathic joint

QUESTION 257

Neurological sequaelae of infection with the HIV virus include

A. Meningitis
B. CNS lymphoma
C. Transverse myelitis
D. Hydrocephalus
E. Mononeuropathy

QUESTION 258

Creutzfeld-Jakob disease

A. Was described by Creutzfeld in 1920
B. Is transmitted by proteinaceous infectious particles
C. Has a short incubation period
D. Causes cerebellar ataxia
E. Death occurs within two years from onset of symptoms

QUESTION 259

Tumours commonly producing cerebral metastases

A. Colon
B. Bronchus
C. Breast
D. Stomach
E. Prostate

QUESTION 260

Raised intracranial pressure

A. Herniation of the temporal lobe causes a third nerve lesion
B. False localising signs are unimportant
C. Masses in the posterior fossa produce symptoms earlier than those above the tentorium
D. Tachycardia is common
E. Technetium brain scan is helpful

QUESTION 261

Benign intracranial hypertension

A. The ventricles are increased in size
B. Steroid therapy is indicated
C. Thiazide diuretics reduce intracranial pressure
D. Weight reduction improves outcome
E. CT scan commonly shows a mass lesion

QUESTION 262

The following features occur with migraine

A. Hemiplegia
B. Unilateral facial weakness
C. Scotomata
D. Dysarthria
E. Third nerve palsy

QUESTION 263

Features of giant cell arteritis include

A. Tender pulsatile superficial temporal artery
B. Jaw claudication
C. Occlusion of ciliary artery
D. Polymyalgia rheumatica
E. Erythema nodosum

QUESTION 264

Causes of anterior spinal artery occlusion include

A. Decompression sickness
B. Polyarteritis nodosa
C. Dissecting aneurysm of the descending aorta
D. Cervical spondylosis
E. Endocarditis

QUESTION 265

Syringomyelia

A. Commonly occurs in association with the Arnold-Chiari malformation
B. Results in loss of all sensation below the syrinx
C. Upper limb reflexes are preserved
D. Gait is normal
E. Wasting of the small muscles of the hands occurs

QUESTION 266

Features of motor neurone disease include

A. Strabismus
B. Tremor
C. Loss of temperature and pain sensation
D. Scanning speech
E. Fasciculation

WITHDRAWN

QUESTION 267

The following neurological syndromes are transmitted by autosomal dominant inheritance

A. Sydenham's chorea
B. Ataxia telangiectasia
C. Tuberose sclerosis
D. Neurofibromatosis
E. Von Hippel-Lindau syndrome

QUESTION 268

Features of Friedreich's ataxia include

A. Cardiomyopathy
B. Kyphoscoliosis
C. Pes cavus
D. Adenoma sebaceum
E. Nystagmus

QUESTION 269

Sites at which peripheral nerves are frequently compressed

A. Common peroneal nerve – neck of fibula
B. Radial nerve – surgical neck of humerus
C. Posterior interosseous nerve – supinator muscle
D. Sural nerve – flexor retinaculum
E. Lateral cutaneous nerve of thigh – inguinal ligament

QUESTION 270

Autonomic neuropathy occurs in

A. Hypothyroidism
B. Guillain-Barré syndrome
C. Wernicke-Korsakoff syndrome
D. Amyloidosis
E. Porphyria

QUESTION 271

Important drug-associated peripheral neuropathies include

A. Gentamicin
B. Chloramphenicol
C. Vincristine
D. Isoniazid
E. Amphotericin

QUESTION 272

The following occur in the Wernicke-Korsakoff syndrome

A. Carpal tunnel syndrome
B. Absent response to caloric stimulation
C. Spinal stenosis
D. Nystagmus
E. Confabulation

QUESTION 273

Features of subacute combined degeneration of the cord include

A. Macrocytosis
B. Treatment with vitamin B12 reverses CNS damage
C. Pyridoxine deficiency
D. Muscle fasciculation
E. Proximal muscle weakness

QUESTION   274

Features of polymyositis

A. Proximal muscle wasting
B. Microcytic anaemia
C. Elevated creatine phosphokinase
D. Spiky polphasic action potentials on EMG
E. Infiltration of muscle by polymorphonuclear cells

QUESTION   275

Myasthenia gravis

A. Thymectomy improves outcome
B. Cardiomyopathy is a common cause of death
C. Constipation should be treated with magnesium sulphate enemas
D. The ESR is elevated
E. Is associated with small-cell carcinoma of the bronchus

QUESTION   276

With regard to Duchenne muscular dystrophy

A. It is linked to a defect on chromosone 21
B. Suxamethonium is contraindicated
C. Cardiomyopathy is a recognised feature
D. Kyphoscoliosis is commonly found
E. Patients should have a nasogastric tube inserted perioperatively

QUESTION   277

Features of dystrophia myotonica

A. Weakness is worsened by a carbohydrate meal
B. Regional anaesthesia blocks the myotonic response
C. Cardiac conduction defects are common
D. Increased motor conduction velocity is diagnostic
E. Competitive muscle relaxants should be reversed at the end of surgery

QUESTION   278

Recognised features of neuromuscular junction disease include

A. Distal muscles usually more affected than proximal muscles
B. Ptosis
C. Diplopia
D. Distal sensory loss
E. Dysphagia

QUESTION 279

Drugs that worsen neuromuscular diseases include

A. Lithium
B. Lignocaine
C. Propranolol
D. Chlorpromazine
E. Quinidine

QUESTION 280

Tests used in the diagnostic evaluation of neuromuscular junction diseases include

A. Serum creatine kinase
B. Tensilon test
C. Acetylcholine receptor antibody
D. Beta-adrenergic receptor antibody
E. Repetitive stimulation on EMG

QUESTION 281

Myotonic dystrophy

A. Has an autosomal recessive mode of inheritance
B. Is associated with diabetes mellitus
C. Is associated with hypogammaglobulinaemia
D. Has a characteristic EMG pattern
E. Results in type I respiratory failure

QUESTION 282

Recognised causes of peripheral neuropathy include

A. Amyloid
B. Diabetes mellitus
C. Alcohol
D. Porphyria
E. Vincristine

QUESTION 283

Central causes of vertigo include

A. Ménière's
B. Benign positional vertigo
C. Acoustic neuroma
D. Vestibular neuronitis
E. Multiple sclerosis

QUESTION 284

A small pupil is characteristic of

A. IIIrd nerve palsy
B. Horner's syndrome
C. Tabes dorsalis
D. Optic neuritis
E. Holmes–Adie pupil

QUESTION 285

The following statements are true regarding TIAs

A. Approx. 30% will have only one episode
B. Approx. 30% will continue to have TIAs alone
C. Approx. 30% will have a completed stroke within 3 years
D. Approx. 30% with carotid territory TIAs will have only minor carotid disease on angiography
E. Approx. 30% are associated with intracranial haemorrhage

QUESTION 286

Drugs used in the treatment of Parkinson's disease include

A. Amantadine
B. Benztropine
C. Chlorpromazine
D. Selegiline
E. L-DOPA

QUESTION 287

The following are recognised features of classical neurofibromatosis

A. Scoliosis
B. Axillary freckles
C. Low IQ
D. Hamartomas of the iris
E. Cerebral gliomas

QUESTION 288

Motor neurone disease

A. Commonly presents with upper limb wasting and lower limb spasticity
B. Is more common in women than men
C. Responds to treatment with beta-interferon
D. May involve the brainstem without clinical limb involvement
E. Is associated with a painful sensory neuropathy

QUESTION 289

Recognised causes of episodic disturbances in consciousness include

A. Spontaneous hypoglycaemia
B. Vertebrobasilar ischaemia
C. Basilar artery migraine
D. Transient global ischaemia
E. Epilepsy

QUESTION 290

Complex partial epilepsy

A. Is the most common form of epilepsy following prolonged febrile convulsions as a child
B. Frequently presents in childhood
C. Is best treated with sodium valproate
D. May have an aura of abdominal discomfort
E. Is a form of petit mal

QUESTION 291

The following are causes of intracranial calcification on skull X-ray

A. Hyperparathyroidism
B. Sturge-Weber syndrome
C. Meningioma
D. Chromophobe pituitary adenoma
E. Myeloma

QUESTION 292

Intracranial aneurysms

A. Are linked to the presence of hypertension in the majority of patients
B. Are seldom familial
C. Are associated with polycystic kidney disease
D. Are multiple in approx. 10-20% of patients
E. Are most frequently found on the posterior communicating artery

QUESTION 293

Lesions of the hypothalamus

A. Are a cause of hypothermia
B. Can cause hypoprolactinaemia
C. Can cause anorexia
D. May be associated with bitemporal hemianopia
E. Are seen with neurosarcoidosis

QUESTION 294

After recovery of consciousness following a closed head injury

A. The patient may not remember the blow on the head
B. The period of retrograde amnesia shrinks as the recovery continues
C. The period of post-traumatic amnesia shrinks as recovery continues
D. Permanent anosmia is a recognised complication
E. If no fits occur in the first 3 months following injury, there is no risk of post-traumatic epilepsy

QUESTION 295

The following are associated with a raised CSF protein

A. Pyogenic meningitis
B. Parkinson's disease
C. Guillian-Barré syndrome
D. Benign intracranial hypertension
E. Carcinomatosis

ENDOCRINE

QUESTION 296

The following are features of primary hypothyroidism in the adult

A. Raised serum creatinine kinase
B. Pleural effusions
C. Malignant change within the thyroid
D. Fibrosis of the thyroid
E. Circulating thyroid autoantibodies

QUESTION 297

In myxoedema coma

A. Patients are usually known to be hypothyroid
B. Treatment should be started with 2.5-5 μg of T3 intravenously every 8 hours
C. Corticosteroids should be given
D. Mortality is >70%
E. Hypoglycaemia is common

QUESTION 298

Concerning thyroid storm

A. Propranolol is contraindicated if there are signs of cardiac failure
B. Carbimazole should be started early
C. Oral potassium iodide should be given
D. Steroids may be of value
E. Radioactive iodine is an effective treatment in this setting

QUESTION 299

de Quervain's thyroiditis is characterised by

A. An elevated ESR
B. A bacterial aetiology
C. Increased technetium-99 uptake on radioisotope scanning
D. Transient hypothyroidism
E. Circulating anti-thyroid antibodies

QUESTION 300

Exophthalmic Graves' disease

A. Is always associated with thyrotoxicosis
B. Is best assessed by CT scan of the orbits
C. Is usually associated with circulating antithyroid antibodies
D. Occurs in at least 50% of patients with thyrotoxic Graves' disease
E. Orbital radiotherapy may be of some help

QUESTION 301

Concerning Graves' disease in pregnancy

A. Fetal hyperthyroidism is caused by maternal T4 crossing the placenta
B. Propylthiouracil may cause neonatal goitre
C. Radioiodine may be used as it does not cross the placenta
D. Transient neonatal hypothyroidism is common
E. Propranolol may be used for control of tachycardia

QUESTION 302

Adrenal failure may be associated with

A. Pallor
B. Vitiligo
C. Diabetes
D. Hypocalcaemia
E. Hypercalcaemia

QUESTION 303

In Cushing's syndrome

A. Profound hypokalaemia is usually associated with an adrenal tumour
B. Failure to suppress with low-dose dexamethasone supports the diagnosis
C. Patients with ectopic ACTH usually suppress with high-dose dexamethasone
D. The most useful screening test is a 24-hour urinary free cortisol
E. Metyrapone inhibits 11-beta-hydroxylase and reduces cortisol production

QUESTION 304

In Cushing's syndrome due to adrenal carcinoma

A. Virilization is common
B. Diurnal variation in cortisol levels remains
C. Plasma ACTH may be normal
D. There is an exaggerated ACTH response to corticotrophin releasing factor (CRF)
E. Metyrapone should be administered pre-operatively

QUESTION 305

Adrenal tumours

A. May be associated with multiple endocrine neoplasia type I
B. When found incidentally are usually non-functioning
C. Are usually malignant if >2 cm in diameter
D. Plasma sodium is useful in screening for hormone production
E. Are incidential findings in ~1% of CT scans

QUESTION 306

The following are features of multiple endocrine neoplasia type 2

A. Hypoglycaemia
B. Recurrent goitre
C. Hypertension
D. Facial flushing
E. Raised urinary cyclic AMP levels

QUESTION 307

The following cause a rise in serum renin levels

A. Standing upright from being supine
B. Angiotensin II infusion
C. Treatment with thiazide diuretics
D. Cortisol
E. Hypertension

QUESTION 308

Congenital adrenal hyperplasia

A. Is most commonly due to 11-hydroxylase deficiency
B. Causes precocious puberty in girls
C. Due to 21-hydroxylase deficiency is associated with hypertension
D. May be treated with dexamethasone
E. Is characterised by high cortisol levels

QUESTION 309

The following are recognised risk factors for developing cataracts

A. Hyperparathyroidism
B. Diabetes mellitus
C. Wilson's disease
D. Chronic uveitis
E. Hypomagnesaemia

QUESTION 310

In primary hyperparathyroidism

A. Hypercalcaemia may be associated with a normal PTH level
B. >80% of patients have a solitary parathyroid adenoma
C. Hypertension is a recognised association
D. Pancreatitis is a recognised complication
E. Cutaneous moniliasis is a recognised association

QUESTION 311

In acromegaly

A. There is an increased risk of malignancy
B. Patients often have hypercalcaemia
C. Excessive daytime drowsiness is a recognised association
D. Serum growth hormone is suppressed during an oral glucose tolerance test
E. Cardiovascular disease is a common cause of morbidity

QUESTION 312

Concerning Nelson's syndrome

A. There is marked hyperpigmentation
B. Treatment of choice is bilateral adrenalectomy
C. The patient may present with bitemporal hemianopia
D. It may follow post-partum haemorrhage
E. Recurrent hypoglycaemia is common

QUESTION   313

Lesions of the hypothalamus

A. Are a cause of hypothermia
B. Can cause hypoprolactinaemia
C. Can cause anorexia
D. May be associated with bitemporal hemianopia
E. Are seen with neurosarcoidosis

QUESTION   314

Gestational diabetes mellitus

A. Is associated with an increased risk of fetal cardiac defects
B. Is due to high circulating prolactin levels
C. May not recur with subsequent pregnancies
D. Carries a higher risk of established diabetes mellitus post-partum
E. Is diagnosed by glycosuria

QUESTION   315

Recurrent hypoglycaemia is more common in diabetics with

A. Autonomic neuropathy
B. Adrenal insufficiency
C. Coeliac disease
D. Diabetic nephropathy
E. Acromegaly

QUESTION   316

The following signs are typically found on examination

A. Increased pigmentation in Addison's disease
B. Pretibial myxoedema in Graves' disease
C. Proximal myopathy in thyrotoxicosis
D. Proximal myopathy in Cushing's syndrome
E. Hirsutism in Addison's disease

QUESTION   317

The following results are typical

A. Normal serum aldosterone in Addison's disease
B. Hypokalaemia in Conn's syndrome
C. Normal parathyroid hormone in multiple endocrine neoplasia (MEN) type 1
D. Low urine osmolality and low plasma osmolality in diabetes insipidus
E. Increased circulating ACTH in Cushing's disease

QUESTION 318

In a thyroid crisis

A. Corticosteroids should be given
B. Propranolol inhibits peripheral conversion of T3 to T4
C. Lithium may be useful
D. Atrial fibrillation is common
E. Hyperkalaemia is common

QUESTION 319

Primary hyperparathyroidism

A. Is usually due to parathyroid carcinoma
B. Can cause diabetes insipidus
C. Causes hypophosphataemia
D. The hypercalcaemia is usually suppressed by hydrocortisone
E. Chvostek's sign is usually positive

QUESTION 320

Concerning the adrenal glands

A. Aldosterone is produced in the zona glomerulosa
B. Cushing's disease is caused by a steroid secreting adrenal adenoma
C. Cortisol secretion is reduced in congenital adrenal hyperplasia
D. Catecholamines are produced in the adrenal medulla
E. Mineralocorticoid secretion is mainly controlled by ACTH

QUESTION 321

Cushing's syndrome

A. May be caused by bronchial carcinoma
B. Is a cause of hypoglycaemia
C. May be mimicked by excess alcohol consumption
D. May be associated with purple striae
E. Causes thin skin

QUESTION 322

Growth hormone

A. Stimulates renal production of insulin-like growth factor
B. Is produced in the hypothalamus and secreted from the pituitary
C. Secretion may be stimulated by "Bovril"
D. Secretion is high during REM sleep
E. Excess is usually due to increased growth hormone releasing hormone

QUESTION 323

Acromegaly

A. Is usually associated with an abnormal skull X-ray
B. May be treated with octreotide
C. May cause a large tongue
D. Is associated with hypertension
E. Is associated with diabetes mellitus

QUESTION 324

Concerning the pituitary

A. A large (non-ACTH-secreting) tumour will cause early loss of ACTH secretion
B. Binasal hemianopias are common with large tumours
C. Kallmann's syndrome is caused by pituitary infarction following postpartum haemorrhage
D. Dopamine causes prolactin release from the anterior pituitary
E. Nelson's syndrome may occur after adrenalectomy

QUESTION 325

Hypertension is commonly associated with

A. Cushing's syndrome
B. Acromegaly
C. Polyarteritis nodosa
D. Rheumatoid arthritis
E. Congenital adrenal hyperplasia

QUESTION 326

Phaeochromocytoma

A. 90% are malignant
B. 10% are extra-adrenal
C. Urinary 5HIAA is a useful screening test
D. Metaiodobenzylguanidine (MIBG) scanning may be helpful
E. Treatment should initially be with beta-blockers

QUESTION 327

Nephrogenic diabetes insipidus may be caused by

A. Lithium
B. Amphotericin B
C. Nicotine
D. Hypokalaemia
E. Brain death

QUESTION 328

The following are complications of diabetes mellitus

A. Sixth cranial nerve palsy
B. Kimmelstein Wilson lesions in the eye
C. Loss of sinus arrhythmia
D. Microalbuminuria detectable by dipsticks
E. Gastroparesis

QUESTION 329

Concerning hyperglycaemic emergencies

A. Cerebral oedema during the treatment of diabetic ketoacidosis is more common in the elderly than in the young
B. Long term insulin therapy is always indicated following diabetic ketoacidosis
C. Gastric stasis is common in diabetic ketoacidosis
D. They may be precipitated by loop diuretics
E. Diabetic ketoacidosis has a higher mortality than hyperosmolar non-ketotic hyperglycaemia

QUESTION 330

Addisonian crisis

A. Classically presents with hyponatraemia and hyperkalaemia
B. May be precipitated by ketoconazole
C. Fludrocortisone should be started immediately
D. Diagnosis can be confirmed with a tetracosactrin test
E. Hypoglycaemia is common

METABOLISM/NUTRITION

QUESTION 331

In acute intermittent porphyria

A. There is an increase in urinary 5 amino-laevulinate
B. There is an increase in faecal porphyrins
C. The diagnosis is aided by the estimation of porphobilinogen deaminase
D. Acute attacks are more common in women
E. Skin lesions may occur in the acute phase

QUESTION 332

Acute intermittent porphyria (AIP)

A. Is diagnosed by the presence of excess protoporphyrin in the urine
B. Is classically associated with urine which turns red-brown on addition of Ehrlich's aldehyde
C. Is an autosomal dominant disorder
D. Presents with frank psychosis
E. Presents with a photosensitive bullous rash on the face and hands

QUESTION 333

The following are correctly matched to the metabolic process they are involved in

A. Pyridoxal phosphate (B6) — synthesis of DNA
B. Nicotinic acid — electron transport
C. Cholecalciferol (D3) — calcium metabolism
D. Folic acid — DNA synthesis
E. Thiamine (B1) — synthesis of amino acids

QUESTION 334

Deficiency of

A. Zinc causes poor wound healing
B. Vitamin A causes bone pain and perifollicular bleeding
C. Iron causes brittle nails
D. Niacin causes Casal's necklace
E. Copper causes microcytic hypochromic anaemia

QUESTION 335

During fasting, the following may be used for gluconeogenesis

A. Pyruvate
B. Glycerol
C. Lactate
D. Amino acids
E. Acetyl coenzyme A

QUESTION 336

Recognised features of lactic acidosis include

A. Most commonly due to accumulation of the L-isomer of lactate
B. Complicates metformin therapy
C. Should be suspected in high anion-gap acidosis where there is no uraemia or diabetic ketoacidosis
D. Serum lactate concentrations of >5 mmol/l are diagnostic
E. Associated with short bowel syndrome

QUESTION 337

Regarding the physiology of glucose control

A. A protein meal stimulates glucagon release
B. A protein meal stimulates insulin release
C. Somatostatin infusion induces hypoglycaemia
D. Insulin-like growth factor-I (ILGF-I) secretion by the liver is stimulated by insulin
E. Ketone body synthesis is stimulated by insulin

QUESTION 338

Hyperuricaemia is seen in

A. Renal failure
B. High-dose aspirin therapy
C. Myeloproliferative disease
D. Acute intermittent porphyria
E. Chronic liver disease

QUESTION 339

The following drugs may precipitate an attack of acute intermittent porphyria

A. Alcohol
B. Droperidol
C. Thiopentone
D. Phenytoin
E. Etomidate

QUESTION 340

The following are recognised complications associated with total parenteral nutrition

A. Hypochloraemic metabolic acidosis
B. Central vein thrombosis
C. Hypoglycaemia
D. Hyperphosphataemia
E. Hypermagnesaemia

HAEMATOLOGY

QUESTION 341

The following are normally found in circulating blood

A. Fibrin
B. Plasminogen
C. Factor VIII
D. Factor V
E. Thromboplastin

QUESTION 342

The following are found in circulating blood

A. Plasmin
B. Fibrinogen
C. D–Dimer
D. Thrombin
E. Factor Xa

QUESTION 343

Skin bleeding time is increased in the following conditions

A. Haemophilia
B. Sickle cell disease
C. Idiopathic thrombocytopaenic purpura
D. von Willebrand's disease
E. Renal failure

QUESTION 344

The prothrombin time is prolonged in

A. Haemophilia A
B. Liver failure
C. Vitamin C deficiency
D. Intravascular coagulation
E. von Willebrand's disease

QUESTION 345

The activated partial thromboplastin time is prolonged in the following conditions

A. Haemophilia A
B. Vitamin K deficiency
C. DIC
D. von Willebrand's disease
E. Factor VII deficiency

QUESTION 346

Disseminated intravascular coagulation

A. Is often characterised by a neurological presentation
B. Responds to heparin therapy in the majority of cases
C. May be caused by an ABO incompatible transfusion
D. Is characterised by raised fibrinogen levels
E. Is associated with thrombocythaemia

QUESTION 347

The following are recognised causes of thrombocytopenia

A. Pernicious anaemia
B. Porphyria
C. HIV infection
D. Hereditary telangiectasia
E. Systemic lupus erythematosus

QUESTION 348

Regarding bleeding disorders

A. Prolonged bleeding time is a characteristic feature of Christmas disease
B. DDAVP may be used for the treatment of haemophilia
C. Bleeding in patients with Osler-Weber-Rendu is due to thrombocytopenia
D. Prothrombin time is normal in patients with von Willebrand's disease
E. Alcoholic cirrhosis is associated with hypofibrinoginaemia

QUESTION 349

Prolonged bleeding time is a characteristic feature of

A. Haemophilia
B. Thrombocytopenic purpura
C. von Willebrand's disease
D. Henoch-Schonlein purpura
E. Christmas disease

QUESTION   350

Laboratory findings consistent with a diagnosis of disseminated intravascular coagulation include

A. Prolonged prothrombin time
B. Low fibrinogen levels
C. Reduced factor VIII levels
D. Increased thrombin
E. Decreased platelet count

QUESTION   351

With regard to autoimmune thrombocytopenic purpura

A. Often follows a viral infection in adults
B. Is associated with chronic lymphocytic leukaemia
C. Platelet autoantibodies are always detectable
D. Splenomegaly is rare
E. Prothrombin time may be abnormal

QUESTION   352

Haemophilia A

A. The gene for factor VIII is on chromosome 11
B. There is no family history in one third of cases
C. The prothrombin time is normal
D. Plasma vWF factor is also reduced
E. Clot retraction is abnormal

QUESTION   353

The following would occur with a defect in the intrinsic pathway of the clotting cascade

A. Platelet count – normal
B. Bleeding time – normal
C. Prothrombin time – increased
D. Activated partial thromboplastin time – increased
E. Clot retraction – decreased

QUESTION 354

In the management of haemophilia

A. The analgesic of choice is aspirin
B. A haematoma in soft tissue requires urgent surgical decompression
C. Prior to major surgery, factor VIII or IX levels should be raised to 30% of normal
D. DDAVP may be beneficial
E. Factor VIII needs more frequent replacement than factor IX

QUESTION 355

Vitamin K may be used in the treatment excessive bleeding associated with

A. Scurvy
B. Haemophilia B
C. Heparin overdose
D. Extrahepatic cholestasis
E. Warfarin therapy

QUESTION 356

Ineffective erythropoiesis is a characteristic feature of

A. Pernicious anaemia
B. Sideroblastic anaemia
C. Folate deficiency
D. Fanconi's anaemia
E. Aplastic anaemia

QUESTION 357

The Coombs' test is normally positive in haemolytic anaemias associated with the following conditions

A. Chronic lymphocytic leukaemia
B. Thalassaemia
C. SLE
D. Methyl-dopa therapy for hypertension
E. Haemolytic disease of the newborn

QUESTION 358

The following agents may precipitate megaloblastic anaemia in patients with mild folate deficiency

A. Septrin
B. Methotrexate
C. Phenytoin
D. Chloroquine
E. Pyrimethamine

QUESTION 359

Haemolytic anaemia

A. Precipitated by cold, is usually due to an IgM antibody
B. May complicate malignant hypertension
C. May be associated with splenomegaly
D. Is associated with raised serum haptoglobins
E. Complicating primaquine therapy is typically Coombs' positive

QUESTION 360

Macrocytosis without megaloblastic changes may be caused by

A. Alcoholism
B. Gluten-sensitive enteropathy
C. Methotrexate therapy
D. Hypothyroidism
E. Pregnancy

QUESTION 361

Radiological abnormalities of the skeleton are seen in

A. Sickle cell disease
B. G-6-PDH deficiency
C. Vitamin C deficiency
D. Haemophilia
E. Thalassaemia

QUESTION 362

In sickle cell disease

A. The amino acid mutation is in the alpha chain of haemoglobin
B. Leg ulcers are common
C. Aseptic necrosis of the femoral head is a recognised complication
D. Howell-Jolly bodies are seen in the peripheral blood
E. Nocturia is common

QUESTION 363

In a patient with sickle cell disease, sickling may be precipitated by

A. Infection
B. Dehydration
C. Hypoxia
D. Acidosis
E. Suxamethonium

QUESTION 364

The following statements concerning a patient with sickle cell trait are true

A. HbA levels are usually about 60%
B. Patients are at risk of overwhelming malarial infection
C. Mild anaemia is a characteristic feature
D. The sickle test is positive
E. There is an increased risk of retinopathy

QUESTION 365

Sickle cell disease

A. Occurs only in negroes
B. Is always homozygous for HbS
C. Does not present in the first year of life
D. Is associated with the substitution of valine for glutamic acid at the 6th position of the alpha haemoglobin chain
E. Sickling may be precipitated by sulphonamides

QUESTION 366

The following finding are consistent with acute haemolysis

A. Reticulocytosis
B. Raised urinary urobilinogen
C. Raised plasma unconjugated bilirubin
D. Raised haptoglobins
E. Methaemalbuminemia

QUESTION   367

The following drugs may induce haemolysis in a patient with Glucose-6-Phosphate dehydrogenase deficiency

A. Thiopentone
B. Quinine
C. Primaquine
D. Aspirin
E. Suxamethonium

QUESTION   368

Pyruvate kinase deficiency

A. Is more common than G-6-PDH deficiency
B. Is more common in males
C. Is associated with gall stones
D. Symptoms are less severe than expected for the level of Hb
E. Suxamethonium administration may lead to hyperkalaemia

QUESTION   369

The following are reliable indices of iron deficiency

A. Serum ferritin below 15 μg/l
B. MCHC below 30 g/dl
C. MCH below 25 g/dl
D. Absence of stainable iron in a marrow biopsy
E. Raised free erythrocyte protoporphyrin

QUESTION   370

The following statements are true

A. Basophillic stippling is seen in beta-thalassaemia
B. Target cells occur in hypersplenism
C. Howell-Jolly bodies are a feature of coeliac disease
D. Heinz bodies are characteristic of G-6-PDH deficiency
E. Macrocytosis may be seen in methotrexate therapy

QUESTION   371

The following are recognised associations

A. Thrombocytosis and CLL
B. Thalassaemia major and increased total body iron
C. Aplastic anaemia and Down's syndrome
D. Polycythaemia and hydronephrosis
E. Myelofibrosis and gout

QUESTION 372

The following are associated with venous thromboses

A. Systemic lupus erythematosus
B. Glanzman's syndrome
C. Adenocarcinoma
D. Protein C deficiency
E. Defective fibrinolytic mechanism

QUESTION 373

The following are associated with a Coombs' positive haemolytic anaemia

A. Thalassaemia
B. SLE
C. Methyldopa therapy
D. Chronic lymphocytic leukaemia
E. Primaquine therapy

QUESTION 374

Beta thalassaemia minor

A. Represents the heterozygous state
B. Is associated with gene deletions
C. There is an excess of beta chains
D. May be confused with iron deficiency
E. May occur in association with sickle cell trait

QUESTION 375

Alpha thalassaemia is associated with

A. Hydrops fetalis
B. Splenomegaly
C. Macrocytosis
D. Increased HbA2 levels
E. Normal HbF levels

INFECTIOUS DISEASES

QUESTION   376

Body fluids considered to be high risk for transmission of HIV are

A. Synovial fluid
B. Nasal secretions
C. Urine
D. Vaginal secretions
E. Saliva

QUESTION   377

The following penicillins are active against Pseudomonas infection

A. Azlocillin
B. Pivampicillin
C. Carbenicillin
D. Cloxacillin
E. Phenoxymethylpenicillin

QUESTION   378

The following penicillins are active against penicillinase producing organisms

A. Norfloxacin
B. Piperacillin
C. Temocillin
D. Timentin
E. Cloxacillin

QUESTION   379

Examples of orally active cephalosporins are

A. Cephalexin
B. Cephradine
C. Cefuroxime
D. Cefaclor
E. Cephamandole

QUESTION 380

Vancomycin

A. Is produced by Streptomyces orientalis
B. Is bacteriostatic in action
C. Is given by rapid intravenous bolus
D. May cause pseudomembranous colitis
E. Is an aminoglycoside

QUESTION 381

Advantages of azithromycin over erythromycin include

A. Increased activity against pseudomonas
B. Enhanced activity against gram positive organisms
C. Bactericidal action
D. Increased tissue penetration
E. Fewer gastrointestinal side effects

QUESTION 382

The following are true of beta–lactam antibiotics

A. Beta–lactam antibiotics are bacteriostatic
B. Imipenem is administered in combination with cilastatin
C. Meropenem is partially inactivated in the kidney
D. Aztreonam is active against gram positive and negative bacteria
E. Aztreonam is a monocyclic beta lactam

QUESTION 383

Ciprofloxacin is indicated in severe infections of the gastrointestinal tract caused by

A. *Campylobacter jejuni*
B. *Shigella dysenteriae*
C. *Escherichia coli*
D. *Salmonella typhi*
E. *Helicobactor pylori*

QUESTION 384

Antiviral therapy

A. Ganciclovir is indicated for cytomegalovirus infections in patients with HIV
B. Acyclovir is active against herpes viruses
C. Idoxuridine should be given orally before the onset of herpetic skin lesion
D. Ritonavir inhibits nucleoside reverse transcriptase
E. Tribavarin reduces the mortality from lassa fever

QUESTION 385

Antifungal therapy

A. Amphotericin is absorbed from the gut
B. Griseofulvin should be applied topically for fungal infections of the skin
C. Terfenadine is contraindicated in patients taking imidazole antifungal drugs
D. Fluconazole is indicated for central nervous system infection with *Cryptococcus neoformans*
E. Ketoconazole is nephrotoxic

QUESTION 386

Clinical conditions associated with toxins produced by Staphylococcus aureus

A. Bacterial endocarditis
B. Scalded-skin syndrome
C. Toxic shock syndrome
D. Pneumonia
E. Food poisoning

QUESTION 387

Antibacterial prophylaxis is indicated in patients with prosthetic heart valves undergoing

A. Tooth extractions
B. Tonsillectomy
C. Uncomplicated vaginal delivery
D. Colonoscopy
E. Fibreoptic bronchoscopy

QUESTION 388

Likely pathogens in hospital acquired urinary tract infections are

A. *Bacteroides*
B. *Staphylococcus aureus*
C. *Serratia*
D. *Klebsiella*
E. *Proteus*

QUESTION 389

Modes of action of antimicrobial agents

A. Tetracycline inhibits bacterial cell wall synthesis
B. Imipenem inhibits bacterial protein synthesis
C. Ciprofloxacin inhibits bacterial DNA synthesis
D. Aminoglycosides inhibit bacterial cell wall synthesis
E. Co-trimoxazole inhibits bacterial folate synthesis

QUESTION 390

Patients with the following conditions require antimicrobial prophylaxis when undergoing dental surgery

A. Prosthetic joint implants
B. Indwelling intraperitoneal catheters
C. Post renal transplant
D. Ventricular septal defects
E. Post splenectomy

QUESTION 391

In HIV positive patients

A. *Pneumocystis carinii* is a common cause of pneumonia
B. *Toxoplasma gondii* commonly causes diarrhoea
C. *Cryptosporidium parvum* causes encephalitis
D. *Cryptococcus neoformans* is an important cause of meningitis
E. *Candida albicans* frequently infects the oropharynx

QUESTION 392

The following drugs should be avoided in renal failure

A. Chloramphenicol
B. Erythromycin
C. Fusidic acid
D. Tetracycline
E. Nalidixic acid

QUESTION 393

Enterococci

A. Are alpha haemolytic streptococci
B. Possess Lancefield group D antigen
C. Are gram negative diplococci
D. Are sensitive to cephalosporins
E. Commonly cause endocarditis

QUESTION 394

Tuberculosis

A. Is treated with rifampicin only
B. In adults, it results from primary infection
C. Is a non caseating granulomatous disease
D. There is a high incidence in HIV positive patients
E. Clarithromycin is indicated for resistant organisms

QUESTION 395

The following are various methods of sterilization

A. Boiling in water for 5 minutes
B. Heating to 122°C for 15 minutes at 101.3 kPa
C. Gamma irradiation
D. Immersion in 0.1% chlorhexidine for one hour
E. Heating to 150°C for 10 minutes

QUESTION 396

Human immunodeficiency virus

A. Is a DNA virus
B. Its genome encodes for reverse transcriptase
C. Its primary target cell is the CD8+ T lymphocytes
D. Anti-HIV antibody is detectable 6-12 weeks after exposure
E. Can be cultured from the peripheral blood of infected individuals even before the antibody titre rises

QUESTION 397

Concerning HIV infection

A. Seroconversion can be associated with an acute aseptic meningoencephalitis
B. Persistent generalised lymphadenopathy is usually tender
C. Cryptococcus neoformans is the commonest cause of meningitis in AIDS patients
D. Oral candidiasis in an otherwise asymptomatic individual is a predictor of progression to AIDS
E. Pentamidine is the first drug of choice for preventing PCP infection

QUESTION 398

The following are recognised side effects of antibiotics

A. Metronidazole — painless peripheral neuropathy
B. Ciprofloxacin — arthralgias
C. Amphotericin B — renal tubular acidosis
D. Tetracycline — benign intracranial hypertension
E. Imipenem — seizures

QUESTION 399

Concerning lung manifestations of HIV/AIDS

A. Palatal Kaposi's are strongly associated with intrathoracic Kaposi's sarcoma
B. Reduction in TLCO is the most sensitive marker of Pneumocystis carinii pneumonia
C. Transbronchial biopsy carries a higher risk of complications in HIV-positive individuals
D. Mycobacterium avium intracellulare infection is rare in those with CD4 counts $> 0.1 \times 10^9/l$
E. Cytomegalovirus is an important cause of pneumonitis in HIV-positive individuals

QUESTION 400

Babies born to HIV-positive mothers

A. Have a higher rate of congenital malformations
B. In the UK have a higher risk of prematurity
C. Are more likely to become HIV positive if they are the first of twins to be delivered vaginally
D. Risk infection through breast milk
E. May acquire HIV infection transplacentally

QUESTION 401

Acute infection with the following organisms is associated with a glandular-fever like syndrome

A. Cytomegalovirus
B. Toxoplasma
C. Human herpes virus-6
D. Parvovirus B19
E. Coxsackie A

QUESTION 402

Legionnaire's disease

A. Person-to-person spread is common
B. Is more frequent in smokers
C. Is typically a short, mild illness
D. SIADH is a recognised complication
E. May be caused by *Legionella micdadei*

QUESTION   403

Chlamydial pneumonia

A. Is caused by *Chlamydia trachomatis* in neonates
B. Can be seen in adults with no contact with birds
C. Myocarditis is a recognised complication
D. Is treated with benzylpenicillin
E. Typically produces a lobar pneumonia on CXR

QUESTION   404

The following are deterred from donating blood in the UK

A. Men who have had sex with prostitutes
B. Individuals whose partners are from sub-Saharan Africa
C. Glue-sniffers
D. Individuals whose partners have had sex with prostitutes
E. Those who received blood products before 1982

QUESTION   405

The following are transmitted by blood

A. Malaria
B. Giardia
C. Epstein Barr virus
D. *Treponema pallidum*
E. HTLV-1

PSYCHIATRY

QUESTION   406

The following are inhibitors of monoamine oxidase types A and B

A. Phenelzine
B. Seleginine
C. Tranylcypromine
D. Isocarboxazid
E. Moclobemide

QUESTION 407

The following are selective serotonin reuptake inhibitors

A. Venlafaxine
B. Fluoxetine
C. Nortriptyline
D. Paroxetine
E. Sertraline

QUESTION 408

The following are true of donepezil

A. It is used to treat Alzheimer's dementia
B. Should be avoided in renal impairment
C. Exacerbates the action of suxamethonium
D. Causes tachycardia
E. Increases serum creatine kinase

QUESTION 409

Electroconvulsive therapy is effective in the treatment of

A. Mania
B. Puerperal psychosis
C. Acute schizophrenia with predominantly negative symptoms
D. Depression
E. Acute catatonic states

QUESTION 410

Regarding electroconvulsive therapy

A. Heart rate initially increases
B. Cerebral blood flow remains constant
C. Mortality is 4 per 100,000 treatments
D. Atropine should be given routinely
E. Serum prolactin increases

QUESTION 411

Pathological features of Alzheimer's disease include

A. Lewy bodies
B. Neurofibrillary tangles
C. Argentophil plaques
D. Granulovacuolar degeneration
E. Loss of choline acetyltransferase

QUESTION   412

Illnesses commonly producing the clinical features of depression include

A. Insulinomas
B. Phaeochromocytoma
C. Addison's disease
D. Cushing's syndrome
E. Hyperparathyroidism

QUESTION   413

Good prognostic signs in schizophrenia include

A. Insidious onset
B. Mood disturbance
C. Male sex
D. Negative symptoms
E. Family history

QUESTION   414

Delirium tremens

A. Has a mortality of less than 1%
B. Should be treated with disulfiram
C. Is associated with vestibular disturbances
D. B vitamins should be given parenterally
E. Patients should be nursed in a dark room

QUESTION   415

Psychiatric complications of alcohol abuse include

A. Othello syndrome
B. Dementia
C. Depression
D. Korsakoff's psychosis
E. Cotard's syndrome

QUESTION   416

Features of bulimia nervosa include

A. Metabolic alkalosis
B. Primary amenorrhoea
C. Laxative abuse
D. Erosion of dental enamel
E. Less than 25% ideal body weight

QUESTION 417

Factors indicating an increased risk of suicide in depressed patients are

A. Living alone
B. Alcohol dependence
C. Unemployment
D. Male sex
E. Recent bereavement

QUESTION 418

Puerperal psychosis

A. Occurs once in every 5,000 births
B. Recurrence rate for depressive illness in subsequent puerperium is 15-20%
C. Prognosis is poor
D. Electroconvulsive therapy is contraindicated
E. Onset typically occurs 3 months after delivery

QUESTION 419

The following drugs may cause psychosis

A. Reserpine
B. Prednisolone
C. Amantidine
D. Disulfiram
E. Methyldopa

QUESTION 420

Moclobemide

A. Covalently binds to monoamine oxidase A
B. Causes a hypertensive crisis if cottage cheese is ingested
C. Potentiates the action of sulphonylureas
D. Metabolises adrenaline
E. Needs to be discontinued for two weeks before safely starting tricyclic antidepressants

QUESTION 421

Hyponatraemia is a recognised side effect of

A. Moclobemide
B. Flupenthixol
C. Carbamazepine
D. Fluoxetine
E. Amitriptyline

QUESTION 422

Overdose of ecstasy (methylenedioymethamphetamine) causes

A. Disseminated intravascular coagulation
B. Hypothermia
C. Hypotension
D. Tinnitus
E. Polyuria

QUESTION 423

Indications for antidepressants are

A. Bulimia
B. Bipolar depression
C. Alzheimer's disease
D. Neuropathic pain
E. Schizophrenia

QUESTION 424

Characteristics of hysterical symptoms

A. Produced deliberately
B. Occur in the absence of physical disease
C. Associated with secondary gain
D. Abreaction produces long-term recovery
E. Are affected by cultural beliefs

QUESTION 425

Signs of lithium toxicity include

A. Tremor
B. Hepatitis
C. Ataxia
D. Constipation
E. Oliguria

QUESTION 426

The following are contraindications to ECT

A. Puerpural psychosis
B. Depression with suicidal ideation
C. Manic depression
D. Raised intracranial pressure
E. Severe depression with weight loss

QUESTION 427

The following are recognised features of cocaine abuse

A. Sexual dysfunction in men
B. Increased need for sleep
C. Severe anxiety and paranoid ideation
D. Hallucinations
E. Dilated pupils not reactive to light

QUESTION 428

The following are common side effects of lithium

A. Ataxia
B. Symptomatic hypothyroidism
C. Polyuria
D. Leukocytosis
E. Seizures

QUESTION 429

The following are recognised side-effects of neuroleptic drugs

A. Oculogyric crisis
B. Catatonia
C. Akathisia
D. Tardive dyskinesia
E. Parkinsonism

QUESTION 430

Regarding the neuroleptic–malignant syndrome

A. Profound hyperthermia is typical
B. Concious level remains normal
C. Dantrolene is effective in controlling symptoms
D. Leukocytosis is common
E. Further use of neuroleptics is contraindicated

SUBSTANCE ABUSE

QUESTION 431

In paracetamol overdose

A. The toxic metabolite is N-acetyl-P-benzoquinonimine
B. Decreased conscious level is common on admission
C. A paracetamol level above 200 ng/l at 4 hours after ingestion requires treatment with acetylcysteine
D. Those taking enzyme-inducing drugs are at increased risk
E. After a severe overdose the patient should not take paracetamol again, even in normal therapeutic doses

QUESTION 432

Chronic alcohol abuse can cause

A. Subacute combined degeneration of the cord
B. Macrocytosis
C. Beri-beri
D. Pancreatitis
E. Impaired carbohydrate metabolism

QUESTION 433

When treating poisoning

A. Snake anti-venom has a high risk of anaphylaxis
B. Expired air resuscitation should not be used in cyanide poisoning
C. Forced alkaline diuresis may cause cerebral oedema
D. Penicillamine is useful in treating iron poisoning
E. Glucagon is useful in treating beta-blocker overdose

QUESTION 434

After drug overdose

A. Tricyclic antidepressants delay gastric emptying
B. Charcoal haemoperfusion may be useful in the management of theophylline overdose
C. Salicylate is removed with haemodialysis
D. Ethanol is used in the treatment of methanol poisoning
E. Atropine may be used in organophosphate poisoning

QUESTION   435

Poisoning by

A. Mercury may cause tremor
B. Lithium may be due to co-administration of a diuretic
C. Lithium may be treated with haemodialysis
D. Digoxin may be treated with specific antibodies
E. Cyanide causes a metabolic acidosis

QUESTION   436

Carbon monoxide

A. Levels up to 10% may be found in smokers
B. Affinity for haemoglobin is 24 times that of oxygen
C. Will falsely elevate the readings on a pulse oximeter
D. May cause coma
E. Toxicity is synergistic with cyanide

QUESTION   437

Activated charcoal

A. Increases elimination of digoxin
B. Is ineffective in salicylate overdose
C. Should be repeated 4 hourly for at least 24 hours following cyanide poisoning
D. Is only useful in those drugs with significant enterohepatic circulation
E. Is dangerous if aspirated

QUESTION   438

Poisoning by

A. Organophosphates may occur after skin contact
B. Cyanide inhibits cytochrome oxidase
C. Methanol is due to its metabolites
D. Amanita phalloides is more severe if the mushrooms are cooked rather than eaten raw
E. Paraquat is made worse by giving high oxygen concentrations

QUESTION   439

Tricyclic antidepressant overdose may cause

A. Fixed dilated pupils
B. Extensor plantar responses
C. Metabolic alkalosis
D. Urinary retention
E. Ventricular arrhythmias

QUESTION 440

Salicylic acid

A. Delays gastric emptying
B. Has a pKa of 6.1
C. Is predominantly unionized at a urinary pH > 7
D. Causes a respiratory acidosis
E. Causes hyperpyrexia

IMMUNOLOGY/GENETICS

QUESTION 441

The following statements concerning Immunoglobulin G (IgG) are true

A. The natural haemagglutinins anti-A and anti-B are IgG's
B. IgG is the predominant immunoglobulin in tracheobronchial secretions
C. IgG freely crosses the placenta
D. IgG has a molecular weight of 250,000 Daltons
E. IgG bears a single antigen-binding site

QUESTION 442

With regard to Immunoglobulin M (IgM)

A. It crosses the placenta freely
B. It is a dimeric molecule
C. It is a good marker of intrauterine infection in the newborn
D. It is responsible for haemolytic disease of the newborn
E. It is the antibody of the primary immune response

QUESTION 443

Secretory IgA

A. Is responsible for mucosal immunity
B. Activates compliment via the alternative pathway
C. Crosses the placenta
D. Is not present in the plasma
E. Is important in preventing the attachment of polio virus

QUESTION   444

The following are examples of acute phase proteins

A. C-reactive protein
B. Haptoglobin
C. Fibrinogen
D. Caeruloplasmin
E. Alpha-1-antitrypsin

QUESTION   445

Regarding the human lymphocyte antigens (HLA)

A. The genetic loci are situated on chromosome 12
B. Class I antigens are expressed on red blood cells
C. They are involved in antigen recognition by T cells
D. Inter-racial variation is a recognised feature
E. They form part of the Major Histocompatibility Complex (MHC)

QUESTION   446

Concerning the immune response of premature infants

A. IgM synthesis occurs at 24 weeks gestation
B. IgG synthesis starts immediately after birth
C. Placental transfer of IgG is an active process
D. Antibody levels increase immediately after birth
E. An intact immune response is essential for normal fetal development

QUESTION   447

In X-linked recessive diseases

A. The mother is always the carrier
B. There is a maternal age effect
C. Fathers never pass the affected gene to their sons
D. Women may have variably severe manifestations due to random inactivation
E. Half the daughters of a carrier female will themselves be carriers

QUESTION   448

The following are examples of X-linked recessive disorders

A. Haemophilia A
B. Nephrogenic diabetes insipidus
C. Christmas disease
D. Myotonic dystrophy
E. Glucose-6-phosphate dehydrogenase deficiency

QUESTION 449

The following are examples of autosomal dominant conditions

A. Acute intermittent porphyria
B. Fascioscapulohumeral dystrophy
C. Friedreich's ataxia
D. Neurofibromatosis
E. Beta thalassaemia

QUESTION 450

The following are examples of autosomal recessive disorders

A. Vitamin D resistant rickets
B. Sickle cell disease
C. Wilson's disease
D. Cystic fibrosis
E. Glucose-6-phosphate dehydrogenase deficiency

QUESTION 451

Plasmapheresis is a recognised treatment for

A. Guillain-Barré syndrome
B. Goodpasture's syndrome
C. Von Willebrand's disease
D. Myasthenia gravis
E. Hyperviscosity syndrome

QUESTION 452

Selective IgA deficiency

A. May be associated with transfusion reactions
B. Is an extremely common disorder
C. Is associated with IgG3 subclass deficiency
D. Is associated with other autoimmune disorders
E. Anaphylaxis may occur following gammaglobulin administration

QUESTION 453

Selective IgA deficiency

A. Is associated with bronchiectasis
B. Is associated with malabsorption from the GI tract
C. Intravenous immunoglobulin is the treatment of choice
D. Is associated with an increased incidence of chronic active hepatitis
E. Displays X-linked recessive inheritance

QUESTION 454

Regarding hypersensitivity reactions

A. Type II (membrane-bound antigen) is involved in graft rejection
B. Serum sickness is a type III reaction
C. Tuberculin reaction is a type III reaction
D. C1-esterase deficiency is a type I reaction
E. Contact dermatitis is an example of a type IV reaction

QUESTION 455

Hereditary angio-oedema

A. Is inherited as an autosomal dominant condition
B. Is associated with C1 deficiency
C. May be associated with lymphoproliferative disorders
D. Danazol is a recognised treatment option
E. Antifibrinolytics are used in short term prophylaxis

QUESTION 456

The following cytokines are linked to the appropriate function

A. Interleukin-1 (IL-1) - proliferation of activated B cells
B. Interleukin-2 (IL-2) - released by macrophages
C. Gamma interferon - direct antiviral and tumouricidal activity
D. Interleukin-3 (IL-3) - stimulates growth of most haematopoietic cell lines
E. Tumour necrosis factor (TNF) - induces fever and catabolic state

QUESTION 457

T lymphocytes

A. Are the principle mediators of the type I hypersensitivity reaction
B. Are CD3 positive
C. IL-15 induces T cell activation and TNF production
D. Memory T lymphocytes are CD45RO positive
E. Naive T cells circulate through tissues screening for antigen

QUESTION 458

The major histocompatibility complex

A. Class I antigens are found on erythrocytes
B. Class I and class II antigens are encoded on different chromosomes
C. The CD8 molecule interacts with non-polymorphic regions of HLA class I molecules
D. Non-identical twins have a 1 in 4 chance of being identical in their HLA type
E. Class II molecules are found on sperm

QUESTION 459

With regard to anaphylactic reactions associated with anaesthesia

A. Reactions are more common in female patients
B. Previous history of specific drug exposure is necessary
C. The reported incidence is 1 in 100,000
D. Known allergy to banana and avocado may be significant
E. Latex allergy reactions occur within 5 minutes of exposure

QUESTION 460

Mast cell tryptase

A. Is used in the diagnosis of anaphylactic reactions
B. Is released in anaphylactic but not anaphylactoid reactions
C. Is also present in white blood cell granules
D. In reactions to anaesthetic drugs, it is a sensitive diagnostic test
E. In reactions to anaesthetic drugs, it is a specific diagnostic test

PAEDIATRICS

QUESTION 461

Respiratory problems in the neonate may occur with the following conditions

A. Treacher-Collins syndrome
B. Laryngomalacia
C. Cloacal atresia
D. Pierre-Robin syndrome
E. Eaton-Lambert syndrome

QUESTION 462

Pyloric stenosis is associated with

A. Hypokalaemia
B. Hyperchloraemia alkalosis
C. Hypoglycaemia
D. Male preponderance
E. Preterm neonates more than full term neonates

QUESTION 463

The following may predispose to the development of respiratory distress syndrome in the neonate

A. Premature birth
B. Maternal diabetes
C. Antepartum haemorrhage
D. Pre–eclampsia
E. Congenital heart disease in the fetus

QUESTION 464

Kernicterus is associated with

A. Toxic levels of conjugated bilirubin
B. Hypertonicity
C. Opisthotonus
D. Spasticity
E. Sepsis

QUESTION 465

Concerning tracheo–oesophageal fistulae

A. 30-40% of infants with this condition are born preterm
B. Incidence is about 1 in 35,000 live births
C. 20% have associated cardiovascular anomalies
D. There is a recognised association with oligohydramnios in the mother
E. Tracheo–oesophageal fistula without oesophageal atresia is the most common type

QUESTION 466

Omphalocele

A. Is associated with external herniation of abdominal viscera lateral to the umbilical cord
B. Occurs more commonly in females
C. Incidence is of the order of 1 in 5,000–10,000 live births
D. 75% of patients have other congenital defects
E. Most infants with this condition are born prematurely

QUESTION 467

Gastroschisis

A. Is rarely associated with other congenital abnormalities
B. Is more commonly associated with prematurity than omphalocele
C. The abdominal viscera are covered with a hernia sac
D. Initial fluid requirements are increased
E. Nitrous oxide should not be used

QUESTION   468

The following are features of Reye syndrome

A. Cererbal oedema
B. Splenomegaly
C. Hypoglycaemia
D. Respiratory alkalosis
E. Hyperactive tendon reflexes

QUESTION   469

Nephroblastoma (Wilms tumour)

A. Accounts for about 10% of solid tumours in children
B. May be asymptomatic
C. Is a recognised cause of hypertension in children
D. May be associated with hyperkalaemia
E. Mainly occurs in children under the age of 4

QUESTION   470

With regard to the Apgar score

A. It correlates well with acid-base measurements performed immediately after birth
B. A heart rate below 100 scores 1
C. They should be documented immediately after delivery and at 5 minutes
D. Colour is the least informative criteria
E. An infant who is crying scores 2 for respiratory effort

QUESTION   471

With regard to Haemophilus Influenza type b (Hib)

A. It occurs in 1 in 400 children by their fifth birthday
B. It is rare in children below the age of 3 months
C. 60% of all cases present with meningitis frequently accompanied by bacteraemia
D. Peak incidence occurs at age 3 years
E. The case fatality rate is 4-5%

QUESTION   472

The following are examples of live vaccines

A. Haemophilus influenza type B
B. BCG
C. Polio
D. Meningococci groups A and C
E. Tetanus

QUESTION 473

Regarding maternal rubella infection

A. The risk of damage to the fetus declines to 10-20% by 16 weeks gestation
B. Multiple defects are common if infection occurs in the fist 8-10 weeks of pregnancy
C. Perceptive deafness commonly occurs alone
D. Cataracts are a recognised feature
E. The incubation period is 7-10 days

QUESTION 474

The following factors have been implicated in the aetiology of necrotising enterocolitis

A. Perinatal asphyxia
B. Infection
C. Hyperosmolar feeding
D. Cyanotic congenital heart disease
E. Umbilical artery catherisation

QUESTION 475

In a child the intraosseus route can be used to administer

A. Sodium bicarbonate
B. Adrenaline
C. Blood
D. Lignocaine
E. Calcium

QUESTION 476

Complications of intraosseus cannulation include

A. Osteomyelitis
B. Occur with an incidence of 10%
C. Leukaemia
D. Fat embolus
E. Tibial fracture

QUESTION 477

As an aid to immediate resuscitation of a child

A. Body weight = $2 \times$ (Age in years)
B. Oral endotracheal tube length = (Age in years / 2) + 15
C. Defibrillation charge = 2 joules / kg
D. Endotracheal tube size = (Age in years / 4) + 4
E. 5th centile systolic blood pressure = (Age in years $\times$ 2) + 70

QUESTION 478

Causes of neonatal jaundice include

A. Bruising
B. Swallowed blood
C. Breast milk
D. Thalassaemia
E. Hyperthyroidism

QUESTION 479

The following neonatal haematology values are normal

A. Hb of 16.8 g / dl from a cord blood sample
B. Platelet count of 85,000 on day 1
C. A falling reticulocyte count over the first week of life
D. Presence of nucleated red cells in the first two days following delivery
E. A haematocrit of 30%

QUESTION 480

Normal capillary blood gas values for a 1 day old neonate include

A. pH = 7.45
B. PO_2 = 7.1 kPa
C. PCO_2 = 2 kPa
D. A pH that is equivalent to arterial pH
E. PCO_2 = 35 mmHg

MEDICAL BIOCHEMISTRY

QUESTION 481

The following are true of urinalysis

A. Specific gravity is normally 1.002 – 1.035
B. pH is usually between 5.3 and 7.2
C. A urine sodium of greater than 40 mmol/l differentiates renal from prerenal failure
D. A urine/plasma creatinine ratio of greater than 40 differentiates prerenal from renal failure
E. A protein content of up to 150 g per 24 hrs is normal

QUESTION 482

In congenital pyloric stenosis

A. There is an increase in plasma bicarbonate
B. Urinary bicarbonate loss is increased
C. Hyperkalaemia is common
D. Plasma chloride ion concentration is low
E. The urine is initially acidic

QUESTION 483

With regard to the collection of specimens

A. Plasma protein concentrations may vary with posture
B. Spurious hyponatraemia may be caused by hyperlipidaemia
C. Blood for glucose estimation is collected in a tube containing fluoride
D. Potassium measurement should be performed on heparinised samples
E. Calcium measurement may be performed on blood in EDTA bottles

QUESTION 484

With regard to magnesium

A. Magnesium is a predominately extracellular ion
B. It is highly protein bound
C. Renal excretion is increased by aldosterone
D. Hypomagnesaemia is associated with cytotoxic drug therapy
E. Hypomagnesaemia is associated with intestinal fistulae

QUESTION 485

Hyponatraemia is associated with

A. Excessive fluid intake
B. Cardiac failure
C. Diuretic therapy
D. Chlorpropamide therapy
E. Oxytocin therapy

QUESTION 486

With regard to iron metabolism

A. 10 % of the total body iron is found circulating in the plasma
B. Iron is bound to transferrin in the ferrous form
C. Androgens increase plasma iron concentration
D. Oral contraceptives increase plasma iron concentration
E. Plasma iron is lower in the morning

QUESTION 487

With regard to plasma proteins

A. Electrophoresis separates proteins into five main groups
B. Electophoresis is usually performed on a sample of plasma
C. The most obvious band on an electrophoretic strip is albumin
D. Prolonged venous stasis may lead to falsely low results
E. Total protein estimation is a useful diagnostic tool

QUESTION 488

Albumin

A. Has a biological half life of 20 days
B. Has a molecular weight of 65,000 Daltons
C. Analbuminaemia presents with severe peripheral oedema
D. 60 % of the extracellular albumin is in the plasma compartment
E. Plasma levels vary with posture

QUESTION 489

With regard to thyroid function tests

A. Thyroid binding globulin is increased in patients taking danazol
B. 60% of plasma T4 and T3 is bound to thyroid binding globulin
C. They must be performed in the morning because of circadian variations
D. Serum T3 measurement is a clinically useful indicator of thyroid function
E. TRH assay is a useful first line investigation

QUESTION 490

Hypernatraemia is associated with

A. Cushing's syndrome
B. Mannitol therapy
C. Adrenocortical insufficiency
D. Diabetes insipidus
E. Hypoaldosteronism

QUESTION 491

Hyperuricaemia is associated with

A. Psoriasis
B. Acute starvation
C. Alkalosis
D. Loop diuretics
E. Glucose 6 Phosphatase deficiency

QUESTION 492

With regard to the carcinoid syndrome

A. Argentaffin cells synthesise 5-HT from tryptophan
B. 5 hydroxyindole acetic acid (5-HIAA) is excreted in the urine
C. Hyperkalaemia is a common finding in patients with metastatic disease
D. Nicotinamide synthesis may be affected
E. Parathyroid hormone levels may be decreased

QUESTION 493

Clinically important causes of hypophosphatemia include

A. Insulin treatment of diabetic ketoacidosis
B. Starvation
C. Severe burns
D. Acromegaly
E. Hyperalimentation

QUESTION 494

Causes of hypokalaemia include

A. Hyperglycaemia
B. Conn's syndrome
C. Crush injury
D. Diarrhoea
E. Cushing's syndrome

QUESTION 495

Biochemical features of Addison's disease include

A. Hyperkalaemia
B. Hyperglycaemia
C. Hypercalcaemia
D. Hyponatraemia
E. Increased urea concentration

QUESTION 496

Increased alkaline phosphatase may be found in

A. Pregnancy
B. Preterm neonates
C. Ascorbate deficiency
D. Myeloma
E. Acute hepatitis

QUESTION 497

With regard to amylase

A. Plasma levels are increased in glomerular impairment
B. May be extracted from ovaries
C. Levels may increase following morphine administration
D. Levels are low in infants under 1 year
E. May be increased in patients with a ruptured ectopic pregnancy

QUESTION 498

Biochemical features of Cushing's syndrome include

A. Hyperglycaemia
B. Hyperkalaemia
C. Hyponatraemia
D. Hyperlipidaemia
E. Hypercalciuria

QUESTION 499

With regard to creatine kinase

A. Levels are raised following a myocardial infarction
B. Levels are raised in Duchenne muscular dystrophy
C. Levels are raised in multiple sclerosis
D. The enzyme consists of four protein subunits
E. Levels may be raised in hyperthyroidism

QUESTION 500

The following are associated with hypercalcaemia

A. Hyperparathyroidism
B. Thiazide diuretics
C. Hypothyroidism
D. Osteoporosis
E. Sarcoidosis

QUESTION 501

The following substances can cause peripheral oedema

A. Insulin
B. Diclofenac
C. Oestrogen
D. Nifedipine
E. Metolazone

QUESTION 502

Causes of hyponatraemia with decreased extracellular volume include

A. Sick cell syndrome
B. Hypothyroidism
C. Diabetes Mellitus
D. Renal artery stenosis
E. Nephrotic syndrome

QUESTION 503

Hypernatraemia may result from administration of the following

A. 0.9% saline
B. 8.4% sodium bicarbonate
C. Mannitol
D. Desmopressin
E. Antibiotics

QUESTION 504

The following are associated with hypokalaemia

A. Hypermagnesaemia
B. Metabolic acidosis
C. Adrenocortical insufficiency
D. 'Sine wave' pattern on electrocardiogram
E. Bartter's syndrome

QUESTION 505

Conditions resulting in hypomagnesaemia include

A. Acute pancreatitis
B. Bartter's syndrome
C. Conn's syndrome
D. Diabetic ketoacidosis
E. Alcoholism

QUESTION 506

The following cause metabolic acidosis with an increased anion gap

A. Lactic acidosis
B. Type 4 renal tubular acidosis
C. Diabetic ketoacidosis
D. Hyperparathyroidism
E. Salicylate overdose

QUESTION 507

In hypophosphataemia

A. There is a right shift in the oxyhaemoglobin dissociation curve
B. The diagnosis is made if the serum phosphate is less than 1.2 mmol/l
C. Convulsions may occur
D. Renal failure is a common cause
E. Overtreatment can result in severe hypocalcaemia

QUESTION 508

Hyponatraemia in a 50-year-old man may be due to

A. Conn's syndrome
B. Nephrotic syndrome
C. Small cell lung carcinoma
D. Cirrhosis of the liver
E. Hypopituitarism

QUESTION 509

Hypocalcaemia is a recognised feature of

A. Acute renal failue
B. Acute pancreatitis
C. Hypomagnesaemia
D. Pseudohypoparathyroidism
E. Thryotoxicosis

QUESTION 510

In the following causes of metabolic alkalosis, urinary chloride excretion is low

A. Bartter's syndrome
B. Excessive diuretic abuse
C. Surreptitious vomiting
D. Primary hyperaldosteronism
E. Cushing's syndrome

QUESTION 511

The anion gap

A. Is calculated from plasma concentrations of sodium, bicarbonate and phosphate
B. Is usually < 17 meq/l
C. Is increased with paraproteinaemia
D. Is high in ketoacidosis
E. May be normal in patients with a pancreatic fistula

QUESTION 512

Hypophosphataemia

A. Complicates insulin treatment of diabetic ketoacidosis
B. Occurs with paracetamol overdosage
C. Produces a bleeding disorder by reducing fibrinogen levels
D. Occurs with osteoporosis
E. Accompanies hyperparathyroidism

QUESTION 513

A patient has the following electrolytes. Na 112 mmol/l, K 3.2 mmol/l, urea 3.0 mmol/l, plasma osmolarity 254 mOsm. Urine osmolarity 550 mOsm. Possible causes include

A. Astrocytoma
B. Primary adrenal failure
C. Acute intermittent porphyria
D. Demeclocycline therapy
E. Nephrotic syndrome

QUESTION 514

A 36-year-old woman complains of severe polydipsia and polyuria without glycosuria. A diagnosis of compulsive water drinking is unlikely if

A. The plasma potassium is 2.1 mmol/l
B. There is a visual field defect
C. Urine output is diminished by water deprivation
D. The plasma osmolality is greater than normal
E. The urine osmolality remains at 300 mOsm/kg

QUESTION 515

Urine specific gravity is increased in

A. Proteinuria
B. Glycosuria
C. Antibiotic therapy
D. Mannitol therapy
E. Diuretic therapy

PHARMACOLOGY

QUESTION 516

The antiarrhythmic drug flecainide

A. Reduces mortality in myocardial infarction survivors with high-frequency ventricular extrasystoles
B. Given intravenously can convert 20–30% of patients with acute onset lone atrial fibrillation to sinus rhythm
C. Acts primarily on the slow rectifier potassium channel
D. Exhibits 'use-dependence' in ion-channel binding
E. Reduces tachycardia incidence in Wolff-Parkinson-White syndrome by modulating the conduction within the AV node

QUESTION 517

Genetic polymorphisms of drug metabolism

A. Exhibit inter-ethnic differences
B. Are not associated with adverse effects
C. Are dependent on the pharmacological actions of the drug
D. Are due to altered gene expression
E. Are not clinically important for drugs that are eliminated by the kidney

QUESTION 518

The following statements are true

A. Angiotensin-converting enzyme inhibitors reduce mortality in congestive cardiac failure
B. Angiotensin-converting enzyme inhibitors reduce plasma renin activity
C. Aldosterone can be suppressed in some hypertensive patients by dexamethasone
D. The oedema associated with administration of nifedipine is associated with an increase in body weight
E. In hypertensive patients, measurement of renal vein renin activity is a good predictor of response to captopril

QUESTION 519

The following statements concerning anticoagulants and antithrombotic agents are true

A. Low molecular weight heparins are more likely to stimulate platelet aggregation than standard (unfractionated) heparin
B. Hirudin is a potent inhibitor of thrombin
C. Antibodies to GPIIb/IIIa receptors inhibit platelet aggregation
D. Antibodies to alteplase prevent its re-use within 6 months of receiving it
E. Aspirin is contraindicated in patients receiving thrombolysis

QUESTION 520

The following are recognised complications of oral treatment with amiodarone

A. Pneumonitis
B. Hypotension
C. Photosensitivity
D. Hyperthyroidism
E. Torsade de pointes

QUESTION 521

Concerning calcium antagonists

A. They inhibit the slow calcium efflux of stage 2 of the cardiac action potential
B. Diltiazem increases AV node refractoriness
C. Nifedipine is safe for use in pregnancy
D. Gum hypertrophy is a side effect of the dihydropyridines
E. Verapamil is the treatment of choice for SVT due to digoxin toxicity

QUESTION 522

The following may be used to control the ventricular rate in atrial fibrillation

A. Quinidine
B. Sotalol
C. Digoxin and verapamil
D. Amiodarone
E. Disopyramide

QUESTION 523

Digoxin toxicity is

A. Precipitated by hypomagnesaemia
B. Due to an idiosyncratic reaction to the drug
C. Aggravated by hypokalaemia
D. More likely in patients taking drugs which induce hepatic enzymes
E. Is predictable from the plasma level of the drug

QUESTION 524

In the treatment of cardiogenic shock

A. Enoximone reduces the left ventricular end diastolic pressure
B. Adrenaline increases the systemic vascular resistance
C. Cardiac output is increased by noradrenaline
D. Isoprenaline increases myocardial oxygen consumption
E. Dobutamine increases systemic vascular resistance

QUESTION 525

A patient treated with digoxin is likely to develop digoxin toxicity if also given

A. Amphotericin B
B. Cholestyramine
C. Nifedipine
D. Quinidine
E. Amiodarone

QUESTION 526

Regarding overdose, haemodialysis would be effective in removing the following drugs

A. Digoxin
B. Pethidine
C. Amitryptyline
D. Propranolol
E. Salicylate

QUESTION 527

The following statements about drug metabolism are true

A. First-order metabolism applies to most drugs in clinical use
B. In zero-order kinetics, the half life is independent of drug concentration
C. The rate of metabolism is proportional to drug concentration in first-order metabolism
D. Phenytoin, in the therapeutic dose range, is eliminated by first-order metabolism
E. Alcohol metabolism is an example of zero-order kinetics

QUESTION 528

Adverse drug reactions

A. Most commonly affect the cardiovascular and respiratory systems
B. Are uncommon in patients taking digoxin and diuretics
C. Often affect the gastrointestinal tract and skin
D. Are particularly likely to occur in females over 60 years old
E. Cause up to 3% of admissions to acute medical wards

QUESTION 529

In acute poisoning

A. Activated charcoal increases the elimination of theophylline
B. Haemodialysis is ineffective for antifreeze ingestion
C. Protein-bound drugs are removed effectively by haemodialysis
D. Due to aspirin, simple infusion of sodium bicarbonate is as effective as forced alkaline diuresis
E. Gastric lavage is of no value more than 5 hours after tricyclic ingestion

QUESTION 530

The following are safe in pregnancy

A. Lisinopril
B. Antiepileptics
C. Warfarin
D. Aspirin
E. Methyldopa

QUESTION 531

The following statements regarding antimicrobials are true

A. Flucloxacillin is resistant to beta-lactamases
B. Most cephalosporins are excreted unchanged by the kidney
C. Neomycin used topically may be absorbed sufficiently to cause ototoxicity
D. Sulphonamides may cause the Stevens-Johnson syndrome
E. Co-trimoxazole is the treatment of choice for Pneumocystis pneumonia

QUESTION 532

The following drugs produce metabolically active metabolites

A. Diazepam
B. Amitryptilline
C. Zidovudine
D. Lisinopril
E. Benzyl penicillin

QUESTION 533

The following poisons are matched to the appropriate therapy

A. Carbon monoxide – hyperbaric oxygen
B. Organophosphates – atropine and pralidoxime
C. Beta-blocker – phentolamine
D. Methanol – ethanol
E. Tricyclic antidepressants – phenytoin

QUESTION 534

The following may be used in the treatment of diabetes insipidus

A. DDAVP
B. Chlorothiazide
C. Chlorpropamide
D. Metformin
E. Lithium

QUESTION 535

The following drugs have extensive first-pass metabolism

A. Glyceryl trinitrate
B. Verapamil
C. Chlormethiazole
D. Gentamicin
E. Ciprofloxacin

QUESTION 536

The following are recognised causes of pulmonary fibrosis

A. Amiodarone
B. Erythromycin
C. Methotrexate
D. Daunorubicin
E. Radiotherapy

QUESTION 537

The following drugs are safe for use in acute intermittent porphyria

A. Aspirin
B. Pethidine
C. Chlorpromazine
D. Carbamazepine
E. Co-trimoxazole

QUESTION 538

Regarding the mode of action of the following drugs

A. Nicorandil is a potassium channel opener
B. Losartan is an angiotensin II receptor antagonist
C. Nitroprusside is a nitric oxide donor
D. Gabapentin is a glutamate antagonist
E. Lanzoprazole is a proton pump inhibitor

QUESTION 539

Alpha-adrenergic stimulation results in

A. Decreased insulin secretion in response to a glucose load
B. Axillary sweating
C. Bronchoconstriction
D. Lipolysis
E. Vasodilatation

QUESTION 540

The following statements concerning vasoactive factors are true

A. Endothelin-I is a potent vasoconstrictor with mitogenic properties
B. Endothelin-I is broken down by endothelin-converting enzyme
C. Nitric oxide is synthesised from L-arginine
D. Infusion of nitric oxide antagonists causes vasoconstriction in normal humans
E. Nitric oxide activity is enhanced by cyclic GMP phosphodiesterase inhibitors

RHEUMATOLOGY

QUESTION 541

The following are recognised pulmonary complications of rheumatoid arthritis

A. Pleural effusion
B. Felty's syndrome
C. Caplan's syndrome
D. Rheumatoid nodules
E. Fibrosing alveolitis

QUESTION 542

The following statements about crystal deposition arthropathies are true

A. Calcium pyrophosphate crystals are positively birefringent
B. The presence of brick-shaped, negatively birefringent crystals is diagnostic of gout
C. Renal failure secondary to stone formation is a recognised complication of pseudogout
D. Tophi may occur in both gout and pseudogout
E. Allopurinol is the treatment of choice in pseudogout

QUESTION 543

The following auto-antibodies are associated with the paired diseases

A. Anti-Jo : Polymyositis
B. Anti-cardiolipin : Rheumatoid arthritis
C. Anti-La : Primary Sjögren's syndrome
D. Anti-centromere : CREST syndrome
E. Anti-ds DNA : Reiter's syndrome

QUESTION 544

The following statements are true

A. Rheumatoid arthritis is an asymmetrical pauciarticular arthritis
B. Rheumatoid factor must be present to confirm a case of Rheumatoid arthritis
C. Psoriatic arthropathy may occur without the skin lesions
D. The presence of neutrophils in synovial fluid will differentiate between gout and a septic arthritis
E. Systemic lupus erythematosis is often associated with a characteristic rash

QUESTION 545

Primary osteoarthritis is associated with the following changes in the hands

A. Heberden's nodes
B. Bouchard's nodes
C. Boutonniere deformity
D. Swan neck deformity
E. Osler's nodes

QUESTION 546

The following renal complications occur in Rheumatoid arthritis

A. Retro-peritoneal fibrosis
B. Amyloidosis
C. Renal cell carcinoma
D. Analgesic nephropathy
E. Immune complex - mediated glomerulonephritis

QUESTION 547

The following are all accepted complications of Systemic lupus erythematosis (SLE)

A. Glomerulonephritis
B. Cerebellar ataxia
C. Pericarditis
D. Aseptic necrosis of the hip
E. Restrictive lung defect

QUESTION 548

The following statements are true

A. One third of women who have had more than two spontaneous abortions have antiphospholipid syndrome
B. Oesophageal involvement is almost invariable in systemic sclerosis
C. Systemic lupus erythematosis may occur as a side effect of procainamide
D. A raised antinuclear antibody is diagnostic of systemic sclerosis
E. Systemic sclerosis may lead to a limited mouth opening

QUESTION 549

The following statements about the vasculitides are true

A. Polyarteritis nodosa is commoner in women
B. Polyarteritis nodosa is associated with Hepatitis B antigenaemia
C. Churg-Strauss syndrome is a condition associated with Polyarteritis nodosa
D. Wegener's granulomatosis is a condition of necrotising granulomatous lesions due to immune complex deposition
E. Polymyalgia rheumatica is universally fatal unless treated promptly with steroids

QUESTION   550

The following ocular complications may occur as a result of rheumatological diseases

A. Keratoconjunctivitis sicca
B. Keratoderma blenorrhagica
C. Anterior uveitus
D. Senile cataracts
E. Vitreal haemorrhage

QUESTION   551

Polymyalgia rheumatica

A. Is associated with elevated creatinine kinase
B. Commonly presents with stiffness and tenderness of proximal muscles
C. Serum alkaline phosphatase may be elevated
D. Is associated with temporal arteritis in up to 50%
E. ESR is the single most useful investigation

QUESTION   552

Clinical features of ankylosing spondylitis include

A. Achilles tendonitis
B. Hip disease
C. Conjunctivitis
D. Aphthous ulceration
E. Heart block

QUESTION   553

The following may occur with rheumatoid arthritis

A. Pleural effusions
B. Obliterative bronchiolitis
C. Stridor
D. Cavitating nodules in the lungs
E. Fibrosing alveolitis

QUESTION   554

The following are associated with a reactive arthritis

A. *Campylobacter jejuni*
B. *Chlamydia trachomatis*
C. *Helicobacter pylori*
D. Mycoplasma
E. *Shigella flexneri*

QUESTION 555

Treatment of acute gout includes

A. Intra-articular steroids
B. Colchicine
C. Allopurinol
D. Paracetamol
E. Probenecid

ANSWERS

QUESTION 1

A. FALSE B. FALSE C. FALSE D. FALSE E. TRUE

Fallot's tetralogy is the commonest cyanotic congenital heart condition presenting after the first year of life. The four features that make up the 'tetralogy' are: pulmonary stenosis, ventricular septal defect (VSD), over-riding aorta and right ventricular hypertrophy. Other associations include a right-sided aortic arch, atrial septal defect, absence or hypoplasia of the left main pulmonary artery and aortic incompetence due to a large aortic ring with a subaortic VSD.

On clinical examination, the patients have clubbing and cyanosis. There is a parasternal heave. A2 is usually palpable as the aorta is large and anterior. The second heart sound is single and the sound of pulmonary closure (P2) is absent. The murmur arises from the pulmonary outflow tract (ejection murmur and not pan-systolic). With increasing severity of stenosis the murmur gets quieter (as there is a VSD for the blood to shunt through). If there is aortic incompetence, a diastolic murmur may be audible. Large aorto-pulmonary collaterals may produce a machinery murmur heard over the back.

The degree of stenosis determines the clinical condition as it dictates the degree of shunt through the VSD. Children suffer from 'spells' due to spasms of infundibular stenosis caused by catecholamines, acidosis and hypoxia. Atrial fibrillation is uncommon and associated with clinical deterioration. Most children now undergo radical correction early if the distal pulmonary arteries are of adequate size. Alternatively a shunt is performed with a second-stage total correction later (>2 years). All congenital heart disease is more common with increasing maternal age.

Ref: Oxford Textbook of Medicine, 3rd Ed. Oxford University Press Ch. 15.15.
Kumar & Clark. Clinical Medicine, 3rd Ed. W. B. Saunders. Ch. 11.

QUESTION 2

A. TRUE B. FALSE C. TRUE D. FALSE E. TRUE

Secondary hypertension may be due to one of the following causes; renal, endocrine, cardiovascular, pregnancy and drugs. Primary hypertension is less likely in patients below the age of 35.

Renal causes of secondary hypertension are the commonest form of secondary hypertension although it may be hard to determine which came first - the hypertension or the renal disease (chronic glomerulonephritis, chronic atrophic nephritis and polycystic disease).

Endocrine causes include primary hyperaldosteronism, phaeochromocytoma, Cushing's and acromegaly. Primary hyperaldosteronism is due to adrenal adenomas (Conn's syndrome) in 60% and hyperplasia in 30%, but is rare - contributing to less that 1% of all hypertensive disease. Excessive aldosterone production leads to salt retention, hypertension and hypokalaemia. Acromegaly is due to excess growth hormone after epiphyseal fusion. Symptoms are due to the somatic (increased growth of skin & bone, goitre, cardiomegaly and hypertension), metabolic (glucose intolerance, clinical diabetes mellitus and hypercalcaemia) and the local effects of tumour (headache, visual field defects, hypopituitarism and diabetes insipidus).

Hyperthyroidism causes atrial fibrillation and heart failure but not hypertension.

Pre-eclampsia occurs in 5% of all pregnancies and is thought to be due to an autoimmune reaction against the placenta leading to increased thromboxane and decreased prostacyclin levels leading to vasoconstriction and hypertension.

Persistent PDA may cause pulmonary hypertension and not systemic hypertension.

Ref: Kumar & Clark. Clinical Medicine, 3rd Ed. W. B. Saunders. Ch. 11.
Oxford Textbook of Medicine, 3rd Ed. Oxford University Press. Ch. 13.

QUESTION 3

A. TRUE B. FALSE C. TRUE D. TRUE E. FALSE

The QT interval is taken from the start of the QRS complex to the end of the T wave. The interval varies with heart rate and should be corrected using Bazett's formula.

Corrected QT interval is QT interval divided by the square root of the R-R interval measured in seconds. The normal value is 0.35 - 0.43 seconds. Rate corrected values greater than 0.44 secs represent prolongation of the QT interval.

Causes of a long QT Interval include:

- Congenital syndromes
- Jervell-Lange-Nielsen (autosomal recessive) associated with deafness
- Romano-Ward (autosomal dominant)
- Electrolyte abnormalities - hypokalaemia, hypocalcaemia, hypomagnesaemia
- Drugs   - Quinidine, Amiodarone and other class 1a and 3 antiarrhythmics
               - Tricyclic antidepressants, phenothiazines, Terfenadine, Astemizole
               - Terodiline, Erthyromycin
- Poisons - organophosphorus compounds
- Bradycardia, Mitral valve prolapse, myocardial infarction, Hypothyroidism, anorexia, starvation and liquid protein diets.

Ref: Kumar & Clark. Clinical Medicine, 3rd Ed. W. B. Saunders. Ch. 11.
Oxford Textbook of Medicine, 3rd Ed. Oxford University Press. Ch. 15.8.1.
Oxford Handbook of Clinical Medicine, 3rd Ed. Oxford University Press. p264.

QUESTION 4

A. FALSE B. FALSE C. TRUE D. FALSE E. FALSE

Aortic stenosis may occur at the level of the valve, above (supravalvular) or below the valve (subvalvular). On auscultation, the first heart sound is usually soft. An ejection sound (heard best at the apex) is heard if the valve is mobile and bicuspid and is rarely present in elderly calcified valves. A2 may be inaudible if the valve is calcified and there may be reverse splitting of S2 due to prolonged left ventricular ejection.

Subvalvular stenosis may be due to a discrete fibromuscular ring, septal hypertrophy (as in hypertrophic cardiomyopathy) and anomalous attachment of the mitral valve leaflet and is often associated with aortic regurgitation.

Supravalvular stenosis is associated with Williams' syndrome (autosomal dominant with variable penetrance). Associations are 'elfin' facies, hypercalcaemia and hypervitaminosis D, peripheral pulmonary artery stenosis, pulmonary valve stenosis, aortic regurgitation, mesenteric artery stenosis and thoracic aortic aneurysms.

Unequal upper limb pulses are seen in coarctation of the aorta which is associated with bicuspid aortic valve. However, aortic stenosis does not CAUSE unequal limb pulses. Angina may occur with normal coronary arteries due to an imbalance in myocardial oxygen supply (shorter diastole with longer systole, impaired coronary perfusion, etc.) vs demand (cardiac hypertrophy, increased cardiac work).

Ref: Oxford Textbook of Medicine, 3rd Ed. Oxford University Press. Ch. 15.18.

QUESTION 5

A. FALSE B. TRUE C. TRUE D. TRUE E. TRUE

In utero, blood flows through the ductus arteriosus from the pulmonary artery to the descending aorta because the pulmonary vascular resistance is high. At birth the placental circulation is cut off causing a sudden rise in systemic vascular resistance. The ensuing hypoxia causes the first lung expanding breath and a modest fall in pulmonary vascular resistance which results in a marked increase in pulmonary blood flow. The parallel foetal circulation changes to flow in series. The foramen ovale closes in the first day or two while the ductus arteriosus is usually closed by a week. When the ductus arteriosus remains open a continuous 'machinery' murmur is heard, the pulse volume is large and may result in severe heart failure as blood passes from the aorta into the pulmonary arteries and increases venous return to the left heart. A rise in arterial PaO_2 helps to close the duct. Prostacyclin is used in complex neonatal congenital cardiac disease to maintain ductal patency prior to surgery. Indomethacin is used to help close the duct.

Ref: Ganong. Review of Medical Physiology, 16th Ed. Appleton & Lange. Ch. 32.

QUESTION 6

A. FALSE B. TRUE C. TRUE D. TRUE E. TRUE

Pulmonary hypertension has many causes but can be classified into 5 groups:

1. Unknown aetiology – most commonly seen in women
2. Due to alveolar hypoxia – chronic lung disease
3. Increased flow – left to right intracardiac shunts
4. Pulmonary venous hypertension – atrial myxoma, mitral stenosis or left ventricular failure
5. Obstructive disease – pulmonary embolus and sickle cell disease.

The right atrium becomes dilated and the right ventricle hypertrophied. This leads to the physical findings of a prominent 'a' wave on the JVP, a right ventricular parasternal heave, and a loud pulmonary component to the second heart sound. Tricuspid regurgitation due to right ventricular failure causes a large 'v' wave in the JVP and a pansystolic murmur. Pulmonary incompetence produces an early diastolic murmur (Graham–Steele murmur). The CXR shows a large right ventricle and atrium with prominent pulmonary arteries and oligaemic peripheral lung fields. The ECG changes include right axis deviation and P pulmonale.

Ref: Kumar & Clark. Clinical Medicine, 3rd Ed. W. B. Saunders. Ch. 11.
Oxford Textbook of Medicine, 3rd Ed. Oxford University Press. Ch. 13.

QUESTION 7

A. TRUE B. TRUE C. FALSE D. TRUE E. TRUE

Sinus tachycardia is defined as an accelerated sinus rate to more than 100 bpm. Common causes include fever, anxiety, exercise, emotion, pregnancy and anaemia. It may be a sign of thyrotoxicosis or cardiac failure as well as situations in which there is excess catecholamine release.

In anaesthesia it may represent pain, light anaesthesia with awareness, sepsis, hypovolaemia, hypoxaemia, hypoglycaemia or malignant hyperthermia.

Mitral stenosis is usually associated with atrial fibrillation.

Ref: Kumar & Clark. Clinical Medicine, 3rd Ed. W. B. Saunders. Ch. 11.

QUESTION 8

A. TRUE B. TRUE C. TRUE D. FALSE E. TRUE

Patients requiring procedural antibiotic prophylaxis include:

- Past medical history of endocarditis
- Prosthetic heart valve
- Rheumatic heart disease
- Most congenital heart disease (except ASD)
- Mitral valve prolapse
- HOCM

Prophylaxis is required for most dental, ENT, gynae or abdominal surgery. It may be unnecessary for dental fillings, endoscopy (upper GI), cardiac catheterization and laparoscopy.

Consult a cardiologist and microbiologist if in doubt

Ref: Epstein RJ. Medicine for Examinations, 3rd Ed. Churchill Livingstone.

QUESTION 9

A. TRUE B. FALSE C. FALSE D. FALSE E. FALSE

Bicuspid aortic valve is the commonest congenital abnormality of the heart. The valve may remain functionally normal throughout childhood and adult life but more commonly develops calcific thickening (accounting for up to 50% of calcific aortic stenosis in adults). Associated conditions include aortic dissection (even years after successful aortic valve replacement) and coarctation of the aorta. Occasionally bicuspid valves may develop progressive regurgitation without stenosis.

Patients with Turner's syndrome have an 45XO karyotype generated through chromosomal non-disjunction and clinically appear as pre-pubertal females (unless they receive HRT). Other features that may occur include short-webbed neck (54%), cubitus valgus at the elbow, shield-like chest with wide-spaced nipples, hypoplastic nails, short 4th metacarpals, high arched palate, lymphoedema, renal abnormalities (horse-shoe kidney), hypertelorism, coarctation of the aorta, ASD, VSD and aortic stenosis. Noonan's syndrome has some of the features of the Turner phenotype but patients develop a right-sided cardiac lesion (pulmonary stenosis) and have a 46XX karyotype.

Patients with Marfan's syndrome are at high risk of developing cystic medial degeneration of the aorta leading to progressive dilatation of the aortic root, aortic dissection and aortic regurgitation. Mitral valve prolapse and incompetence may occur. Bicuspid aortic valves are not a feature.

Ref: Oxford Textbook of Medicine, 3rd Ed. Oxford University Press. Ch. 15.18 and 15.28.

QUESTION 10

A. FALSE B. TRUE C. TRUE D. FALSE E. FALSE

Acute cardiac tamponade is the result of rapidly increasing pericardial fluid (serous or blood) preventing effective ventricular filling, reducing cardiac output and eventually blood pressure. The heart sounds are muffled but there may be a pericardial rub. Ascites is not a feature of acute cardiac tamponade, it may be seen in constrictive pericarditis. Reduced right ventricular output prevents the pulmonary vessels becoming engorged. Pulsus paradoxus is normally present in those patients with clinically significant tamponade. However it may be absent or minimal when there is significant constriction or in patients with LVH, severe LVF, ASD or aortic regurgitation. Right heart tamponade due to bleeding after cardiac surgery is not normally associated with pulsus paradoxus. Beware of this type of question!

Ref: Kumar & Clark. Clinical Medicine, 3rd Ed. W. B. Saunders. Ch. 11.
Hinds & Watson. Intensive Care: A Concise Textbook, 2nd Ed. W. B. Saunders. Ch. 4.

QUESTION 11

A. TRUE B. TRUE C. TRUE D. FALSE E. FALSE

Chronic constrictive pericarditis and restrictive cardiomyopathy present with symptoms and signs of right and left ventricular failure. Right-sided signs are prominent with elevation of the JVP (prominent x and y descents, ± Kussmaul's sign), hepatomegaly, ankle oedema and ascites. Atrial fibrillation is found in 30% of patients. A pericardial knock may be audible and is due to rapid and abruptly halted ventricular filling. Causes include cardiac surgery or trauma, infection, pyogenic disease, irradiation, connective tissue disease and chronic renal failure.

Ref: Talley & O'Connor. Clinical Examination. Blackwell Scientific Publications. Ch. 3.

QUESTION 12

A. FALSE B. FALSE C. TRUE D. TRUE E. TRUE

The commonest congenital heart lesion is a VSD which accounts for about 30-40% of all lesions. Secundum ASD and PDA account for about 10% each. PDA is more common in females. Congenital heart disease overall shows a male preponderance. Fallot's has a recognised higher incidence in first degree relatives (4%). The other common forms of congenital heart disease are Fallot's, pulmonary stenosis, aortic stenosis, coarctation of the aorta, transposition of the great vessels, primum ASD and total anomalous pulmonary venous drainage. These common types account for over 90% of all CHD.

Ref: Kumar & Clark. Clinical Medicine, 3rd Ed. W. B. Saunders. Ch. 11.

QUESTION 13

A. FALSE B. FALSE C. FALSE D. TRUE E. TRUE

Sick sinus syndrome (Bradycardia -tachycardia syndrome) is a consequence of ischaemia, infarction or degeneration of the sinus node. It is characterised by long intervals (> 2 seconds) between consecutive P waves. It may present with a wide range of rhythm disturbances and is associated with AV nodal conduction defects, escape rhythms and SVT's. The patient may present with syncopal attacks. Sinus pauses may allow tachydysrhythmias to emerge. Treatment of chronic symptomatic sick sinus syndrome requires permanent pacing supplemented with anti-arrhythmics. Thromboembolism is common and anticoagulation should be considered.

Ref: Oxford Textbook of Medicine, 3rd Ed. Oxford University Press. Ch. 13.

QUESTION 14

A. FALSE B. TRUE C. FALSE D. FALSE E. FALSE

The differential diagnosis of absent P waves includes atrial fibrillation, nodal rhythm with sinoatrial block and severe hyperkalaemia. In atrial flutter there is a saw tooth baseline atrial depolarisation which may be difficult to see if the patient is in 2:1 block.

These are normally known as flutter waves (F waves) but can be regarded as P waves. In nodal tachycardias the QRS complex is usually normal and P waves may occur before, within or after the QRS complex. In ventricular tachycardia disassociated P wave activity may be seen. This occurs in about 30% of cases.

Ref: Kumar & Clark. Clinical Medicine, 3rd Ed. W. B. Saunders. Ch. 11.

QUESTION 15

A. FALSE B. TRUE C. FALSE D. FALSE E. FALSE

Haematuria in infective endocarditis is usually due to immune complex deposition, vasculitis and glomerulonephritis. Bacteria are only found in the kidney following systemic embolization of infected material from the heart and resulting mycotic aneurysm (rare). Complement levels are low in the acute phase and may rise (acute phase response) with treatment. Other immune phenomena include splinter haemorrhages, Osler's nodes, Janeway lesions. Complications include intracardiac abscess, valve destruction, emboli and mycotic aneurysms.

After blood cultures, treatment should be started immediately. Dental treatment should be undertaken early (within 10 days) as there is a risk that oral organisms may become resistant to the antibiotics with time. The timing of surgery depends on the haemodynamics - ideally clear the infection first.

QUESTION 16

A. FALSE B. TRUE C. TRUE D. TRUE E. TRUE

Clinical signs of pulmonary hypertension are raised JVP with prominent a waves and large v waves (especially with coexistent tricuspid regurgitation), parasternal heave, sometimes a palpable pulmonary second sound, and on auscultation, loud P2 sometimes with an ejection click (P2 is closer to A2, not further apart), pansystolic murmur of tricuspid incompetence, right ventricular fourth heart sound and early diastolic murmur of functional pulmonary regurgitation (the Graham-Steele murmur). Atrial fibrillation may occur.

Ref: Kumar & Clark. Clinical Medicine, 3rd Ed. W. B. Saunders. Ch. 11.

QUESTION 17

A. TRUE B. FALSE C. TRUE D. TRUE E. FALSE

Bicuspid aortic valves occur in at least 50% of patients with coarctation of the aorta. Cerebral aneurysms are a recognised finding and may lead to cerebral haemorrhage. Preductal coarctation is associated with heart failure in infancy and patent ductus arteriosus as well as other cardiac defects (VSD, mitral valve malformation). There is no association between Marfan's and coarctation. Coarctation is a recognised feature of Turner's and Noonan's syndrome. It is more common in males.

Ref: Oxford Textbook of Medicine, 3rd Ed. Oxford University Press. Ch. 15.28.3.

QUESTION   18

A. FALSE B. TRUE C. TRUE D. FALSE E. TRUE

Fallot's tetralogy is the commonest form of cyanotic congenital heart disease in children who survive beyond the neonatal period. Incidence is between 5 and 10% of cases of congenital heart disease and it is more common in first degree relatives. Classical features are a VSD, right ventricular outflow tract obstruction, overriding aorta and right ventriclar hypertrophy. There is right to left shunting and the patient is cyanosed. Children with Fallot's present with dysp-noea, fatigue or hypoxic episodes (spells) where there is deep cyanosis and possible syncope associated with exertion. Squatting is a common feature. The rise in SVR reduces the degree of shunting and cyanosis. Cyanosis is usually present from birth but clubbing and poly-cythaemia do not occur until the child is about a year old. Fallot's spells may be treated with beta-blockade. When severe they may require diamorphine to relax the right ventricular out-flow obstruction.

QUESTION   19

A. TRUE B. TRUE C. TRUE D. TRUE E. TRUE

Aortic regurgitation may be due to primary disease of the valve or secondary to stretching of the aortic ring due to dilatation of the aortic root. Congenital AR is seen with bicuspid aortic valves, supravalvular stenosis and high VSDs (loss of support) causing prolapse of the valve leaflets. The valve may be affected by rheumatic fever, infection, SLE or rheumatoid arthritis, collagen vascular diseases such as pseudoxanthoma elasticum and mucopolysaccharidoses. Aortic root diseases causing dilatation include dissection, syphilis, Marfan's, long-standing hypertension, coarctation, seronegative spondyloarthritides (Reiter's, psoriatic, ankylosing spondylitis), relapsing polychondritis and giant cell arteritis.

With chronic aortic regurgitation, the left ventricle will dilate if the patient is not followed up carefully. The diastolic murmur of AR gets shorter with increasing severity as it takes less time for the aortic and left ventricular diastolic pressures to equalise. In acute-onset AR (e.g. infective endocarditis), the patient may experience severe left ventricular failure even with a ventricle of normal size as the chamber does not have time to dilate.

Ref: Oxford Textbook of Medicine, 3rd Ed. Oxford University Press. Ch. 15.18.
Kumar & Clark. Clinical Medicine, 3rd Ed. W. B. Saunders. Ch. 11.

QUESTION 20

A. TRUE B. TRUE C. FALSE D. FALSE E. TRUE

Mid-systolic murmurs begin some time after the first heart sound and are crescendo-decrescendo in nature. They are usually due to turbulent flow across a restriction or increased flow through normal sized valve orifices. Recognised causes include aortic stenosis, pulmonary stenosis, HOCM, pulmonary flow murmur associated with an ASD and Fallot's.

Pan-systolic murmurs begin at the first heart sound and extend to the second heart sound and are due to mitral or tricuspid reflux and VSD.

Late systolic murmur may be caused by mitral valve prolapse or papillary muscle dysfunction and coarctation or the aorta. However a mid systolic murmur may be audible over the precordium and back in coarctation. This may be due to blood flow through collateral vessels.

Ref: Talley & O'Connor. Clinical Examination. Blackwell Scientific Publications. Ch. 3. Kumar & Clark. Clinical Medicine, 3rd Ed. W. B. Saunders. Ch. 11.

QUESTION 21

A. FALSE B. FALSE C. FALSE D. FALSE E. TRUE

Congenital cardiac malformations occur in about 1% of live births. There is an overall male preponderance. Some lesions occur more commonly in females (ASD and PDA). Clubbing is a feature of cyanotic congenital heart disease. Overall VSD account for about 40% of all lesions, ASD 10%, PDA 10% and pulmonary stenosis, coarctation, aortic stenosis and Fallot's about 6-7% each. Down's syndrome in associated with endomyocardial cushion defects leading to ostium primum ASD's and abnormalities of the tricuspid and mitral valves.

Ref: Kumar & Clark. Clinical Medicine, 3rd Ed. W. B. Saunders. Ch. 11.

QUESTION 22

A. TRUE B. FALSE C. TRUE D. TRUE E. TRUE

Causes of a pericardial effusion include:

- Cardiac rupture or trauma (myocardial infarction, iatrogenic e.g. post cardiac surgery, catheterization, pacing, etc.)
- Aortic dissection
- Spontaneous bleed (anticoagulation, uraemia, thrombocytopenia)
- Malignant disease
- Idiopathic pericarditis
- Uraemia
- Infections (bacterial, tuberculosis, viral, fungal)
- Radiation
- HYPOthyroidism
- SLE
- Chronic salt and water retention of any cause (heart failure, nephrotic syndrome, hepatic cirrhosis)
- Pregnancy
- Idiopathic

Ref: Kumar & Clark. Clinical Medicine, 3rd Ed. W. B. Saunders. Ch. 11.

QUESTION 23

A. FALSE B. TRUE C. FALSE D. FALSE E. TRUE

In the uncomplicated PDA the shunt is from the aorta into the pulmonary artery as pulmonary hypertension has not supervened. Classical features are a collapsing pulse with sharp upstroke and a low diastolic blood pressure leading to a wide pulse pressure. The apex beat is hyperkinetic. Small shunts are associated with a single heart sound. Large shunts may be associated with reversed splitting of the second heart sound due to delayed A2. There is a continuous and loud machinary murmur maximal at the left first interspace. An apical late diastolic murmur may occur due to flow over the mitral valve. Cyanosis and clubbing are not features of an uncomplicated PDA.

Ref: Talley & O'Connor. Clinical Examination. Blackwell Scientific Publications. Ch. 3.

QUESTION 24

A. FALSE B. TRUE C. TRUE D. FALSE E. TRUE

With increasing severity of mitral stenosis, it takes longer to fill the left ventricle in diastole and the murmur gets longer. The closer the opening snap to the second heart sound, the more severe the stenosis. In addition, signs of pulmonary hypertension, functional pulmonary valve incompetence (Graham-Steele murmur) suggest long-standing mitral valve disease. Indications for surgery for mitral stenosis include significant symptoms not responding to medical therapy, an episode of left ventricular failure without an obvious precipitating cause, recurrent emboli and pulmonary oedema in pregnancy. Signs of severe mitral stenosis are present when the valve area is less than 1 cm². This may be assessed by an echocardiogram along with the mid-diastolic closure rate of the anterior leaflet of the mitral valve.

Ref: Oxford Textbook of Medicine, 3rd Ed. Oxford University Press Ch. 15.18.
Kumar & Clark. Clinical Medicine, 3rd Ed. W. B. Saunders. Ch. 11.

QUESTION 25

A. TRUE B. FALSE C. TRUE D. TRUE E. FALSE

The P wave is normally upright in lead I and represents depolarization of the atria of the normal heart towards the left arm . It is classically inverted in reversal of the limb leads when seen in association with normal chest lead morphology. Inverted T wave and dominant S wave in lead I are the other diagnostic criteria. In limb lead reversal the morphology of aVR and aVL appear to be reversed. Nodal rhythm may be associated with retrograde P wave conduction which may be seen as an inverted P wave in lead I. In dextrocardia inversion of the lead I P wave is seen in association with a dominant R wave in V1. The P wave is normal in HOCM and absent in 70% of patients with ventricular tachycardia.

Ref: Epstein RJ. Medicine for Examinations. 3rd Ed. Churchill Livingstone. Ch. 2.

QUESTION   26

A. TRUE B. TRUE C. FALSE D. TRUE E. TRUE

First degree heart block is characterised by a PR interval greater than 0.22 seconds (5 small squares on the ECG). Ventricular beats are not dropped.

Second degree heart block describes the heart that does not conduct all P waves to the ventricle. In Mobitz type I (Wenckebach phenomenon) there is progressive prolongation of the PR interval until one fails to conduct to the ventricle. In Mobitz type II there is also failure to conduct to the ventricle but this does not follow an increasing PR interval. When this is regular it is said to be a 3:1 or 4:1 block depending on the number of conducted P waves.

Third degree block (complete heart block) describes the heart that fails to conduct any P waves to the ventricle. Cardiac output is maintained by a ventricular escape rhythm which may be narrow or wide. Narrow QRS complexes denote disease in the AV node or the proximal bundle of His. It occurs in congenital heart disease, inferior MI, diphtheria, rheumatic fever and toxic levels of digoxin, verapamil or beta-blockers. Apart from treating drug toxicity, asymptomatic patients only rarely need pacing. However a broad QRS complex complete heart block (indicating Purkinje system disease) always requires permanent pacing even when asymptomatic because of the significant reduction in mortality.

Ref: Kumar & Clark. Clinical Medicine, 3rd Ed. W. B. Saunders. Ch. 11.
Oxford Textbook of Medicine, 3rd Ed. Oxford University Press. Ch. 13.

QUESTION   27

A. TRUE B. FALSE C. TRUE D. FALSE E. FALSE

In patients with mixed mitral valve disease it is often difficult to distinguish clinically the dominant lesion. The factors favouring mitral incompetence are a displaced, volume overload (thrusting) apex beat and a soft first heart sound. In addition, the presence of a third heart sound is incompatible with any degree of mitral stenosis. A loud first heart sound and a tapping, non-displaced apex beat suggest predominant stenosis. Usually cardiac catheterization is necessary to resolve the issue (and will usually be required prior to surgery). A parasternal heave suggests pulmonary hypertension and right ventricular hypertrophy. This may occur with either lesion.

Ref: Talley & O'Connor. Clinical Examination. Blackwell Scientific Publications. Ch. 3.

QUESTION   28

A. TRUE B. TRUE C. FALSE D. TRUE E. TRUE

The signs and symptoms of a PE are related to the size of the embolus. Onset of symptoms is sudden with larger emboli and include pleuritic pain, haemoptysis and dyspnoea. In life threatening PE the patient will have severe central chest pain, shock, tachycardia and tachypnoea. Cardiovascular collapse may be sudden and irreversible. Signs include right ventricular heave, prominent 'a' wave on CVP trace, gallop rhythm, variable second heart sound (loud in pulmonary hypertension, soft if cardiac output is greatly reduced). Evidence of DVT is present in 50% of cases.

Ref: Kumar & Clark. Clinical Medicine, 3rd Ed. W. B. Saunders. Ch. 11.

QUESTION 29

A. FALSE B. TRUE C. TRUE D. FALSE E. TRUE

In patients with ischaemic heart disease, myocardial oxygen demand exceeds supply. With prolonged angina, there is impaired diastolic relaxation and eventually impaired systolic contraction resulting in overall reduction in left ventricular function. Clinical evidence of heart failure develops when the remainder of the normal myocardium is unable to maintain cardiac output. However, dyspnoea on exercise does not suggest severe left ventricular disease, but may just reflect severe reduction in exercise-induced vasodilatation and a limited residual coronary flow reserve. A fall in BP on exercise occurs for similar reasons. The patients may develop a third heart sound during episodes of angina as the ventricle is 'stiffer'. Tachycardia from any cause can precipitate angina.

QUESTION 30

A. FALSE B. TRUE C. FALSE D. FALSE E. TRUE

Enterococci are sensitive to penicillins but not highly so and require treatment with other agents, e.g. aminoglycosides. *Streptococcus bovis* is frequently associated with colonic tumours. Indolent infection is usually due to *Staph. epidermidis*. Anticoagulation does not reduce the risk of embolic phenomena and increases the risk of bleeding from mycotic aneurysms. Mycotic aneurysms typically affect the cerebral circulation and may rupture late (after many years).

QUESTION 31

A. TRUE B. TRUE C. TRUE D. FALSE E. FALSE

The combination of a long QT interval during sinus rhythm in association with intermittent torsades de pointes tachycardia is known as the long QT syndrome. It may be acquired or congenital. The recognised causes of a long QT interval include:
Drug induced – class 1 and 3 antiarrhythmics, tricyclics, erythromycin, terfenadine and astemizole.
Metabolic– hypothyroidism, starvation, anorexia, liquid protein diets
Electrolyte disturbance – Hypocalcaemia, hypokalaemia, hypomagnesaemia
Bradycardia– sinoatrial disease and AV block
Toxins– organophosphorus drugs and heavy metals
The QT interval is rate dependent and should be corrected using Bazett's formula.
Corrected QT interval = Measured QT interval divided by square root of RR interval in seconds.
Non specific causes of bradycardia increase the QT interval but not when corrected for rate.
The normal corrected QT interval is 0.34-0.43 seconds.

Ref: Oxford Textbook of Medicine, 3rd Ed. Oxford University Press. Ch. 15.8.1.
Kumar & Clark. Clinical Medicine, 3rd Ed. W. B. Saunders. Ch. 11.

QUESTION 32

A. TRUE B. TRUE C. TRUE D. TRUE E. FALSE

Mitral valve prolapse (also known as Barlow's syndrome, floppy mitral valve, etc.) has a prevalence of ~4% in the normal asymptomatic population. It is thought to occur by progressive stretching of the mitral leaflets and weakening with deposition of mucopolysaccharides in the valve tissue. It is associated with ostium secundum ASD, Turner's syndrome, Marfan's syndrome, pseudoxanthoma elasticum, osteogenesis imperfecta, dilated + hypertrophic cardiomyopathy and WPW syndrome (Pre-excitation).

Presenting features include atypical chest pain, palpitations, infective endocarditis, dyspnoea and progressive mitral incompetence, stroke (from emboli), re-entry tachyarrhythmias, VT and sudden death. Ventricular ectopic beats are benign and usually do not require therapy. If treatment is necessary beta-blockers frequently are successful in reducing both chest pains and palpitations.

Ref: Oxford Textbook of Medicine, 3rd Ed. Oxford University Press Ch. 15.18.
Kumar & Clark. Clinical Medicine, 3rd Ed. W. B. Saunders. Ch. 11.

QUESTION 33

A FALSE B. TRUE C. TRUE D. TRUE E. FALSE

Withdrawal of digoxin increases hospital admissions and reduces quality of life in patients with heart failure who were on it, but no study as yet has demonstrated any effect on overall survival. Despite extensive use in pregnancy there is no reported teratogenicity. It is effective in 50-60% of fetal tachyarrhythmias. Digoxin is a steroid analogue and digoxin-like substances from the placenta may interfere with assays – it is not known if these have any digoxin-like activity. Digoxin has little impact on heart rate during exercise as its actions on the AV node can be overridden by sympathetic stimulation. Verapamil and beta-blockers provide better rate control in this situation.

QUESTION 34

A. FALSE B. TRUE C. FALSE D. TRUE E. TRUE

The QT interval is taken from the start of the QRS complex to the end of the T wave. The interval varies with heart rate and should be corrected using Bazett's formula.

Corrected QT interval is QT interval divided by the square root of the R-R interval measured in seconds. The normal value is 0.35 - 0.43 seconds. Rate corrected values greater than 0.44 secs represent prolongation of the QT interval.

Causes of a long QT Interval include:

• Congenital syndromes
• Jervell-Lange-Nielsen (autosomal recessive) associated with deafness
• Romano-Ward (autosomal dominant)

- Electrolyte abnormalities – hypokalaemia, hypocalcaemia, hypomagnesaemia
- Drugs   – Quinidine, Amiodarone and other class 1a and 3 antiarrhythmics
          – Tricyclic antidepressants, phenothiazines, Terfenadine, Astemizole
          – Terodiline, Erthromycin
- Poisons   – organophosphorus compounds

- Bradycardia, Mitral valve prolapse, myocardial infarction, hypothyroidism, anorexia, starvation and liquid protein diets.

Ref: Kumar & Clark. Clinical Medicine, 3rd Ed. W. B. Saunders. Ch. 11.
Oxford Textbook of Medicine, 3rd Ed. Oxford University Press. Ch. 15.8.1.
Oxford Handbook of Clinical Medicine, 3rd Ed. Oxford University Press. p264.

QUESTION 35

A. TRUE B. TRUE C. FALSE D. TRUE E. TRUE

Risk factors for developing dissection of the thoracic aortic aneurysm include: hypertension, trauma, coarctation of the aorta, pregnancy, connective tissue disorders (Marfan's, Ehlers-Danlos), SLE, relapsing polychondritis, congenitally bicuspid aortic valve, Turner's or Noonan's syndromes, and syphilis.

Dissecting thoracic aortic aneurysms carry a very high mortality. If untreated 50% die within 48 hours, up to 70% within 1 week and 90% within 3 months. Patients are commonly men aged 40-70 years (Afrocarribean > Caucasian). Clinical features may point to the site of dissection. Aortic incompetence, inferior infarction on the ECG (right coronary ostial involvement), cardiac tamponade and Marfanoid habitus suggest ascending aortic involvement. Asymmetric upper limb pulses and stroke suggest arch involvement. Descending aortic involvement results in haemothorax or pleural effusions, absent or reduced femoral pulses and renal failure.

QUESTION 36

A. TRUE B. FALSE C. FALSE D. TRUE E. TRUE

Metabolic predispositions to digoxin toxicity include:

- General – old age, low body weight, pre-existing myocardial disease
- Renal impairment – due to reduced clearance
- Metabolic abnormalities – hypokalaemia, hypomagnesaemia, hypercalcaemia, hypothyroidism and hypoxia (especially cor pulmonale)
- Cardiac amyloidosis

Ref: Epstein RJ. Medicine for Examinations. 3rd Ed. Churchill Livingstone Ch. 2.

QUESTION 37

A. FALSE B. FALSE C. FALSE D. TRUE E. FALSE

Prominent T waves are classically associated with hyperkalaemia. Hypothermia is associated with the development of J waves which are positive deflections occurring at the end of the QRS complex. They are clinically insignificant. Hypokalaemia is associated with ST segment depression, QT and PR prolongation and T wave inversion. There may also be U waves. Hypocalcaemia prolongs the QT interval but does not affect the size of the T wave. Hypomagnesaemia does not affect the size of the T wave.

Ref: Yentis, Hirsch & Smith. Anaesthesia A to Z. Butterworth Heineman.

QUESTION 38

A. TRUE B. FALSE C. TRUE D. TRUE E. TRUE

The long standing hypoxia seen in chronic lung disease is the trigger for cor pulmonale. It leads to pulmonary vasoconstriction, a rise in the afterload of the right ventricle and pulmonary hypertension. Subsequently this leads to right ventricular hypertrophy (causing a parasternal heave) and right ventricular failure. As right ventricular failure progresses tricuspid incompetence develops leading to a large 'v' wave in the JVP. A large 'a' wave is seen in cor pulmonale in association with pulmonary hypertension and ventricular hypertrophy. The ECG changes include right axis deviation and p pulmonale (large p wave in leads II & III).

Ref: Kumar & Clark. Clinical Medicine, 3rd Ed. W. B. Saunders. Ch. 11.
Oxford Textbook of Medicine, 3rd Ed. Oxford University Press. Ch. 13.

QUESTION 39

A. FALSE B. TRUE C. TRUE D. FALSE E. TRUE

An opening snap is a high pitched sound occurring a variable distance after the second heart sound. It occurs in mitral stenosis and tricuspid stenosis. It is due to the sudden opening of the valve and may be followed by a diastolic murmur. It may be confused with a third heart sound or a widely split second heart sound. However it occurs later in diastole than either and is best heard at the lower left sternal edge with the diaphragm of the stethoscope. The earlier the sound occurs in diastole the greater is the severity of the stenosis. This is due to the increased left atrial pressure in mitral stenosis. There is no respiratory variation associated with opening snaps.

Ref: Talley & O'Connor. Clinical Examination. Blackwell Scientific Publications. Ch. 3.
Kumar & Clark. Clinical Medicine, 3rd Ed. W. B. Saunders. Ch. 11.

QUESTION 40

A. FALSE B. TRUE C. FALSE D. TRUE E. TRUE

Nicorandil is a potassium channel activator used to treat angina. It causes a fall in preload and afterload by vascular smooth muscle relaxation. It has a direct affect on coronary blood vessels which dilate without provoking a "steal phenomenon" leading to improved myocardial oxygen delivery. It is well absorbed with minimal first pass metabolism and is minimally bound to plasma proteins. There have been no reports of serious interactions although its antihypertensive effect may be augmented by other vasodilators, tricyclic antidepressants or alcohol. The side effect profile is small but headache is recognised at the start of treatment.

QUESTION 41

A. TRUE B. FALSE C. TRUE D. TRUE E. TRUE

Hypertrophic cardiomyopathy is usually familial with autosomal dominant transmission with a high degree of penetrance. Many mutations can produce hypertrophic cardiomyopathy (HCM) - beta-myosin heavy chain gene on chr 14 (~20-30%), cardiac troponin T on chr 1, alpha-tropomyosin on chr 15. 50% of pedigrees evaluated have mutations in the genes mentioned. It appears to be a disease of sarcomeric contractile proteins. Adults have a 2-3% risk of sudden death and non-sustained VT is the only marker proven to be of predictive value (7 fold increased risk). The risk in children and adolescents is 4-6%. ACE gene polymorphism occurs with increased frequency in those families where there is an increased incidence of sudden death. Mitral regurgitation is a common finding. Thiamine deficiency is related to beri-beri and a dilated cardiomyopathy.

Ref: Oxford Textbook of Medicine, 3ʳᵈ Ed. Oxford University Press Ch. 15.14.1.
Kumar & Clark. Clinical Medicine, 3ʳᵈ Ed. W. B. Saunders. Ch. 11.

QUESTION 42

A. TRUE B. FALSE C. FALSE D. FALSE E. FALSE

Angiotensinogen is cleaved by renin (produced in the kidneys in response to decreased renal perfusion) to produce angiotensin I. Angiotensin converting enzyme (ACE) acts on angiotensin I to form angiotensin II, which causes vasoconstriction and stimulates the adrenal gland to produce aldosterone. Renal perfusion is increased and the stimulus for renin production is reduced. Thus the system is kept in balance.

Losartan is a specific angiotensin II receptor (type AT1) antagonist and blocks the ability of angiotensin II to cause vasoconstriction and release aldosterone. As negative feedback of angiotensin II on renin secretion is removed there is increased plasma renin activity. ACE inhibitors (e.g. captopril) cause an increase in bradykinin levels which are responsible for the dry cough – however Losartan does not cause a rise in bradykinin and therefore cough is not a side effect. As with ACE inhibitors, Losartan should be avoided when K sparing diuretics are being administered as K levels may rise dangerously. Losartan is metabolised to a single active metabolite and many inactive metabolites.

QUESTION 43

A. FALSE B. TRUE C. FALSE D. TRUE E. FALSE

The first heart sound is caused by the closure of the mitral and tricuspid valves. It is usually single in nature but when split may be confused with a fourth heart sound or ejection click. It is best heard at the apex. The sound is loud in thin patients and when the diastolic filling time is reduced in tachycardias (anaemia and thyrotoxicosis) or any other cause of a short atrioventricular conduction time. The sound is also loud when the cusps of the valves are widely open at the end of diastole and close forcefully at the start of systole. This occurs in mitral and tricuspid stenosis.

The first heart sound is soft in patients with obesity, pericardial effusions and emphysema where the transmission of the sound is impaired. It may also be soft in first or second degree heart block (prolonged diastolic filling), LBBB (delayed onset of LV systole) and mitral reflux due to a failure of the leaves to close normally.

Ref: Talley & O'Connor. Clinical Examination. Blackwell Scientific Publications. Ch. 3.

QUESTION 44

A. FALSE B. FALSE C. TRUE D. FALSE E. TRUE

The QRS complex corresponds to ventricular depolarisation and with the phase of isovolumetric contraction. The ST segment and T wave correspond to ventricular repolarisation. It is the QT interval that is prolonged in tricyclic poisoning and the QRS complex is widened along with AV block and intraventricular conduction disturbances. RBBB is characteristic.

A normal Q wave is <0.04 seconds wide and <25% of the total QRS complex.

Pathological Q waves are seen with transmural myocardial injury (myocardial infarction, myocarditis or cardiac trauma) hypertrophic cardiomyopathy and Wolff-Parkinson-White syndrome.

Artefactual Q waves are seen with dextrocardia (other clues include: decreasing size of QRS complex across the chest leads, rightward axis) or reversed limb leads (other clues: lead I looks like reversed polarity, leads II and III as well as aVR and aVL appear as if they have been swapped around).

Ref: Epstein RJ. Medicine for Examinations. 3rd Ed. Churchill Livingstone. Ch. 2.
Hinds & Watson. Intensive Care: A Concise Textbook. 2nd Ed. W. B. Saunders. Ch. 18.

QUESTION 45

A. TRUE B. TRUE C. TRUE D. TRUE E. TRUE

The third heart sound is a low pitched mid-diastolic sound due to rapid ventricular filling in diastole as soon as the mitral and tricuspid valves open. Physiological left ventricular third sounds are heard in children and young adults due to very fast ventricular diastolic filling. This is best heard at the apex in the left lateral position. In patients over the age of 40 the sound is normally pathological and represents reduced ventricular compliance. Pathological left ventricular S3 is best heard at the apex in expiration and represents heart failure or volume overload (LVF, AR, MR, VSD and PDA). Pathological right ventricular S3 is best heard at the left sternal edge and is louder in inspiration. It occurs in patients with right ventricular dysfunction or constrictive pericarditis.

Ref: Talley & O'Connor. Clinical Examination. Blackwell Scientific Publications. Ch. 3. Kumar & Clark. Clinical Medicine, 3rd Ed. W. B. Saunders. Ch. 11.

QUESTION 46

A. TRUE B. TRUE C. FALSE D. FALSE E. TRUE

Coarctation of the aorta has a male to female ratio of 2:1. Most are post ductal in origin and are less severe than preductal lesions which present with heart failure in infancy and are associated with a patent ductus arteriosus and a variety of other cardiac defects (VSD and mitral valve lesions). It is associated with both Turner's and Noonan's syndrome. At least 50% of patients have a bicuspid aortic valve which may lead to problems in later life. There is a recognised association with cerebral artery aneurysm. Proximal vasculature hypertension leads to the formation of large collateral arteries in the first few years of life. There may be dilatation of the aorta both immediately before and after the coarctation leading to the 3 sign on a chest X-ray. The murmurs associated with a coarct are an ejection systolic murmur at the aortic valve with or without some aortic regurgitation. Turbulence at the coarct itself may lead to a systolic murmur best heard in the back and systolic or continuous bruits from collaterals.

Ref: Oxford Textbook of Medicine, 3rd Ed. Oxford University Press. Ch. 15.28.3.

QUESTION 47

A. FALSE B. TRUE C. TRUE D. TRUE E. FALSE

The jugular venous pulse consists of three peaks (a, c, v waves) and two troughs (x, y descent). The a wave reflects atrial systole, and coincides with the first heart sound. It precedes the carotid pulse. The v wave corresponds to atrial filling against a closed tricuspid valve during ventricular systole. The x descent is a trough caused by atrial relaxation. The c wave occurs during the x descent and is due to the transmission of the carotid impulse. It coincides with tricuspid valve closure. During the y descent there is rapid ventricular filling following the opening of the tricuspid valve. It is measured from the manubriosternal angle with the patient at about 45° to the horizontal. The normal value is usually less than 3 cm of H_2O which is equivalent to a right atrial pressure of 8 mmHg.

A steep x descent is associated with constrictive pericarditis and acute cardiac tamponade. It is absent in atrial fibrillation. A steep y descent is associated with severe tricuspid regurgitation as well as constrictive pericarditis and right ventricular failure. It is slow in tricuspid stenosis and right atrial mxyoma.

The JVP normally falls on inspiration unless there is impaired right ventricular filling when the JVP rises on inspiration due to the increased venous return to the heart. This is known as Kussmaul's sign

Ref: Talley & O'Connor. Clinical Examination. Blackwell Scientific Publications. Ch. 3.
Kumar & Clark. Clinical Medicine, 3rd Ed. W. B. Saunders. Ch. 11.

QUESTION 48

A. FALSE B. FALSE C. FALSE D. TRUE E. FALSE

The ECG records potential differences at the surface of the skin generated by the activity of the heart. These differences are of the order of 1mV at the body surface and create the familiar QRST pattern of the normal ECG. The ECG represents the vector sum of the depolarization and repolarization potentials of all the myocardial cells. Myocardial cells have a resting intracellular potential difference of -90mV when compared to the extracellular space and this is maintained by a high intracellular potassium concentration. Recording from three mutually perpendicular axes is required to represent the three dimension spatial vector correctly. This is not practicable with the shape of the human body. ECG machines therefore record 12 projections of the vector. These are the so called conventional leads.

Ref: Kumar & Clark. Clinical Medicine, 3rd Ed. W. B. Saunders. Ch. 11.

QUESTION 49

A. TRUE B. TRUE C. FALSE D. FALSE E. FALSE

The T wave does represents ventricular repolarization however it is both the ST segment and T wave that truly represent the repolarization phase in the ECG. The T wave is normally less than 5 mm in amplitude in the standard leads and 10mm in the precordial leads. Digoxin is associated with ST depression and T wave flattening. T wave inversion may occur in digoxin toxicity. Increased T wave amplitude is a characteristic feature of hyperkalaemia.

80% of patients have an upright T wave in V1. It is inverted or flattened in the other 20% which can therefore not be regarded as an abnormality. Only 5% of patients have an inverted T wave in V2. An inverted T wave in V2 is abnormal if the T wave is upright in V1. T wave inversion may be seen in V3 in black people. T wave inversion in V4 is always abnormal. The T wave is usually abnormal if inverted in I, II or V4-6. A small Q wave in association with T wave inversion may be normal in lead III. This may disappear if the ECG is repeated in deep inspiration.

Ref: Kumar & Clark. Clinical Medicine, 3rd Ed. W. B. Saunders. Ch. 11.
Oxford Textbook of Medicine, 3rd Ed. Oxford University Press. Ch. 15.4.2.
Oxford Handbook of Clinical Medicine, 3rd Ed. Oxford University Press. p264.

QUESTION 50

A. TRUE   B. TRUE   C. TRUE   D. FALSE   E. TRUE

The ECG in hypothermia indicates reduced conductivity. The characteristic signs are prolongation of the PR and QT interval, widening of the QRS complex, ST depression and J waves. J waves are almost always present when the core temperature is below 31°C. Rhythm disturbances are common. Sinus rhythm is maintained in moderate hypothermia. Atrial flutter or fibrillation with or without ventricular premature beats may develop in more serious cases. As the body temperature falls, atrial activity may disappear and an idioventricular rhythm develop. There is a risk of VF below 30°C often precipitated by hypoxia, hypotension or stimulating procedures. If the core temperature falls to below 28°C there is a pronounced tendency to develop VF.

Ref: Hinds & Watson. Intensive Care: A Concise Textbook. W. B. Saunders. Ch. 19.

QUESTION 51

A. FALSE   B. FALSE   C. FALSE   D. TRUE   E. TRUE

In patients presenting with broad complex tachycardias the main problem is differentiating VT from SVT with aberrant conduction. 75% of broad complex tachycardias are ventricular in origin. VT is commoner after myocardial infarction or in the presence of ischaemic heart disease.

Features of the ECG in favour of an SVT are:

* The presence of P wave directly associated with the QRS complex (note that in VT the P waves are dissociated from the QRS!)
* Absence of fusion or capture beats which are diagnostic of VT.
* Classical LBBB or RBBB QRS morphology
* QRS < 0.14 secs
* Normal QRS axis

Ref: Oxford Handbook of Clinical Medicine. Oxford University Press. p 292.

QUESTION 52

A. TRUE   B. FALSE   C. TRUE   D. TRUE   E. FALSE

In the normal second heart sound the aortic component occurs before the pulmonary component. A2-P2. Normal physiological splitting increases with inspiration due to the increased venous return to the right ventricle. It is best heard in the pulmonary area or left sternal edge as P2 is softer than A2 and may not be heard throughout the precordium. In reverse splitting of the second heart sound, the aortic component occurs after the pulmonary component P2-A2. Splitting occurs in expiration and is reduced in inspiration as the pulmonary component of the second heart sound approaches the aortic component.

Causes include:

- Delayed LV depolarisation - LBBB
- Delayed LV emptying - severe aortic stenosis, coarctation, LVF
- Increased LV volume load - large PDA

Ref: Talley & O'Connor. Clinical Examination. Blackwell Scientific Publications. Ch. 3.

QUESTION 53

A. TRUE B. TRUE C. TRUE D. FALSE E. TRUE

Right bundle branch block produces late activation of the right ventricle. The QRS complex is characteristically greater than 120 msecs in duration with the classic rSR or rR pattern in V1. Secondary changes include deep slurred S waves in leads I, aVL, V4-6 and T wave changes in V1-3.

RBBB is a normal finding in about 1% of adults and 5% of elderly patients. The main causes are:

- Congenital heart disease - ASD, VSD, Fallot's and Pulmonary stenosis.
- Pulmonary disease - Cor pulmonale and Pulmonary embolism
- Myocardial disease - Acute MI, Cardiomyopathy, Conduction system fibrosis
- Drugs - Hyperkalaemia and Class 1a antiarrhythmics
- Right ventriculotomy

Ref: Kumar & Clark. Clinical Medicine, 3rd Ed. W. B. Saunders. Ch. 11.
Oxford Textbook of Medicine, 3rd Ed. Ch. 15.4.2.

QUESTION 54

A. FALSE B. TRUE C. FALSE D. TRUE E. FALSE

The third heart sound is a low pitched mid-diastolic sound due to rapid ventricular filling in diastole as soon as the mitral and tricuspid valves open. Physiological left ventricular third sounds are heard in children and young adults due to very fast ventricular diastolic filling. This is best heard at the apex in the left lateral position. In patients over the age of 40 the sound is normally pathological and represents reduced ventricular compliance. Pathological left ventricular S3 is best heard at the apex in expiration and represents heart failure or volume overload (LVF, AR, MR, VSD and PDA). Pathological right ventricular S3 is best heard at the left sternal edge and is louder in inspiration. It occurs in patients with right ventricular dysfunction or constrictive pericarditis.

Ref: Talley & O'Connor. Clinical Examination. Blackwell Scientific Publications. Ch. 3.
Kumar & Clark. Clinical Medicine, 3rd Ed. W. B. Saunders. Ch. 11.

QUESTION 55

A. TRUE B. TRUE C. FALSE D. TRUE E. TRUE

The QT interval is taken from the start of the QRS complex to the end of the T wave. The interval varies with heart rate and should be corrected using Bazett's formula.

Corrected QT interval is QT interval divided by the square root of the R-R interval measured in seconds. The normal value is 0.35 - 0.43 seconds. Rate corrected values greater than 0.44 secs represent prolongation of the QT interval. There is no abnormal atrio-ventricular pathway. The long QT syndrome is the association of a prolonged QT interval in sinus rhythm with intermittent torsades de pointes (atypical ventricular tachycardia)

Causes of a long QT Interval include:

* Congenital syndromes
* Jervell-Lange-Nielsen (autosomal recessive) associated with deafness
* Romano-Ward (autosomal dominant)
* Electrolyte abnormalities - hypokalaemia, hypocalcaemia, hypomagnesaemia
* Drugs   - Quinidine, Amiodarone and other class 1a and 3 antiarrhythmics
                  - Tricyclic antidepressants, phenothiazines, Terfenadine, Astemizole
                  - Terodiline, Erthyromycin
* Poisons - organophosphorus compounds
* Bradycardia, Mitral valve prolapse, myocardial infarction, Hypothyroidism, anorexia, starvation and liquid protein diets.

Ref: Kumar & Clark. Clinical Medicine, 3rd Ed. W. B. Saunders. Ch. 11.
Oxford Textbook of Medicine, 3rd Ed. Oxford University Press. Ch. 15.8.1.
Oxford Handbook of Clinical Medicine, 3rd Ed. Oxford University Press. p264.

QUESTION 56

A. FALSE B. TRUE C. TRUE D. FALSE E. TRUE

The fourth heart sound (S4) is a late diastolic sound caused by the rapid ventricular filling that accompanies atrial contraction. It is never physiological but may be a normal finding in elderly patients. It can sometimes be palpated and usually indicates reduced ventricular compliance. It is known as the sound of cardiac stress (S3 = sound of cardiac distress).

Left ventricular S4 is associated with aortic stenosis, acute mitral regurgitation, systemic hypertension, ischaemic heart disease or advanced age. Right ventricular S4 is associated with reduced right ventricular compliance in pulmonary hypertension or pulmonary stenosis. Note that volume overload is normally associated with a third heart sound.

Ref: Talley & O'Connor. Clinical Examination. Blackwell Scientific Publications. Ch. 3.
Kumar & Clark. Clinical Medicine, W. B. Saunders. Ch. 11.

QUESTION 57

A. TRUE B. TRUE C. FALSE D. TRUE E. TRUE

Diastolic murmurs are usually associated with cardiac disease. Early diastolic murmurs are decrescendo in nature and are normally due to regurgitation through the aortic or pulmonary valves. Pulmonary hypertension secondary to mitral stenosis may lead to pulmonary regurgitation. This is known as the Graham Steele murmur which is best heard at the left sternal edge.

Mid-diastolic murmurs occur later in diastole and may extend right up to the first heart sound. They are due to impaired flow during ventricular filling. The main causes are mitral or tricuspid stenosis and rarely atrial myxomas where there is partial obstruction of the valve orifice. Severe aortic incompetence may be associated with a mid-diastolic murmur known as an Austin Flint murmur. The regurgitant jet causes the anterior leaflet of the mitral valve to shudder. High cardiac output states may be associated with benign flow murmurs.

Presystolic accentuation of diastolic murmurs may occur due to atrial contraction increasing the blood flow across the valve.

The Carey-Coombs murmur is described as a mid-diastolic murmur that occurs in acute rheumatic carditis.

Rafi Talley & O'Connor. Clinical Examination. Blackwell Scientific Publications. Ch. 3. Kumar & Clark. Clinical Medicine, 3rd Ed. W. B. Saunders. Ch. 11.

QUESTION 58

A. TRUE B. FALSE C. FALSE D. FALSE E. TRUE

Pregnancy is associated with marked haemodynamic changes. The blood volume increases substantially. The heart rate, stroke volume and cardiac output increase while systemic blood pressure and vascular resistance fall (diastolic BP > systolic producing a wide pulse pressure). Patients with mitral stenosis may deteriorate significantly during gestation due to the fixed flow obstruction. The increased heart rate and cardiac output with the decrease in colloid osmotic pressure predispose to pulmonary oedema. Aggressive diuretic therapy is contraindicated as it may decrease uterine perfusion pressure. VSD and ASD are usually well tolerated in pregnancy even among patients with large left-right shunts. However, the degree of pulmonary hypertension should guide management as marked reduction in blood pressure during or after delivery may result in reversal of the shunt. Aortic regurgitation is also well tolerated (as is mitral regurgitation) probably because the systemic vascular resistance falls. Pregnancy in patients with primary pulmonary hypertension is associated with a high mortality, probably due to right ventricular ischaemia and failure, increased arrhythmias and pulmonary embolism.

QUESTION 59

A. TRUE B. TRUE C. FALSE D. FALSE E. FALSE

The strain phase of the Valsalva manoeuvre decreases preload. The following occur:-

- HOCM - louder murmur (reduced ventricular filling and greater obstruction)
- Mitral valve prolapse - longer murmur (occurs earlier)
- Aortic stenosis - softer murmur (fall in stroke volume and blood pressure)
- Mitral regurgitation - softer murmur

There is no effect on the fourth heart sound which is due to rapid ventricular filling accompanying atrial systole.

Ref: Talley & O'Connor. Clinical Examination. Blackwell Scientific Publications. Ch. 3.
Kumar & Clark. Clinical Medicine, 3rd Ed. W. B. Saunders. Ch. 11.

QUESTION 60

A. FALSE B. TRUE C. TRUE D. FALSE E. FALSE

Beta-blockers without intrinsic sympathomimetic activity have been shown to reduce mortality, probably by preventing cardiac rupture. They are contraindicated in patients with asthma, pulmonary oedema and hypotension. In ISIS-2, aspirin alone reduced mortality from 13.2% to 10.7% and thrombolysis with streptokinase alone reduced mortality from 13.2% to 10.4%. The combination of these two agents reduced mortality to 8%. The recent GUSTO trial showed a small benefit of 'front-loaded' tPA over SK overall, the effect being most marked for those patients with anterior MI. LIMIT-2 suggested iv magnesium given within 24 hours reduced mortality by 24%. Data from the larger ISIS-4 trial did not confirm this. Several trials have shown that ACE inhibitors (with the possible exception of enalapril in the CONSENSUS II trial) given after 24 hours reduce mortality. Intravenous nitrates were shown to be safe for patients with acute MI but conferred no survival benefit according to the ISIS-4 trial. Direct PTCA has recently been shown to reduce mortality and in the GUSTO IIb trial was shown to confer a short-term survival benefit over tPA. Diltiazem and verapamil have been shown, in small trials, to reduce mortality in patients provided LV function was normal. There is no evidence that nifedipine reduces mortality.

QUESTION 61

A. TRUE B. TRUE C. FALSE D. FALSE E. FALSE

The Lown-Ganong-Levine syndrome is associated with an accessory pathway known as the bundle of James. It is an intranodal bypass that connects the atria to the bundle of His. It does not activate the ventricular muscle directly. The P wave is normal but the PR interval is short as in WPW. There is no pre-excitation and therefore no delta wave. The QRS complex is of normal width. Atrial flutter or fibrillation is associated with this syndrome, although these patients are often asymptomatic. Patients with symptoms should be referred to a cardiologist.

Ref: Oxford Textbook of Medicine, 3rd Ed. Oxford University Press Ch. 15.8.1.
Kumar & Clark. Clinical Medicine, 3rd Ed. W. B. Saunders. Ch. 11.

QUESTION 62

A. TRUE B. FALSE C. FALSE D. TRUE E. FALSE

VSD's constitute up to 40% of all congenital cardiac defects, and occur commonly with ASD's and atrio-ventricular valve defects in Down's syndrome. The shunt is initially left to right due to the pressure gradient but as the right ventricular output and pressure rises obliterative pulmonary vascular changes occur and pulmonary hypertension develops. When right exceeds left ventricular pressure the shunt reverses (Eisenmenger's syndrome) and hypoxia and cyanosis ensue. Large VSD's should be surgically corrected early because pulmonary hypertension may develop within 6 to 9 months of birth. The murmur of a VSD is systolic and varies with the size of the defect.

Ref: Kumar & Clark. Clinical Medicine, 3rd Ed. W. B. Saunders. Ch. 11.

QUESTION 63

A. FALSE B. FALSE C. TRUE D. TRUE E. TRUE

The fourth heart sound (S4) is a late diastolic sound caused by the rapid ventricular filling that accompanies atrial contraction. It is never physiological but may be a normal finding in elderly patients. It can sometimes be palpated and usually indicates reduced ventricular compliance It is known as the sound of cardiac stress (S3 = sound of cardiac distress).

Left ventricular S4 is associated with aortic stenosis, acute mitral regurgitation, systemic hypertension, ischaemic heart disease or advanced age. Right ventricular S4 is associated with reduced right ventricular compliance in pulmonary hypertension or pulmonary stenosis.

Ref: Talley & O'Connor. Clinical Examination. Blackwell Scientific Publications. Ch. 3. Kumar & Clark. Clinical Medicine, 3rd Ed. W. B. Saunders. Ch. 11.

QUESTION 64

A. FALSE B. TRUE C. FALSE D. FALSE E. TRUE

Rheumatic fever is an autoimmune inflammatory disease triggered by Group A Streptococcus. All three layers of the heart are affected. Carditis is manifest by new or changed murmurs, cardiac enlargement or failure, pericardial effusion and ECG changes of pericarditis or myocarditis. The Carey-Coombs murmur is a transient diastolic murmur caused by mitral valvulitis. Non cardiac features include fever with excessive tachycardia, a fleeting polyarthritis of the large joints, Sydenham's chorea, and skin manifestations (erythema marginatum and subcutaneous nodules). About half the patients who have acute carditis progress to chronic rheumatic valvular disease. Of these, 50% have mitral involvement, 40% have combined mitral and aortic involvement, 5% have mitral, aortic and tricuspid involvement and 2% have aortic involvement alone.

Ref: Kumar & Clark. Clinical Medicine, 3rd Ed. W. B. Saunders. Ch. 11.

QUESTION 65

A. FALSE B. TRUE C. TRUE D. TRUE E. TRUE

Mitral valve prolapse (also known as Barlow's syndrome, floppy mitral valve, etc.) has a prevalence of ~4% in the normal asymptomatic population. It is thought to occur by progressive stretching of the mitral leaflets and weakening with deposition of mucopolysaccharides in the valve tissue. It is associated with ostium secundum ASD, Turner's syndrome, Marfan's syndrome, pseudoxanthoma elasticum, osteogenesis imperfecta, dilated + hypertrophic cardiomyopathy and WPW syndrome (Pre-excitation).

Presenting features include atypical chest pain, palpitations, infective endocarditis, dyspnoea and progressive mitral incompetence, stroke (from emboli), re-entry tachyarrhythmias, VT and sudden death. Ventricular ectopic beats are benign and usually do not require therapy. If treatment is necessary beta-blockers frequently are successful in reducing both chest pains and palpitations.

Ref: Oxford Textbook of Medicine, 3rd Ed. Oxford University Press Ch. 15.18.
Kumar & Clark. Clinical Medicine, 3rd Ed. W. B. Saunders. Ch. 11.

QUESTION 66

A. TRUE B. TRUE C. TRUE D. TRUE E. TRUE

Constrictive pericarditis may occur in association with TB, haemopericardium and acute pericarditis (viral, bacterial or rheumatic). The central venous system becomes congested and ascites, dependent oedema and hepatomegaly develop. Pulsus paradoxus, Kussmaul's sign (increased JVP during inspiration) and Friedreich's sign (diastolic collapse of JVP) are all present. Atrial fibrillation is present in approximately 30% of patients. The ECG shows low voltage QRS complexes and T wave inversion. The CXR reveals a small heart often with calcification seen on the lateral film. Treatment is the surgical removal of a significant amount of pericardium

Ref: Kumar & Clark. Clinical Medicine, 3rd Ed. W. B. Saunders. Ch. 11.

QUESTION 67

A. FALSE B. TRUE C. FALSE D. TRUE E. TRUE

In the normal second heart sound the aortic component occurs before the pulmonary component. A2-P2. Normal physiological splitting increases with inspiration due to the increased venous return to the right ventricle. It is best heard in the pulmonary area or left sternal edge as P2 is softer than A2 and may not be heard throughout the precordium. In reverse splitting of the second heart sound, the aortic component occurs after the pulmonary component P2-A2. Splitting occurs in expiration and is reduced in inspiration as the pulmonary component of the second heart sound approaches the aortic component.

Causes include:

- Delayed LV depolarisation - LBBB
- Delayed LV emptying - severe aortic stenosis, coarctation, LVF
- Increased LV volume load - large PDA

Ref: Talley & O'Connor. Clinical Examination. Blackwell Scientific Publications. Ch. 3.

QUESTION 68

A. FALSE B. FALSE C. TRUE D. TRUE E. TRUE

The normal PR interval should be >0.11 s and <0.20 s. A short PR interval is seen with pre-excitation (e.g. Wolff-Parkinson-White or Lown-Ganong-Levine syndrome). The normal QRS axis is -30 to +90°. Left axis deviation is seen with left anterior hemiblock, inferior MI, pre-excitation (WPW or LGL), hyperkalaemia, tricuspid atresia, ostium primum atrial septal defect and right ventricular pacing. Right axis deviation is seen with RV hypertrophy, acute pulmonary embolism, cor pulmonale, secundum ASD, RBBB, Fallot's tetralogy and total anomalous pulmonary venous drainage. Right axis deviation is also seen in left posterior hemiblock where the QRS complex is normal.

Voltage criteria for left ventricular hypertrophy (none is absolute): R wave (aVF) > 20 mm, S(V1) + R (V6) >35 mm, R wave in V4, V5 or V6 >27 mm, S wave in V1, V2 or V3 >30mm, any R + any S >45.

RBBB is a normal finding in up to 10% of individuals. A normal Q wave is <0.04 s wide and <25% of the total QRS complex.

Ref: Oxford Textbook of Medicine, 3rd Ed. Oxford University Press. Ch. 15.4.2.

QUESTION 69

A. TRUE B. FALSE C. FALSE D. TRUE E. FALSE

Variation of RR interval is typically seen in SVTs (varying vagal tone on the AV node) but minor variation (up to 20 ms) may also occur in VT. Absence of pre-excitation in sinus rhythm does not exclude atrioventricular re-entry tachycardia ('hidden' accessory pathway).

Features strongly suggestive of VT are:-
- Fusion beats or capture beats (diagnostic);
- Evidence of AV dissociation (seen in ~25%);
- Evidence of atrial capture, i.e. VA conduction with 2:1 or 3:1 VA block;
- QRS concordance in chest leads. If the predominant deflection of the QRS is positive this is highly suggestive of VT. Negative concordance is less so;
- QRS >140 ms (3.5 small sq) especially with normal duration in sinus rhythm;
- Marked left axis deviation (negative in II);
- In patients with previous LBBB or RBBB, a different QRS morphology in tachycardia suggests VT.

Ref: Oxford Textbook of Medicine, 3rd Ed. Oxford University Press. Ch. 15.8.1.

QUESTION 70

A. TRUE B. FALSE C. TRUE D. FALSE E. TRUE

Recognised toxic effects of digoxin include:

- GI symptoms – nausea, vomiting, abdominal pain, diarrhoea;
- Central effects – confusion, convulsions and depression;
- Visual effects – Xanthopsia, halo and visual blurring;
- Rare effects – facial pain, gynaecomastia, hyperkalaemia and muscle necrosis;
- Arrhythmias – bradycardia, heart block and ventricular ectopics including bi- and trigemini;
- ECG effects – prolonged PR interval and heart block, T wave inversion, ST depression (reverse tick), reduction in T wave amplitude, shortening of the QT interval;
- Beware of the difference between digoxin effects which may be normal at therapeutic doses and digoxin toxicity;

At therapeutic levels digoxin causes ST depression, reduction in size of the T wave and shortening of the QT interval. At toxic levels the T wave may become inverted and any arrhythmia may occur. The most common are sinus bradycardia, PAT with block, AV block, VE's, ventricular bigeminy and VT.

Ref: Epstein RJ. Medicine for Examinations. 3rd Ed. Churchill Livingstone. Ch. 2. Houghton & Gray. Making sense of the ECG. Arnold. Ch. 9.

QUESTION 71

A. TRUE B. TRUE C. TRUE D. FALSE E. FALSE

Digoxin prolongs the PR interval on the ECG. First degree heart block is associated with toxic levels of digoxin therapy. U waves occur in hypokalaemia which may potentiate the effects of toxic levels of digoxin. Shortening of the QT interval, T wave flattening and the reverse tick phenomenon are recognised ECG abnormalities in patients taking digoxin.

Ref: Drugs in Anaesthesia and Intensive Care, 2nd Ed. Sasada and Smith. Oxford University Press.

QUESTION 72

A. TRUE B. FALSE C. FALSE D. FALSE E. FALSE

Coronary artery stents are used to treat dissections during balloon angioplasty and to improve the results of conventional angioplasty. Stent occlusion is much commoner in arteries of <3 mm diameter. Short-term anticoagulation (3 months) was originally used but current protocols show that aspirin alone or aspirin + ticlopidine (another antiplatelet agent) are as effective as warfarin in preventing stent occlusion acutely with less bleeding complications and reduced hospital stay. MRI is not contraindicated, but artefacts may occur due to the metal of the stent. Most stents are very difficult to see on conventional CXR.

QUESTION 73

A. TRUE B. TRUE C. FALSE D. TRUE E. FALSE

The coarctation is a narrowing of the aorta. This is most commonly distal to the origin of the left subclavian artery where the ductus arteriosus attaches to the aorta. Up to 80% have an associated bicuspid aortic valve. Collateral arterial channels develop to bypass the coarctation and dilated intercostal arteries may erode the underside of the ribs ('rib notching'). Renal hypoperfusion leads to activation of the renin-angiotensin system which results in generalised hypertension and a tendency to intracranial haemorrhage and epistaxis. Routine examination in the neonatal period revealing absent femoral pulses may lead to early diagnosis. Following surgical correction the blood pressure should be kept 'low' to avoid excessive stress on aortic suture lines.

Ref: Kumar & Clark. Clinical Medicine, 3rd Ed. W. B. Saunders. Ch. 11.

QUESTION 74

A. TRUE B. FALSE C. TRUE D. TRUE E. FALSE

Rheumatic fever accounts for at least 50% of mitral stenosis, although this is decreasing. The normal valve orifice area is 5 cm², a drop to 1 cm² represents severe stenosis and an increased probability of progressing through the ensuing pathological changes. Initially left atrial pressure rises and the left atrium becomes dilated (seen on CXR). Subsequently pulmonary pressure rises leading to raised right heart pressures and right ventricular failure. Pulmonary oedema may develop but alveolar and capillary thickening partially prevent this. Pulmonary artery wedge pressure reflects left ventricular end diastolic pressure poorly because the stenotic valve situated between these two sites has a pressure gradient across it.

Ref: Kumar & Clark. Clinical Medicine, 3rd Ed. W. B. Saunders. Ch. 11.

QUESTION 75

A. FALSE B. TRUE C. TRUE D. TRUE E. FALSE

Common abnormalities of the second heart sound include:

1. Loud A2: Tachycardia, hypertension, transposition;
2. Loud P2: Pulmonary hypertension;
3. Single S2: Fallot's tetralogy, severe pulmonary or aortic stenosis, pulmonary valve atresia, Eisenmenger's complex, large ventricular septal defect;
4. Widely split S2: RBBB, pulmonary stenosis, deep inspiration, mitral incompetence, ventricular septal defect;
5. Reversed split S2: LBBB, aortic stenosis, patent ductus arteriosus (PDA), right ventricular pacing;
6. Fixed split S2: Atrial septal defect.

Common abnormalities of the first heart sound include:
1. Loud S1: Mitral stenosis, tachycardia, short PR interval (e.g. WPW);
2. Soft S1: Delayed ventricular ejection (e.g. aortic stenosis), long PR interval (i.e. first- or second-degree heart block);
3. Wide split S1: RBBB, LBBB, ventricular ectopic beats, ventricular tachycardia;
4. Variable intensity S1: atrial fibrillation, nodal tachycardia, ventricular tachycardia, complete heart block.

Ref: Talley & O'Connor. Clinical Examination. Blackwell Scientific Publications. Ch. 3.

QUESTION 76

A. TRUE B. FALSE C. TRUE D. TRUE E. TRUE

Tall R waves in V1 are associated with right ventricular hypertrophy. An R wave amplitude greater than 7mm in V1 is recognised as a diagnostic criteria. The diagnosis is supported by the presence of T wave inversion in the other right ventricular precordial leads V1-4 suggesting right ventricular strain.

It is important to exclude other causes of a tall R wave in V1. Recognised causes include:
• Right bundle branch block
• Pulmonary embolism (acute)
• Dextrocardia
• WPW syndrome type A
• True Posterior infarction (the upside-down Q wave)
• Hypertrophic cardiomyopathy
• Friedreich's ataxia

Ref: Epstein RJ. Medicine for Examinations. 3rd Ed. Churchill Livingstone. Ch. 2.

QUESTION 77

A. FALSE B. FALSE C. TRUE D. TRUE E. TRUE

Vagal discharge increases AV nodal conduction time and AV nodal recovery time. During vagal discharge atrial arrhythmias may be revealed as the ventricular response is reduced or for arrhythmias that involve circus movement sinus rhythm may be restored. The vagal manoeuvres used are carotid sinus massage (CSM), ocular pressure, immersion of the face in cold water, and the Valsalva manoeuvre (which is said to be the most effective). When performing CSM it is important to ensure the absence of a carotid bruit as circular pressure over atheroma may precipitate an embolic stroke. Generally right sided CSM slows the sinus rate while left sided CSM will impair AV nodal conduction.

Ref: Kumar & Clark. Clinical Medicine, 3rd Ed. W. B. Saunders. Ch. 11.

QUESTION 78

A. TRUE B. TRUE C. FALSE D. TRUE E. FALSE

The clinical findings associated with an atrial septal defect are a right ventricular heave, fixed and wide splitting of the second heart sound (loud P2), mid-systolic pulmonary flow murmur reflecting increased flow through the right heart and the presence of a diastolic tricuspid flow murmur. The chest X-ray shows prominent pulmonary ARTERIES and pulmonary plethora. There may be right ventricular enlargement. Ostium primum ASD are associated with mitral and tricuspid regurgitation or a VSD.

Ref: Talley & O'Connor. Clinical Examination. Blackwell Scientific Publications. Ch. 3. Kumar & Clark. Clinical Medicine, 3rd Ed. W. B. Saunders. Ch. 11.

QUESTION 79

A. FALSE B. TRUE C. TRUE D. TRUE E. FALSE

Alcoholic cardiomyopathy commonly presents with left-sided failure (breathlessness on exertion, orthopnoea, paroxysmal nocturnal dyspnoea). Beri-beri due to thiamine deficiency presents with high output cardiac failure and right-sided signs ('wet' beri-beri). Peripartum cardiomyopathy - recurrence risk 20% even with complete resolution. Dilated cardiomyopathy is seen in 1-2% of patients on doxorubicin and 4-5% on daunorubicin. Classically occurs with anthracycline doses >450 mg/m2 but may occur with less. Cardiomyopathy is the presenting feature in 1% of HIV infected patients and about 10% develop dilated cardiomyopathy and up to 50% have cardiac involvement on investigation. There is recognised association with selenium deficiency.

Ref: Epstein RJ. Medicine for Examinations. Churchill Livingstone. Ch. 2.

QUESTION 80

A. FALSE B. TRUE C. TRUE D. TRUE E. FALSE

The second heart sound marks the end of systole. It is formed by the closure of the aortic and pulmonary valves. In normal circumstances the pulmonary valve closes later than the aortic valve. It is best heard in the pulmonary area or left sternal edge. Physiological splitting is greater in inspiration due to increased venous return to the right ventricle. Increased splitting of the second heart sound occurs when there is any delay in right ventricular emptying. Common causes include right bundle branch block, pulmonary stenosis (delayed RV ejection), VSD (increased RV volume load), and mitral regurgitation (earlier aortic valve closure due to more rapid LV emptying).

ASD's are associated with a wide and fixed split second heart sound due to a combination of some degree of RBBB and left to right shunting. In tetralogy of Fallot, the second heart sound is usually single.

Ref: Talley & O'Connor. Clinical Examination. Blackwell Scientific Publications. Ch. 3. Kumar & Clark. Clinical Medicine, 3rd Ed. W. B. Saunders. Ch11.

QUESTION 81

A. TRUE B. FALSE C. TRUE D. FALSE E. FALSE

WPW syndrome may be associated with an accessory bundle anywhere in the atrio-ventricular ring. The classical features are a short PR interval, delta wave and wide QRS complex. The QT interval is normal. If the accessory bundle is left sided the QRS complex is positive in V1 and this is known as type A (most common form). Digoxin should be avoided as it shortens the relative refractory period of the accessory bundle which may lead to pre-excitation atrial fibrillation and sudden death in patients with WPW. The delta wave is lost in tachydysrhythmias due to orthodromic conduction through the AV node and antidromic conduction through the accessory pathway.

Ref: Oxford Textbook of Medicine, 3ʳᵈ Ed. Oxford University Press Ch. 15.8.1.
Kumar & Clark. Clinical Medicine, 3ʳᵈ Ed. W. B. Saunders. Ch. 11.

QUESTION 82

A. TRUE B. TRUE C. FALSE D. TRUE E. FALSE

Arising from the anterior aortic sinus, the right coronary artery passes forwards between the pulmonary trunk and right atrium descending in the right part of the AV groove to anastomose with the left coronary at the inferior interventricular groove. It has two branches, the marginal (passing along the inferior boarder of the heart) and the interventricular branch (passing along the inferior interventricular groove towards the apex of the heart where it anastomoses with the interventricular branch of the left coronary artery). The right coronary artery supplies the sino atrial node in 65% and the atrioventricular node in 80% of the population. It supplies the right ventricle except for the upper anterior border.

Ref: Ellis & Feldman. Anatomy for Anaesthetists, 6th Ed. Blackwell Scientific Publications p83.

QUESTION 83

A. TRUE B. TRUE C. FALSE D. TRUE E. TRUE

Atrial myxomas are the most common primary cardiac tumour. They are usually left sided and polypoid with a gelatinous structure attached by a pedicle to the atrial septum. The tumour may cause obstruction of the mitral valve and is associated with embolic phenomenon. Patients often present with shortness of breath, PND, syncope, mild fever and atrial arrhythmias. Clinical signs include a loud first heart sound, apical diastolic murmur, tumour plop and signs of systemic emboli. The ESR and serum Immunoglobulins are raised. The diagnosis is confirmed on echocardiography.

Ref: Kumar & Clark. Clinical Medicine, 3ʳᵈ Ed. W. B. Saunders. Ch. 11.
Oxford Textbook of Medicine, 3ʳᵈ Ed. Oxford University Press. Ch. 15.19.

QUESTION 84

A. FALSE B. FALSE C. TRUE D. TRUE E. FALSE

The classical findings in hypertrophic obstructive cardiomyopathy are:

- Jerky carotid pulse;
- Double apical impulse;
- Ejection systolic murmur - may be late systolic;
- Pan-systolic murmur at the apex due to mitral regurgitation;
- Fourth heart sound which may be palpable;
- Normal chest X-ray;
- ECG - LVH and strain with ST and T wave changes;
- Intraventricular conduction delay is common. 20% have left axis deviation and 5% a right bundle block pattern. The PR interval is either normal or may be short and similar to that seen in WPW;
- Echo - Septal hypertrophy and abnormal anterior motion of the mitral valve in systole.

Ref: Talley & O'Connor. Clinical Examination. Blackwell Scientific Publications. Ch. 3.
Oxford Textbook of Medicine, 3rd Ed. Oxford University Press. Ch. 15.14.1.
Kumar & Clark. Clinical Medicine, 3rd Ed. W. B. Saunders. Ch. 11.

QUESTION 85

A. FALSE B. FALSE C. FALSE D. TRUE E. FALSE

Atrial septal defects can occur in a number of different positions. Patients with secundum ASD (90%) are often asymptomatic in childhood and are not diagnosed until middle age. Primum ASD (10%) is a much more severe defect often involving the AV canal (VSD or abnormal mitral or tricuspid valves producing a pan-systolic murmur). Both types of ASD produce fixed splitting of the second heart sound with an ejection murmur over the pulmonary valve. A diastolic flow murmur over the tricuspid may be audible. Right atrial enlargement is not common (pulmonary plethora more common). On the ECG, both types of ASD produce a RBBB pattern on the ECG (rSR pattern in V1): primum ASD is associated with left axis deviation while secundum ASD is associated with right axis deviation.

Associated conditions:
1. *Secundum ASD* - Floppy mitral valve, anomalous pulmonary venous drainage, mitral stenosis (Lutembacher's syndrome);
2. *Primum ASD* - Down's syndrome, Klinefelter's syndrome, Noonan's syndrome, renal abnormalities, common atrium, pulmonary stenosis, coarctation of the aorta.

Ref: Oxford Textbook of Medicine, 3rd Ed. Oxford University Press Ch. 15.15.
Kumar & Clark. Clinical Medicine, 3rd Ed. W. B. Saunders. Ch. 11.

QUESTION 86

A. TRUE B. TRUE C. FALSE D. FALSE E. FALSE

The jugular venous pulse consists of three peaks (a, c, v waves) and two troughs (x, y descent). The a wave reflects atrial systole, and coincides with the first heart sound. It precedes the carotid pulse. In effect it also coincides with a right ventricular S4 which is due to atrial contraction. The v wave corresponds to atrial filling against a closed tricuspid valve during ventricular systole. The x descent is a trough caused by atrial relaxation. The c wave occurs during the x descent and is due to the transmission of the carotid impulse. It coincides with tricuspid valve closure. During the y descent there is rapid ventricular filling following the opening of the tricuspid valve.

A dominant a wave is seen in situations where there is right ventricular hypertrophy due to pulmonary stenosis or pulmonary hypertension. It may also occur in patients with tricuspid stenosis if the patients remain in sinus rhythm. If the patient is in AF there is no a wave in the JVP. Tricuspid stenosis is also associated with a slow y descent. Tricuspid regurgitation is associated with giant v waves as right ventricular pressure is transmitted directly to the right atrium and great veins.

Very large Cannon 'a' are seen in complete heart block and VT or paroxysmal nodal tachycardia with retrograde conduction or AV dissociation. These are not strictly speaking a waves as they occur when the atrium contracts against a closed tricuspid valve.

Ref: Talley & O'Connor. Clinical Examination. Blackwell Scientific Publications. Ch. 3. Kumar & Clark. Clinical Medicine, 3rd Ed. W. B. Saunders. Ch. 11.

QUESTION 87

A. FALSE B. TRUE C. FALSE D. TRUE E. TRUE

Atrial flutter is nearly always associated with organic heart disease. The atrial rate is classically 300 bpm but this will vary. If each atrial beat is conducted through the AV node to the ventricles the filling time is too small to allow an effective cardiac output. When a conduction ratio of 2:1 or 3:1 exists the ventricular rate becomes approximately 150 or 100 and cardiac output will be greater. Adenosine, verapamil or carotid sinus massage will temporarily block AV conduction and reveal the characteristic sawtooth atrial wave on the ECG. DC shock is useful in acute paroxysms of atrial flutter.

Ref: Kumar & Clark. Clinical Medicine, 3rd Ed. W. B. Saunders. Ch. 11.

QUESTION 88

A. TRUE B. TRUE C. FALSE D. TRUE E. TRUE

Atrial fibrillation is common, occurring in up to 10% of patients over 65yrs. The atrial rate is between 350 and 600 per minute which are seen as 'f' waves on the ECG. However because the AV node is rarely able to conduct beyond 200 impulses per minute the ventricular rate is limited. The atrium usually helps to complete ventricular filling but during atrial fibrillation this is lost and may seriously reduce the cardiac output particularly in the presence of mitral stenosis. Before pharmacological (chemical) attempts are made to convert atrial fibrillation, any obvious precipitating pathology should be treated. This includes chest infection, thyrotoxicosis and electrolyte imbalance (K^+ and Mg^{2+}). Class Ia, Ib, III drugs and digoxin have all been used. Patients should be anticoagulated before and after elective DC cardioversion due to the risk of systemic embolisation - usually from the left atrial appendage.

Ref: Kumar & Clark. Clinical Medicine, 3ʳᵈ Ed. W. B. Saunders. Ch. 11.

QUESTION 89

A. FALSE B. TRUE C. TRUE D. TRUE E. FALSE

Hypertrophic cardiomyopathy is usually familial with autosomal dominant transmission with a high degree of penetrance. Many mutations can produce hypertrophic cardiomyopathy (HCM) - beta-myosin heavy chain gene on chr 14 (~20-30%), cardiac troponin T on chr 1, alpha-tropomyosin on chr 15. It appears to be a disease of sarcomeric contractile proteins. The outflow tract gradient is dynamic and may improve with pacing. As the LV is stiff, atrial activity is important and dual chamber pacing is preferred. Adults have a 2-3% risk of sudden death and non-sustained VT is the only marker proven to be of predictive value (7 fold increased risk). The risk in children and adolescents is 4-6%. Squatting (passive leg elevation, handgrip) reduces the murmur by increasing the afterload. Standing from squatting, GTN, etc, increases the murmur due a decrease in afterload and reduction in venous return.

Ref: Oxford Textbook of Medicine, 3ʳᵈ Ed. Oxford University Press Ch. 15.14.1.
Kumar & Clark. Clinical Medicine, 3ʳᵈ Ed. W. B. Saunders. Ch. 11.

QUESTION 90

A. FALSE B. FALSE C. TRUE D. TRUE E. FALSE

In a normal ECG the first deflection is the low amplitude slow deflection caused by atrial depolarization - P wave. Depolarization of the sinus node is not seen. The initial deflection in V1 is positive due to the depolarization of the septum from left to right. This is also seen as a small Q wave in V6 with depolarisation of the septum occurring away from the electrode. The T wave represents ventricular repolarization and therefore is normally negative in aVR. The R wave represents the first +ve deflection of the ECG wave form. It is normally smaller than the S wave except in right ventricular hypertrophy where the R:S ratio is greater than 1.

Ref: Kumar & Clark. Clinical Medicine, 3ʳᵈ Ed. W. B. Saunders. Ch. 11.

QUESTION 91

A. FALSE B. FALSE C. TRUE D. TRUE E. TRUE

The axis of the ECG is calculated using the hexaxial reference system in the frontal plane. Leads I,II and III are mainly used and supplemented with the augmented limb leads as required. The normal QRS axis is between -30 and + 90° although some texts extend this to

+120°. Right posterior hemiblock is diagnosed from the ECG when there is right axis deviation in association with a normal QRS complex. In left axis deviation the cardiac vector is rotated anti-clockwise and the main deflection in lead three is away from the electrode which leads to a dominant S wave in this lead. The PR interval represents the time taken for the impulse to travel from the sinus node, through the AV node and His-Purkinje system. Atrial repolarization is not normally seen in the ECG because it is a low voltage wave hidden within the QRS complex. Biphasic P waves in V1 are associated with left atrial hypertrophy.

Ref: Kumar & Clark. Clinical Medicine, 3rd Ed. W. B. Saunders. Ch. 11.
Oxford Handbook of Clinical Medicine, 3rd Ed. Oxford University Press. Ch. 7.

QUESTION 92

A. FALSE B. FALSE C. FALSE D. FALSE E. FALSE

WPW is a congenital condition with an abnormal connection between the atria and ventricles (bundle of Kent). This conducts electricity faster than the AV node such that pre-excitation of the ventricles occurs. The PR interval is short and the QRS complex has a slurred upstroke known as the delta wave. Type A is associated with a left sided connection and a QRS above the isoelectric line in V1. Type B is associated with a right sided bundle and a QRS below the isoelectric line in V1. Delta waves occur in both. There is a recognised association with MVP, HOCM, Ebstein's anomaly and Secundum ASD. Supraventricular dysrhythmias are much more common than ventricular. PSVT is the most frequent. The ventricular rate may be uncontrolled in patients who develop AF and this may lead to ventricular fibrillation or sudden death. Digoxin should be avoided as it may decrease the refractory period of the accessory pathway leading to a rapid ventricular response.

Ref: Oxford Textbook of Medicine, 3rd Ed. Oxford University Press Ch. 15.8.1.
Kumar & Clark. Clinical Medicine, 3rd Ed. W. B. Saunders. Ch. 11.

QUESTION 93

A. TRUE B. TRUE C. TRUE D. FALSE E. FALSE

The JVP is described as having two positive waves (a and v) separated by two descents (x and y). The a wave occurs due to atrial systole (just prior to the carotid pulse). Large a waves are seen in conditions with a raised RVEDP (e.g. pulmonary hypertension). 'Cannon' a waves are produced by atrial contraction against a closed tricuspid valve and are seen in complete heart block, ventricular ectopics, junctional tachycardia. The a wave is absent in atrial fibrillation. The x descent is due to a fall in atrial pressure during ventricular systole as the base of the heart moves caudally. The v wave is a rise in venous pressure due to atrial filling before the tricuspid valve opens. The y descent reflects opening of the tricuspid valve and fall in atrial pressure. The third heart sound is in time with the y descent. Other waves described are the c wave (the effect of tricuspid closure – not visible) and the s wave (fusion of the x descent and v wave due to tricuspid regurgitation with a prominent y descent). Fixed elevation of the JVP is seen in SVC obstruction.

QUESTION   94

A. FALSE B. FALSE C. TRUE D. TRUE E. FALSE

ASD is commoner in women. Shunting is left to right because the right heart is very compliant and pulmonary vascular resistance is low. If left uncorrected there will be (depending on the size of shunt) a large increase in right ventricular output, pulmonary vascular resistance and pulmonary hypertension. Atrial arrhythmias are common at this stage. Due to right ventricular overloading the second heart sound is widely split and fixed. The increased right ventricular output results in an ejection systolic pulmonary flow murmur, and a right ventricular impulse can often be felt. The CXR may show prominent pulmonary arteries and right ventricular enlargement. The ECG often shows a degree of right bundle branch block and right axis deviation which are the usual features of ostium secundum defects. Left axis deviation is a feature of ostium primum ASD. ASD is often present in combination with other complex congenital abnormalities.

Ref: Kumar & Clark. Clinical Medicine, 3rd Ed. W. B. Saunders. Ch. 11.

QUESTION   95

A. FALSE B. TRUE C. TRUE D. TRUE E. FALSE

WPW is due to an anatomical connection between atria and ventricles and is not an acquired condition following rheumatic fever. Type B is associated with a right sided accessory pathway and a QRS complex below the isoelectric line in V1. Sudden death is a recognised complication associated with pre-excitation atrial fibrillation which may lead to ventricular fibrillation. There is a recognised association with MVP, HOCM, Ebstein's anomaly and secundum ASD. The most common tachydysrhythmia is atrio-ventricular re-entry tachycardia which is ortho-dromic in origin. Antidromic tachycardias occur rarely when the refractory period of the AV node exceeds that of the accessory pathway.

Ref: Oxford Textbook of Medicine, 3rd Ed. Oxford University Press Ch. 15.8.1.
Kumar & Clark. Clinical Medicine, 3rd Ed. W. B. Saunders. Ch. 11.

QUESTION   96

A. TRUE B. FALSE C. TRUE D. TRUE E. TRUE

In tricuspid atresia there must be an ASD to allow the systemic venous return to reach the left side of the heart. The right ventricle is underdeveloped while the left ventricle becomes hypertrophied. Associated abnormalities exist such as transposition of the great vessels and pulmonary atresia (both of which are associated with cyanosis) or a VSD which in the absence of pulmonary atresia may not be associated with cyanosis. Eisenmenger's syndrome occurs in the setting of pulmonary hypertension where the shunt direction is reversed to become right to left. Such individuals are cyanosed and become fatigued easily. Approximately 8% of those with ostium primum ASD may develop Eisenmenger's syndrome if left uncorrected. Those with Fallot's are cyanosed due to the combination of an obstructed pulmonary outflow tract, VSD and overriding aorta. The shunt direction in a PDA is left to right and will not result in cyanosis. Reversal of the shunt may lead to cyanosis in the lower limbs only.

Ref: Oxford Textbook of Medicine, 3rd Ed. Oxford University Press. Ch. 13.

QUESTION 97

A. TRUE   B. TRUE   C. FALSE   D. TRUE   E. FALSE

The jugular venous pulse consists of three peaks (a, c, v waves) and two troughs (x, y descent). The a wave reflects atrial systole, and coincides with the first heart sound. It precedes the carotid pulse. The v wave corresponds to atrial filling against a closed tricuspid valve during ventricular systole. The x descent is a trough caused by atrial relaxation. The c wave occurs during the x descent and is due to the transmission of the carotid impulse. It coincides with tricuspid valve closure. During the y descent there is rapid ventricular filling following the opening of the tricuspid valve.

A dominant a wave is seen in situations where there is right ventricular hypertrophy due to pulmonary stenosis or pulmonary hypertension. It may also occur in patients with tricuspid stenosis if the patients remain in sinus rhythm. If the patient is in AF there is no a wave in the JVP. Tricuspid stenosis is also associated with a slow y descent.

Very large Cannon 'a' are seen in complete heart block and VT or paroxysmal nodal tachycardia with retrograde conduction or AV dissociation. These are not strictly speaking a waves as they occur when the atrium contracts against a closed tricuspid valve.

Ref: Talley & O'Connor. Clinical Examination. Blackwell Scientific Publications. Ch. 3. Kumar & Clark. Clinical Medicine, 3rd Ed. W. B. Saunders. Ch. 11.

QUESTION 98

A. FALSE   B. TRUE   C. TRUE   D. TRUE   E. TRUE

Hypothermia is associated with J waves which are positive deflections at the end of the QRS complex. Hypokalaemia is associated with U waves as well as T wave flattening, inversion, and prolongation of the PR and QT intervals. U waves may also be a normal finding and be associated with both hypercalcaemia and hyperthyroidism. A short QT interval is a recognised sign of hypercalcaemia. Biphasic P waves in V1 represent left atrial enlargement and are associated with P mitrale where the P wave is bifid in lead II. Hypothyroidism is associated with low voltage complexes, bradycardia and T wave flattening or inversion.

Ref: Oxford Handbook of Clinical Medicine, 3rd Ed. Oxford University Press. Ch. 7. Houghton & Gray. Making sense of the ECG. Arnold. Ch. 12.

QUESTION 99

A. TRUE   B. FALSE   C. TRUE   D. TRUE   E. TRUE

Ostium primum ASD are associated with the same physiological disturbance as ostium secundum ASD. There may be in addition to this mitral or tricuspid incompetence or a VSD due to

the endomyocardial cushion defect. The ECG in ostium primum ASD shows left axis devia
tion and there may be prolongation of the PR interval.

Ref: Kumar & Clark. Clinical Medicine, 3rd Ed. W. B. Saunders. Ch. 11.
Oxford Textbook of Medicine, 3rd Ed. Oxford University Press. Ch. 15.15.

QUESTION 100

A. TRUE B. TRUE C. FALSE D. TRUE E. TRUE

Recognised toxic effects of digoxin include:

- GI symptoms - nausea, vomiting, abdominal pain, diarrhoea;
- Central effects - headaches, confusion, convulsions and depression;
- Visual effects - Xanthopsia, halo and visual blurring;
- Rare effects - facial pain, gynaecomastia, hyperkalaemia and muscle necrosis;
- Arrhythmias - bradycardia, heart block and ventricular ectopics including bi- and trigemini;
- ECG effects - prolonged PR interval and heart block, T wave inversion, ST depression (reverse tick), reduction in T wave amplitude, shortening of the QT interval.

Beware of the difference between digoxin effects which may be normal at therapeutic doses and digoxin toxicity.

At therapeutic level digoxin causes ST depression, reduction in size of the T wave and shortening of the QT interval. At toxic levels the T wave may become inverted and any arrhythmia may occur. The most common are sinus bradycardia, PAT with block, AV block, VE's, ventricular bigeminy and VT.
Hypokalaemia precipitates digoxin toxicity.

Ref: Epstein RJ. Medicine for Examinations. 3rd Ed. Churchill Livingstone. Ch. 2.
Houghton & Gray. Making sense of the ECG. Arnold. Ch. 9.

QUESTION 101

A. TRUE B. TRUE C. TRUE D. FALSE E. FALSE

The trachea starts at the inferior border of the cricoid cartilage at the level of C6 and runs downwards until it bifurcates at the carina. The carina is at the level of T4 in the cadaver but T5 (and T6 on full inspiration) in the erect live subject. The left main bronchus is 5 cm long and passes under the aortic arch in front of the oesophagus and descending aorta and has the left pulmonary artery lying superior and then anterior to it. There are about 25 divisions between the trachea and the 300 million alveoli in each lung. The alveolus comprises type I & II pneumocytes. Type I cells make up the bulk of the epithelial lining and are very thin thereby facilitating gas exchange; type II cells produce surfactant helping to maintain the structural integrity of the alveolus. The pores of Kohn are holes that allow communication between adjacent lobules.

Ref: Kumar & Clark. Clinical Medicine, 3rd Ed. W. B. Saunders. Ch. 12.
Ellis & Feldman. Anatomy for Anaesthetists, 6th Ed. Blackwell Scientific Publications. p51.

QUESTION 102

A. FALSE B. FALSE C. TRUE D. TRUE E. FALSE

The lungs reflect the shape of the pleural cavity within which they lie, being attached at the hilum. The right lung has two fissures; the oblique (also seen in the left lung) and the transverse fissure. Sibson's fascia is a strong fibrous layer covering both apices and inserting onto the medial side of the first rib and the transverse process of C7. There are two pulmonary veins for each lung. Tributaries are derived from capillaries of both pulmonary and bronchial arteries and lie between the lung segments providing useful surgical landmarks.

Ref: Ellis & Feldman. Anatomy for Anaesthetists, 6th Ed. Blackwell Scientific Publications. p56–73.

QUESTION 103

A. TRUE B. FALSE C. TRUE D. FALSE E. TRUE

FEV1 (the maximum volume expired in one second from vital capacity) is greater than 70% of the forced vital capacity (FVC) in the normal subject. A low FEV1/FVC ratio indicates obstructive lung disease while a normal or raised FEV1/FVC ratio indicates restrictive disease. As the Functional Residual Capacity (FRC) is the sum of the Expiratory Reserve Volume (ERV) and the Residual Volume (RV) it cannot be measured by spirometry. Body plethysmography and Helium dilution are used to measure the FRC. Peak Expiratory Flow Rate (PEFR) is very effort dependent and provided that muscle weakness has been excluded a low PEFR indicates a reduction in lung recoil or intrinsic lung disease. Compliance can be measured during airflow (dynamic) or without airflow (static). Height, age, sex and race (but not weight) are involved in the interpretation of PEFR.

Ref: Kumar & Clark. Clinical Medicine, 3rd Ed. W. B. Saunders. Ch. 12.
West. Respiratory Physiology – The Essentials. 5th Ed. Williams & Wilkins. Ch. 10.

QUESTION 104

A. FALSE B. FALSE C. FALSE D. TRUE E. FALSE

Tracheal deviation becomes easier to palpate as the underlying pathology becomes more exaggerated. Isolated thyroid tumours may deviate the trachea while a nodular goitre has a non specific effect on tracheal deviation. Intrathoracic pathology may cause mediastinal displacement thus deviating the trachea. The following cause no tracheal movement; lobar consolidation, generalised fibrosis (e.g. cryptoenic fibrosing alveolitis), asthma and COAD. Deviation towards the lesion occurs in major lobar collapse and localised fibrosis. Deviation away from the lesion occurs in large pneumothorax and effusion.

Ref: Kumar & Clark. Clinical Medicine, 3rd Ed. W. B. Saunders. Ch. 12.

QUESTION 105

A. TRUE B. TRUE C. TRUE D. FALSE E. FALSE

The physical signs of consolidation are: reduced chest wall movement, a dull percussion note, bronchial breathing, increased vocal resonance and fine crackles. There is no mediastinal movement. Expiratory polyphonic wheeze is characteristic of asthma.

Ref: Kumar & Clark. Clinical Medicine, 3rd Ed. W. B. Saunders. Ch. 12.

QUESTION 106 WITHDRAWN

A. TRUE B. TRUE C. FALSE D. FALSE E. TRUE

Tension pneumothorax is a life threatening medical emergency. As the tension increases within the thorax, venous return is diminished to a critical level and the reduced cardiac output is unable to sustain organ function and death is rapid. Rapid decompression of the pneumothorax is required. The signs are deviation of the trachea and mediastinum away from the tension, hyperresonance to percussion and reduced air entry. The patient will be hypotensive and cyanotic.

Ref: Kumar & Clark. Clinical Medicine, 3rd Ed. W. B. Saunders. Ch. 12.

QUESTION 107

A. TRUE B. FALSE C. TRUE D. FALSE E. FALSE

Acute severe asthma kills up to 3 per 100,000 people per year in NZ and Australia with slightly lower rates in the UK, Europe and North America. Signs of life threatening asthma include tachycardia above 120, tachypnoea, cyanosis, silent chest, unable to speak in sentences, pulsus paradoxus >10 mmHg, and a rising $PaCO_2$ as the patient becomes exhausted. Although PEFR values need to be assessed against the age, sex and height of the patient, 350 L/min is at the lower limit for an average normal female patient. Patients with a PEFR < 30% predicted or 150 L/min should be admitted to hospital and started on oxygen. Treatment in these patients involves oxygen, beta agonists, aminophylline, steroids, rehydration (and antibiotics if specifically indicated). A rising $PaCO_2$ or an exhausted patient would be reasons to consider artificial ventilation.

Ref: Kumar & Clark. Clinical Medicine, 3rd Ed. W. B. Saunders. Ch. 12.

QUESTION 108

A. TRUE B. TRUE C. TRUE D. TRUE E. FALSE

Finger clubbing is present when the normal angle between the base of the nail and the nail fold is no longer present. Increased vascularity of the nail bed leads to a fluctuant nail bed but telangiectasia is not a feature. There is swelling of the finger pulp causing expansion at the end of the digit.

Ref: Oxford Textbook of Medicine, 3rd Ed. Oxford University Press. Ch. 15.

QUESTION   109

A. FALSE B. TRUE C. TRUE D. TRUE E. FALSE

While the conditions associated with finger clubbing are widely known the exact cause is still a mystery. Three categories of thoracic causes are recognised:

1. Suppurative lung disease
2. Fibrosing lung disease
3. Malignant disease

Cardiac causes include cyanotic heart disease and subacute bacterial endocarditis (clubbing develops over months and so cyanotic neonates and patients with acute bacterial endocarditis do not exhibit clubbing initially). Inflammatory bowel disease and occasionally liver disease also cause clubbing. Congenital clubbing is recognised where the is no disease association.

Ref: Kumar & Clark. Clinical Medicine, 3rd Ed. W. B. Saunders. Ch. 12.
Oxford Textbook of Medicine, 3rd Ed. Oxford University Press. Ch. 15.

QUESTION   110

A. TRUE B. FALSE C. TRUE D. FALSE E. FALSE

Cyanosis is a blue discoloration of tissues when they contain hypoxaemic blood. Its assessment is subjective but traditionally 5g/dl of blood should be deoxygenated. It is more readily seen in the polycythaemic patient as a smaller fraction of blood need be deoxygenated to achieve visual recognition. Patients with fibrosing alveolitis develop progressive breathlessness and cyanosis as lung fibrosis worsens - pulmonary hypertension, cor pulmonale and clubbing are also present. SVC obstruction is characterised by early morning headache, facial congestion, oedema of the arms, distended jugular veins and prominent veins over the chest representing collateral circulation with abdominal veins. Cyanosis is not a feature.

Peripheral rather than central cyanosis may develop in hypothermia. Ankylosing spondylitis restricts chest expansion due to fusion of the costovertebral joints. However functional impairment is rare despite developing upper lobe fibrosis.

QUESTION   111

A. TRUE B. FALSE C. FALSE D. TRUE E. FALSE

The signs of collapsed lung differ depending on the extent of collapse. This question deals with a major collapse. Chest wall movement is reduced and there will be mediastinal movement towards the right. 'Stony dull' is a phrase reserved for pleural effusions and the percussion note in collapse is said to sound just 'dull'. Breath sounds and vocal resonance will be diminished or absent (but for a minor or peripheral collapse would be bronchial and increased respectively). Major collapse has no added sounds but a minor or peripheral collapse may demonstrate coarse crackles.

Ref: Kumar & Clark. Clinical Medicine, 3rd Ed. W. B. Saunders. Ch. 12.

QUESTION 112

A. TRUE B. TRUE C. FALSE D. TRUE E. FALSE

Staphylococcal pneumonia is most commonly seen after a viral influenzal illness. Areas of patchy consolidation develop which progress to abscesses and then cysts. Pneumothoraces, empyemas and effusions are common. The illness may progress very rapidly resulting in death. *Chlamydia psittaci* is typical in those who work closely with birds and symptoms include malaise, fever, cough and muscle pains. *Legionella pneumophila* is strongly suggested by the following features; prodromal viral illness, dry cough, diarrhoea, lymphopenia without marked leucocytosis and hyponatraemia.

Ref: Kumar & Clark. Clinical Medicine, 3rd Ed. W. B. Saunders. Ch. 12.

QUESTION 113

A. TRUE B. TRUE C. FALSE D. FALSE E. TRUE

Cystic fibrosis is an inherited disease resulting in generalised exocrine dysfunction particularly affecting the lungs and gut. There is alteration in the viscosity and tenacity of mucus production. The classical form includes bronchopulmonary infections and pancreatic insufficiency associated with high sweat sodium and chloride concentrations. Inheritance is autosomal recessive and the carrier rate is 1 in 20 for Caucasians resulting in a homozygous rate of 1 in 2,000 births. Recurrent chest infections are characteristic and physiotherapy and antibiotics are central to therapy. Finger clubbing is frequently present while nasal polyps may develop later in childhood. Males are infertile because the vas deferens and epididymis fail to develop. Females often develop secondary amenorrhoea but are able to conceive.

85% of patients have steatorrhoea. Children may be born with meconium ileus and develop the meconium ileus equivalent syndrome and intestinal obstruction in later life. Gallstones occur with increased frequency. Diagnosis is based on a family history, a high sweat sodium concentration (>60mmol/L), absent vas deferens/epididymis in males and decreased immunoreactive trypsin.

There is a gene mutation on the long arm of chromosome 7 leading to a defect in the cystic fibrosis transmembrane conductance regulator (CFTR).

Ref: Kumar & Clark. Clinical Medicine, 3rd Ed. W. B. Saunders. Ch. 12.

QUESTION 114

A. FALSE B. TRUE C. TRUE D. TRUE E. TRUE

Primary tuberculosis represents the first infection by Mycobacterium tuberculosis. It usually resides in the mid to upper zones. After as little as 3 weeks typical granulomatous lesions with a central necrotic area (caseation) surrounded by epithelial cells and Langhans' giant cells are present in the regional hilar lymph nodes. Many of these lesions become calcified and some contain dormant tubercle bacilli. Reactivation leads to a post-primary complex, often resulting in upper zone cavitation. Primary tuberculosis is essentially symptomless although erythema nodosum and transient pleural effusions may occur which represent allergic manifestations of the infective process.

Ref: Kumar & Clark. Clinical Medicine, 3rd Ed. W. B. Saunders. Ch. 12.
Oxford Textbook of Medicine, 3rd Ed. Oxford University Press. Ch. 5.

QUESTION 115

A. FALSE B. FALSE C. TRUE D. TRUE E. TRUE

Miliary tuberculosis is the result of acute diffuse dissemination of the tubercle bacilli via the blood. It is always fatal if untreated. The onset may be slow and may present with features of meningitis. Hepatosplenomegaly is a late feature. Choroidal tubercles can be seen in the eyes. They are small, slightly raised pale lesions and vary in number. The CXR appearances vary from normal to lesions up to 10mm in diameter. Staphylococcal, mycoplasma pneumonia and sarcoidosis may mimic miliary TB. The Mantoux test is usually positive but in severe disease it may be negative.

Ref: Kumar & Clark. Clinical Medicine, 3rd Ed. W. B. Saunders. Ch. 12.
Oxford Textbook of Medicine, 3rd Ed. Oxford University Press. Ch. 5.

QUESTION 116

A. TRUE B. TRUE C. TRUE D. FALSE E. TRUE

Pulmonary fibrosis occurs in the end stages of many diseases and may be focal or generalised. Widespread fibrosis results in the typical 'honeycomb' lung when seen on CXR representing thick walled cysts between 0.5 to 2cm in diameter. Causes of honeycomb lung include;
Localised honeycombing: systemic sclerosis, sarcoidosis, TB, asbestosis, berylliosis
Generalised honeycombing: Cryptogenic fibrosing alveolitis, rheumatoid arthritis, drugs (bleomycin, busulphan and cyclophosphamide), Histiocytosis X, Neurofibromatosis.

Ref: Kumar & Clark. Clinical Medicine, 3rd Ed. W. B. Saunders. Ch. 12.

QUESTION 117

A. TRUE B. FALSE C. TRUE D. TRUE E. TRUE

Bronchial carcinoma is the commonest malignant tumour in the Western world. It has been divided into two categories based on cell type.

The *"non-small cell" type* is further divided into three, 1) Squamous 2) Large cell and 3) Adenocarcinoma which account for 40%, 25% and 10% of all carcinomas respectively. The *"small cell" type* (or *oat cell*) accounts for the remaining 25%. Presenting symptoms are cough, chest pain, haemoptysis and weight loss.

There are a number of extrapulmonary manifestations most of which are uncommon apart from weight loss and anorexia which are universal at some stage. Endocrine manifestations include ectopic ACTH secretion, SIADH, hypercalcaemia (particularly squamous carcinoma) and more rarely thyrotoxicosis and gynaecomastia. The neurological manifestations include encephalopathies, neuropathies and muscular disorders (polymyopathy and Eaton-Lambert myasthenic syndrome). While clubbing is present in 30% of patients the cutaneous manifestations of dermatomyositis, acanthosis nigricans and herpes zoster are much rarer. There are a variety of very rare vascular and haematological associations.

Ref: Kumar & Clark. Clinical Medicine, 3rd Ed. W. B. Saunders. Ch. 12.

QUESTION 118

A. TRUE B. FALSE C. TRUE D. TRUE E. FALSE

Legionella pneumophila causes the illness "Legionnaires' disease". It is so named because of the outbreak of a serious respiratory infection in members of the American Legion attending a hotel in Philadelphia in 1976 with a mortality of 15%. It causes outbreaks in previously fit young people who are staying at institutions with contaminated water systems. Men are affected more commonly than women. Maintaining water temperature below 25°C centigrade with adequate chlorination prevents the growth of Legionella. Characteristic features of the illness include malaise, myalgia, rigors and a pyrexia of up to 40°C. Diarrhoea and vomiting are common. Haematuria may occur and rarely renal failure. Initially the cough is dry but usually progresses to being productive. Cavitation is rare. Diagnosis is confirmed by a change in antibody titre but is quicker by direct immunofluorescence of the organisms in pleural fluid, sputum or bronchial washings. Culture takes 3 weeks. Erythromycin or rifampicin are effective antibiotics. The mortality may be up to 30% in elderly patients. Lymphopenia without leucocytosis and hyponatraemia are common findings.

Ref: Kumar & Clark. Clinical Medicine, 3rd Ed. W. B. Saunders. Ch. 12.

QUESTION 119

A. TRUE B. TRUE C. TRUE D. FALSE E. TRUE

Pickwickian syndrome is seen in obese snoring men who indulge in alcohol. There is a decrease in pharyngeal muscle tone causing upper airway obstruction and apnoea particularly in REM sleep. Hypoxia causes the subject to rouse from sleep and the cycle is repeated. While PaO_2 and $PaCO_2$ are often abnormal at night it is also seen during the day and polycythaemia and cyanosis may develop. Sudden death is most commonly associated with patients who have coexisting chronic airway disease.

Treatment includes avoiding alcohol and other sedative agents, weight reduction and continuous nasal positive airway pressure at night which helps prevent upper airway collapse, apnoea and hypoxia.

Ref: Kumar & Clark. Clinical Medicine, 3rd Ed. W. B. Saunders. Ch. 12.
Oxford Textbook of Medicine, 3rd Ed. Oxford University Press. Ch. 15.

QUESTION   120

A. TRUE B. FALSE C. FALSE D. FALSE E. FALSE

Sarcoidosis is a multi-system granulomatous disease which presents most commonly with bilateral hilar lymphadenopathy, pulmonary infiltration and skin or eye lesions. Histologically there are granulomas with epithelioid cells, macrophages and T lymphocytes. The disease is most common in females in the 3rd decade of life and appears to be most severe in American blacks. Pulmonary manifestations are common and produce a restrictive pattern (decreased TLC, FEV1, FVC and a decrease in gas transfer). Erythema nodosum is often the first sign of sarcoidosis and when seen with bilateral hilar lymphadenopathy is diagnostic. Eye manifestations include anterior uveitis, conjunctivitis and retinal lesions. Hypercalcaemia and hypercalciuria are important as they may lead to renal stones. Hypercalcaemia is due to high circulating vitamin D3 levels due to 1 alpha hydroxylation occurring in sarcoid macrophages as well as the kidney. Cardiac involvement is rare causing ventricular arrhythmias, conduction defects and cardiomyopathy.

Ref: Kumar & Clark. Clinical Medicine, 3rd Ed. W. B. Saunders. Ch. 12.

QUESTION   121

A. FALSE B. TRUE C. TRUE D. TRUE E. TRUE

Arterial blood gas estimation is vital in the assessment and monitoring of many forms of disease. Classically [H+] has been expressed in a logarithmic fashion using pH. This has the potential to hide the huge alterations in H+ that occur. For example a pH of 7.4 = [H+] of 40 nmol/L; pH of 7.0 = [H+] of 100 nmol/L; pH of 7.6 = [H+] of 25 nmol/L. Bicarbonate values are calculated using the Henderson-Hasslebach equation and not measured directly. The actual bicarbonate is the calculated value using the measured $PaCO_2$ while the standard bicarbonate assumes a normal $PaCO_2$.

A low $PaCO_2$ is seen in aspirin overdose as the respiratory centre is stimulated and a respiratory alkalosis is induced. However the picture may be complicated by a metabolic acidosis. The contention that all patients with chronic obstructive airway disease depend on a hypoxic drive for respiration is unfounded and oxygen should not be withheld when they become acutely ill. However the phenomenon does exist particularly in those who have chronic CO_2 retention.

Ref: Watson & Hinds. Intensive Care: A Concise Textbook 2nd Ed. W. B. Saunders. Ch. 5.

QUESTION   122

A. FALSE B. FALSE C. FALSE D. TRUE E. FALSE

The diagnosis of ARDS is based on a precipitating event, refractory hypoxia, CXR appearance of bilateral diffuse pulmonary infiltrates, PAOP < 16 mmHg and a low thoracic compliance. It occurs after a wide range of insults to the body including, shock, trauma, infection (the commonest at 30%), aspiration, inhalational injury, DIC, amniotic fluid embolism, cardiopulmonary bypass, pancreatitis and high altitude. There is epithelial injury and haemorrhagic, protein rich alveolar oedema with inflammatory infiltrates (mainly neutrophils). Surfactant is denatured which leads to atelectasis. Subsequently there is fibroblast infiltration and collagen proliferation which may lead to generalised fibrosis. Physiologically there is increased shunt and PA-aO$_2$ gradient. Pulmonary vascular resistance is increased for a number of reasons. Blood vessels may become obstructed by oedema.

Catecholamines, 5-HT, thromboxane and hypoxia cause vasoconstriction. The FRC and compliance decrease. Mortality is variable depending on the aetiology, 90% where it is caused by severe sepsis but only 10% where the cause is fat embolus. There is no prospective, randomised, controlled evidence that treatment with nitric oxide improves outcome in adult respiratory distress syndrome.

Ref: Watson & Hinds. Intensive Care: A Concise Textbook 2nd Ed. W. B. Saunders. Ch. 6.
Intensive Care Medicine (1997) 23:121–1218. UK guidelines for the use of NO in adult ICUs.

QUESTION 123

A. FALSE B. TRUE C. TRUE D. FALSE E. TRUE

Chrysolite or white asbestos is less fibrogenic than crocidolite or blue asbestos which is resistant to chemical destruction. While Asbestosis will produce a severe restrictive pattern the CXR appearances are diffuse streaky shadows or honeycomb lung rather than being limited to the upper lobes. Crocidolite is the most important in the development of all forms of asbestosis especially mesothelioma and bronchial carcinoma. Sputum eosinophilia is found in allergic disease (e.g. asthma), aspergillosis, vasculitides and parasitic disorders.

Ref: Kumar & Clark. Clinical Medicine, 3rd Ed. W. B. Saunders. Ch. 12.
Oxford Textbook of Medicine, 3rd Ed. Oxford University Press. Ch. 15.

QUESTION 124

A. FALSE B. FALSE C. TRUE D. TRUE E. TRUE

Bordetella pertussis causes whooping cough, the typical whoop being caused by a violent inspiration against a narrowed glottis. The incubation period is 10 to 14 days and predominantly affects those below the age of 5. The catarrhal phase presents as an upper respiratory tract infection, and the paroxysmal or coughing phase occurs later. Most children do not require treatment but early erythromycin may be helpful in the initial catarrhal phase and limit spread. Bronchitis, pneumonia and fits are common while rectal prolapse and inguinal herniation occur less frequently. Immunized children can contract a milder form of the disease.

Ref: Kumar & Clark. Clinical Medicine, 3rd Ed. W. B. Saunders. Ch. 12.
Oxford Textbook of Medicine, 3rd Ed. Oxford University Press. Ch. 5.
Collier & Longmore. Oxford Handbook of Clinical Specialities. 2nd Ed. Oxford University Press. p278.

QUESTION 125

A. TRUE B. FALSE C. TRUE D. FALSE E. FALSE

Acute laryngotracheobronchitis (croup) is a childhood illness and may be hard to distinguish from whooping cough or epiglottitis. However while all three have inspiratory stridor, a history and examination should secure the diagnosis. Croup is not accompanied by coughing fits or the acute toxic picture seen in epiglottitis. The illness develops over a few days, rarely causes a pyrexia or drooling and stridor is often present only when the child becomes anxious. It is usually caused by respiratory syncitial (RSV) or parainfluenza viruses. Secondary bacterial infection may follow. Treatment is aimed at relieving symptoms and ensuring adequate humidified oxygen. Steroids have not been shown to improve the outcome.

Ref: Oxford Textbook of Medicine, 3rd Ed. Oxford University Press. Ch. 5.
Collier & Longmore. Oxford Handbook of Clinical Specialities. 2nd Ed. Oxford University Press. p276.

QUESTION 126

A. TRUE B. TRUE C. FALSE D. FALSE E. TRUE

In rheumatoid arthritis the development of lung involvement may very occasionally precede that of joint involvement. Lung involvement falls into 4 main groups:

1. Pleural effusion
2. Interstitial fibrosis
3. Pulmonary nodules
4. Obliterative bronchiolitis

Pleural effusion is seen most commonly. It is sterile with an elevated protein content, lymphocytosis and reduced C3 levels. It also contains ragocytes (macrophages containing IgM inclusions. Stridor occurs as a manifestation of involvement of the crico-arytenoid joints. Pulmonary nodules are rare and may cavitate and give rise to a pleural effusion or pneumothorax. Caplan's syndrome is due to a combination of dust inhalation and the altered immune status seen in rheumatoid arthritis. The typical lesions are round and of variable size and may become incorporated into areas of fibrosis. Pulmonary eosinophilia is seen commonly in asthma and less commonly in simple pulmonary eosinophilia (Loffler's syndrome) and polyarteritis nodosa. Rheumatoid disease is not associated with bronchogenic carcinoma.

Ref: Kumar & Clark. Clinical Medicine, 3rd Ed. W. B. Saunders. Ch. 12.
Oxford Textbook of Medicine, 3rd Ed. Oxford University Press. Ch. 15.

QUESTION 127

A. TRUE B. FALSE C. TRUE D. TRUE E. FALSE
Bronchiectasis develops from the combined destructive action of bronchial obstruction and bronchial infection with associated inflammation when these episodes are prolonged. The classic circumstance for post infective bronchiectasis has been severe respiratory infection in childhood including whooping cough (Bordetella pertussis), measles, tuberculosis and

cystic fibrosis. Hilar lymphadenopathy in TB causing obstruction of mainly the middle lobe bronchus may rarely cause bronchiectasis. An inhaled peanut may also cause obstruction and gross suppurative lung disease. Achalasia patients commonly have pulmonary complications. These are mainly aspiration pneumonias.

Ref: Kumar & Clark. Clinical Medicine, 3rd Ed. W. B. Saunders. Ch. 12.
Oxford Textbook of Medicine, 3rd Ed. Oxford University Press. Ch. 15.

QUESTION   128

A. FALSE B. TRUE C. TRUE D. TRUE E. FALSE

Mycoplasma pneumoniae is the commonest atypical pneumonia, occurring in about 20% of all pneumonias in the UK. There is an incubation period of 10 - 14 days. The chest signs may be hard to detect clinically and the CXR often bears little correlation to the clinical state. Extrapulmonary signs are rare but varied – they include; myocarditis and pericarditis, rashes, erythema multiforme, haemolytic anaemia, thrombocytopenia, myalgia, neurological symptoms, diarrhoea and vomiting. The white cell count is usually not raised. 80% have a significant rise in antibody titre. Treatment is erythromycin. Subphrenic abscesses are usually due to an intra-abdominal cause but very rarely may be secondary to the cavitating pneumonias (Staphlococcus or Klebsiella pneumoniae).

Ref: Kumar & Clark. Clinical Medicine, 3rd Ed. W. B. Saunders. Ch. 12.

QUESTION   129

A. TRUE B. FALSE C. FALSE D. TRUE E. FALSE

Spontaneous pneumothorax can be divided into 2 categories. The first has no apparent lung pathology and is 5 times more common in men, between 20 and 40 years or age. On further investigation there is often a small apical bullous. The second is associated with much more serious lung disease. The symptoms and signs include pleuritic chest pain, dyspnoea, reduced breath sounds, hyper-resonant percussion note and decreased chest movement on the affected side. The upper lobes collapse before the lower lobes in the erect subject because the pneumothorax rises and compresses the lung apex. When pneumothorax is recurrent pleuradesis or pleurectomy should be considered. Recurrence after these procedures is low.

Ref: Kumar & Clark. Clinical Medicine, 3rd Ed. W. B. Saunders. Ch. 12.
Oxford Textbook of Medicine, 3rd Ed. Oxford University Press. Ch. 15.

QUESTION   130

A. TRUE B. TRUE C. TRUE D. TRUE E. TRUE

Pneumocystis is by far the most common infection in patients with AIDS. The typical X ray appearance is a diffuse bilateral alveolar shadowing spreading out from the hilar. Other appearances include localized infiltrates, nodules, cavities and pneumothoraces. Other organisms that produce shadowing in AIDS patients include:

- Cytomegalovirus
- M. avium intracellulare
- M. tuberculosis
- L. Pneumophila
- Cryptococcus
- Pyogenic bacteria
- Kaposi's sarcoma
- Lymphoid interstitial pneumonia and non-specific pneumonitis

Ref: Kumar & Clark. Clinical Medicine, 3rd Ed. W. B. Saunders. Ch. 12.

QUESTION 131

A. TRUE B. FALSE C. FALSE D. FALSE E. FALSE

Acute altitude sickness is produced by a combination of hypoxaemia, respiratory alkalosis, pulmonary hypertension (secondary to hypoxia) and pulmonary oedema, and cerebral oedema. Avoidance is the best policy – slow ascent, controlled oxygen delivery, acetazolamide and nifedipine are effective preventive measures. Treatment: increasing inspired O_2 and CO_2 (to combat alkalosis), dexamethasone for cerebral oedema, return to lower altitude. There are some differences in the clinical features and complications of inhalation of sea water (hypertonic) and fresh water (hypotonic) but no practical difference in the speed of drowning. 'Bends' are caused by bubbles of nitrogen coming out of solution in plasma on rapid ascent from a dive. Divers require rapid recompression and acetazolamide plays no role in therapy.

QUESTION 132

A. TRUE B. FALSE C. FALSE D. TRUE E. TRUE

Other non–metastatic manifestations include: ectopic ACTH and PTH secretion, SIADH, hypercalcaemia (squamous cell), thyrotoxicosis, encephalopathy, motor neurone disease and myelopathy, peripheral neuropathy, thrombophlebitis migrans, TTP, DIC, hypertrophic pulmonary osteoarthropathy, dermatomyositis and acanthosis nigricans.

Ref: Kumar & Clark. Clinical Medicine, 3rd Ed. W. B. Saunders. Ch. 12.

QUESTION 133

A. FALSE B. FALSE C. TRUE D. TRUE E. FALSE

The risk of adenocarcinoma is increased by exposure to petroleum products, chromium, iron oxide, arsenic, coal tar and radiation. Small-cell lung carcinoma (SCLC or oat cell tumours) and squamous cell tumours are more radiosensitive than adenocarcinoma. 10-15% of patients who undergo radiotherapy develop radiation pneumonitis within 3 months of treatment. Most develop fibrosis but this takes years to develop. Squamous tumours metastasise late in the natural history while SCLC and large-cell cancers (poorly differentiated) spread early.

QUESTION 134

A. FALSE B. TRUE C. TRUE D. TRUE E. FALSE

Cigarette smoking has been linked to an increased risk of carcinoma of lung, cervix, bladder and oesophagus. Passive smoking increases the risk of carcinoma of the lung by 1.5 times.

QUESTION 135

A. FALSE B. FALSE C. TRUE D. FALSE E. TRUE

Pleural plaques imply exposure to asbestos and are not pre-malignant. Other markers of exposure include recurrent pleural effusions, mesothelioma, primary lung carcinoma or interstitial lung disease (asbestosis). Interstitial fibrosis affects the mid and lower lung zones and may be accompanied by finger clubbing. Nodules are rarely (if ever) seen with asbestosis. Asbestos exposure is associated with an increased risk of adenocarcinoma of the lung and the risk is markedly increased in smokers as compared to non-smokers.

QUESTION 136

A. FALSE B. TRUE C. TRUE D. FALSE E. TRUE

Sarcoidosis is a non-caseating granulomatous disorder of unknown aetiology. On the basis of radiology it is divided into 4 stages (0 = normal CXR, 1 = bilateral hilar lymphadenopathy (BHL), 2 = BHL and infiltration of lung parenchyma, 3 = pulmonary infiltration without BHL). Any organ system may be affected; heart failure is usually due to cardiac infiltration.

Lofgren's syndrome is the association of BHL, erythema nodosum, anterior uveitis and joint pains and up to 80% will show spontaneous remission. Heerfordt syndrome is bilateral parotid enlargement, facial palsy and uveitis. Lacrimal involvement gives sicca syndrom12

Diagnosis: serum ACE is raised in 65% of patients with active disease and correlates with disease activity, but it is non-specific and is raised in a number of other conditions also (TB, asbestosis, silicosis, lymphoma). The CD4:CD8 ratio is increased. Tuberculin test is negative in most patients and the Kveim test is positive in 85% of acute disease and 35% of chronic disease (and up to 40% of patients with Crohn's disease). Transbronchial biopsy is positive in the majority of patients with BHL. Hypercalcaemia is due to increased production of 1, 25-vitamin D3 by the sarcoid macrophages.

Treatment: corticosteroids are indicated for uveitis, CNS sarcoidosis, significant pulmonary involvement. Hypercalcaemia also responds to steroids. Benefits in cardiac sarcoid are variable.

QUESTION 137

A. TRUE B. TRUE C. FALSE D. TRUE E. FALSE

Interstitial nodules on CXR may also be due to miliary TB, mitral stenosis, malignancy (teratoma), hydatid disease, lymphangitis carcinomatosis, alveolar cell carcinoma, pneumoconiosis. Granulomata are seen in Wegener's, Churg-Strauss, other fungal pneumonias and histiocytosis X.

QUESTION 138

A. TRUE B. TRUE C. FALSE D. TRUE E. TRUE

Other causes include tuberculosis, pneumoconiosis, sarcoidosis, eggshell calcification in lymph nodes in silicosis and malignancy.

QUESTION 139

A. TRUE B. TRUE C. TRUE D. FALSE E. FALSE

Other causes include tuberculosis, staphylococcal infection, Klebsiella, actinomyces, vasculitis (PAN, Wegener's) and malignancy (squamous cell carcinoma).

QUESTION 140

A. FALSE B. FALSE C. TRUE D. TRUE E. FALSE

Upper zone lung infiltrates are also seen with tuberculosis, Aspergillus infection, Klebsiella pneumoniae, silicosis, radiation, chronic extrinsic allergic alveolitis and coal workers pneumoconiosis.

Lower zone lung fibrosis is a feature of bronchiectasis, asbestosis, rheumatoid arthritis, scleroderma, radiation, drugs (busulphan, nitrofurantoin, bleomycin, methotrexate, chronic high oxygen, chloramphenicol, amiodarone and melphlan), cryptogenic fibrosing alveolitis, sarcoidosis, tuberose sclerosis and neurofibromatosis.

QUESTION 141

A. TRUE B. TRUE C. TRUE D. FALSE E. FALSE

Causes of a transudate (protein content <30 g/l): constrictive pericarditis, Meig's syndrome, any cause of congestive cardiac failure, hypoproteinaemia (cirrhosis, nephrotic syndrome, protein-losing enteropathy, etc.), beri-beri (thiamine deficiency), myxoedema and dialysis.

Causes of an exudate (protein >30 g/l, pleural fluid: serum protein ratio >0.5, pleural LDH >200 U): infection (TB, pneumonia, subphrenic abscess), connective tissue diseases, pulmonary infarction, acute pancreatitis, familial Mediterranean fever, Dresslers' syndrome, mesothelioma, sarcoid, yellow nail syndrome (lymphoedema) and neoplasia.

Pleural fluid glucose is reduced in rheumatoid arthritis, empyema, TB and malignancy.

QUESTION 142

A. TRUE B. TRUE C. TRUE D. FALSE E. TRUE

Other features include flapping tremor, hyporeflexia, muscle twitching, sweating, headache, bounding pulse, retinal vein distension; if CO_2 >120 mmHg, then coma and extensor plantars.

QUESTION 143

A. TRUE B. FALSE C. TRUE D. TRUE E. FALSE

An elevated $PaCO_2$ is not synonymous with respiratory failure. Respiratory failure is defined as PaO_2 <8 kPa; type I is essentially ventilation-perfusion mismatch and $PaCO_2$ is <6.5 kPa; while in type II, $PaCO_2$ is raised and the problem is due to pure hypoventilation.

Clinical signs of CO_2 retention include papilloedema, miosis, hypertension, flapping tremor, hyporeflexia, muscle twitching, sweating, headache, bounding pulse and retinal vein distension; if CO_2 >120 mmHg, then coma and extensor plantars.

QUESTION 144

A. FALSE B. TRUE C. FALSE D. FALSE E. FALSE

Long-term oxygen therapy has been shown to prolong survival of patients with cor pulmonale or severe COAD. Department of Health guidelines: patients with PaO_2 <7.3 kPa on air, $PaCO_2$ >6 kPa, FEV1 <1.5 and FVC <2 litres, on two occasions at least 3 weeks apart after appropriate bronchodilators have been administered. There is no evidence for low-flow oxygen therapy for other disorders.

QUESTION 145

A. FALSE B. TRUE C. FALSE D. TRUE E. FALSE

Cystic fibrosis is an autosomal recessive disorder with a carrier frequency of 1:25 of the Caucasian population. The defect is a mutation on chromosome 7 in the gene encoding a chloride channel. The most common identified (68%) mutation is called delta F 508 (amino acid number 508 mutated in the protein sequence). This results in defective transport of Cl and water across epithelia in the body. The presenting feature in neonates is often meconium ileus or chest infections. Diabetes mellitus occurs in 5%, steatorrhoea in 85% and cirrhosis in 5%. Sweat sodium >60 mEq/l in children. Men are infertile (azospermic) as the vas and epididymis do not develop and females are fertile but go on to develop secondary amenorrhoea. Colonisation with Pseudomonas cerpacia heralds clinical decline as the organism is very difficult to eradicate.

QUESTION 146

A. TRUE B. TRUE C. TRUE D. TRUE E. FALSE

Pickwickian syndrome (obstructive sleep apnoea) is seen in patients with severe obesity. Symptoms include morning headache (due to carbon dioxide retention) and disorientation, snoring, nocturnal choking, nightmares and hallucinations, excessive daytime drowsiness (often having led to an accident at work or when driving), depression and impotence. It is associated with hypothyroidism and acromegaly. Complications include hypertension, ischaemic heart disease, arrhythmias and if left untreated cor pulmonale and pulmonary hypertension.

Treatment options: weight loss, nocturnal CPAP, medroxyprogesterone acetate, uvulo-palato-pharyngoplasty and protryptiline.

QUESTION   147

A. FALSE B. TRUE C. FALSE D. FALSE E. TRUE

Respiratory failure is defined as PaO_2 <8kPa. Type I is characterised by ventilation perfusion mismatch and patients have a $PaCO_2$ <6.5kPa while type II is characterised by alveolar hypoventilation and patients have a $PaCO_2$ >6.5 kPa. Often both coexist. Hypoxia results in confusion, cyanosis and eventually coma. Hypercapnoea produces papilloedema, miosis, hypertension, flapping tremor, hyporeflexia, muscle twitching, sweating, headache, bounding pulse, retinal vein distension and eventually coma with extensor plantars. Lactic acidosis is a common finding due to anaerobic metabolism within tissues. Treatment should be directed at the precipitant as well as supportive therapy. 100% oxygen is unsafe in patients with COAD. Artificial ventilation or doxapram are the mainstay. Diphtheria produces neuromuscular paralysis and can precipitate respiratory failure. Other causes of neuromuscular respiratory failure include: myasthenia gravis, motor neurone disease, polymyositis, muscle dystrophies (e.g. myotonic), polio, multiple sclerosis, stroke, encephalitis, etc.

QUESTION   148

A. TRUE B. FALSE C. TRUE D. TRUE E. TRUE

Anaerobic lung infections are predominantly caused by microaerophillic streptococci, and bacteroides species and nocardia. Risk factors include diabetes, alcoholism, old age, poor dentition, carcinomatosis, mechanical ventilation (ITU patients), achalasia and neuromuscular swallowing difficulties. Treat with penicillin and metronidazole.

QUESTION   149

A. TRUE B. FALSE C. TRUE D. FALSE E. FALSE

Pneumonia caused by the organism Mycoplasma pneumoniae usually has a long incubation period and presents as an URTI and tracheobronchitis that later progresses to a lower respiratory tract infection. The extrapulmonary manifestations include headaches (sometimes aseptic meningitis), arthralgia, ear pain (bullous myringitis), erythema multiforme, myocarditis, and pericarditis. 'Cold' haemolytic anaemia occurs due to anti-I autoantibody. Diagnosis is by serology (complement-fixing antibody). The organism is resistant to beta-lactams.

QUESTION   150

A. TRUE B. TRUE C. TRUE D. FALSE E. FALSE

Legionnaire's disease is caused by Legionella pneumophila. The organism thrives in water-containing reservoirs and the outbreak in Philadelphia that claimed the lives of several members attending a Foreign Legion convention was traced to the air-conditioning unit. There is no documented person-to-person spread. Clinical features include high fever, gastrointestinal upset, headache and encephalopathy. LFTs are abnormal and patients develop hyponatraemia, hypophosphataemia and renal failure. Diagnosis is by direct fluorescence on pleural fluid or lung biopsy or silver stain on sputum or retrospectively by serology (takes 2 weeks). Pontiac fever is a self-limiting tracheobronchitis caused by the same organism. Treatment: erythromycin +/- rifampicin for 2 weeks.

QUESTION 151

A. TRUE B. TRUE C. TRUE D. FALSE E. TRUE

Alkalosis results from loss of HCl in the vomitus although acidosis may supervene if dehydration and circulatory collapse occur. Urinary chloride excretion falls in response to the lowered concentration of NaCl delivered to the distal tubule; urinary excretion of sodium is initially increased, although this exacerbates the hyponatraemia seen as a result of loss of Na in vomitus. As dehydration continues the kidney conserves sodium leading to increased loss of potassium and hydrogen ions in the urine. Hypokalaemia causes hydrogen ions to move into cells in exchange for potassium.

Ref: Katz, Benumof & Kadis. Anesthesia and Uncommon Diseases. 3rd Ed. W. B. Saunders. Ch10.

QUESTION 152

A. TRUE B. FALSE C. TRUE D. TRUE E. FALSE

Achalasia is a disease of unknown aetiology characterised by aperistalsis in the body of the oesophagus and failure of relaxation of the lower oesophageal sphincter on initiation of swallowing. Along with dysphagia, regurgitation occurs and may result in aspiration pneumonia. Patients may complain of retro-sternal chest pain from vigorous non-peristaltic contraction of the oesophagus. Treatment options include X-ray guided dilatation, surgical cardiomyotomy and in older patients, sub-lingual nifedipine may be effective. There is a 5-10% risk of oesophageal carcinoma in treated and untreated cases.

Ref: Kumar & Clark. Clinical Medicine, 3rd Ed. W. B. Saunders. Ch 4.

QUESTION 153

A. FALSE B. FALSE C. FALSE D. FALSE E. TRUE

Peptic ulceration is seen in hyperparathyroidism as calcium stimulates gastric acid secretion. Duodenal ulcers are two to three times commoner than gastric ulcers with 15% of the population suffering from a duodenal ulcer at some time. Misoprostil is a synthetic analogue of prostaglandin E1 which inhibits gastric acid production via action on intracellular cAMP; its main role is as a cytoprotective agent against NSAID-associated gastric ulcers. Gastric ulcers can occur anywhere in the stomach but are most commonly found on the lesser curve. Helicobacter pylori infection causes acute and chronic gastritis; peptic ulcer disease may develop as a result. Eradication treatment is an important part of medical management of peptic ulceration and may become first-line therapy for duodenal ulceration.

Ref: Kumar & Clark. Clinical Medicine, 3rd Ed. W. B. Saunders. Ch. 4.

QUESTION 154

A. TRUE B. FALSE C. TRUE D. TRUE E. FALSE

Zollinger-Ellison syndrome arises when a slow growing, but malignant tumour arises from the G cells in the pancreas. The large amount of gastrin produced by the tumour stimulates excessive gastric acid secretion, and diarrhoea due to the low pH in the upper intestine commonly occurs. It is usually treated with the proton pump inhibitor Omeprazole (octreotide may be used). The tumour may be surgically removed. This tumour may develop as part of a multiple endocrine neoplasia syndrome, thus the association with acromegaly due to a hormone producing pituitary adenoma.

Ref: Kumar & Clark. Clinical Medicine, 3ʳᵈ Ed. W. B. Saunders. Ch. 5.

QUESTION 155

A. TRUE B. TRUE C. FALSE D. FALSE E. FALSE

Coeliac disease or gluten-sensitive enteropathy, is a malabsorption condition characterised by abnormal jejunal mucosa which improves morphologically with a gluten-free diet. It is possible that an immunogenetic mechanism is responsible, the evidence for which includes the 90% of patients with coeliac disease who share a particular haplotype (including HLA-A1, B8, DR3, DR7, DQW2). Howell-Jolly bodies due to splenic atrophy are amongst the haematological features, which also include anaemia, iron deficiency, folate deficiency and abnormal leucocytes. Anti-reticulin antibodies are found in the serum of most cases. There is an association with dermatitis herpetiformis as well as other atopic and autoimmune diseases.

Ref: Kumar & Clark. Clinical Medicine, 3ʳᵈ Ed. W. B. Saunders. Ch. 4.

QUESTION 156

A. TRUE B. FALSE C. FALSE D. TRUE E. FALSE

Carcinoid tumours are relatively rare and usually associated with the gastro-intestinal tract. Many secrete a variety of physiologically active amines and peptides which include 5-HT (5-hydroxytryptamine or serotonin), bradykinin, histamine and prostaglandins. Carcinoid syndrome occurs in about 5% of patients with carcinoid tumours only when liver metastases are present. Acute appendicitis is the presenting feature in 10% of tumours in the appendix. Tricuspid incompetence or pulmonary stenosis is found in up to 50% of those with carcinoid syndrome and is thought to be caused by 5-HT. Pellegra may occur due to diversion of tryptophan metabolism from production of nicotinamide to formation of amines. Cutaneous flushing is a feature of carcinoid syndrome which is probably produced by one of the kinins. Octreotide may be used to moderate symptoms and control a carcinoid crisis.

Ref: Kumar & Clark. Clinical Medicine, 3ʳᵈ Ed. W. B. Saunders. Ch. 4.

QUESTION 157

A. TRUE B. TRUE C. TRUE D. TRUE E. TRUE

Crohn's disease most commonly affects the terminal ileum but may affect any part of the gastro-intestinal tract from mouth to anus. The cause of the disease is unknown. Typical features include diarrhoea (intermittent or continuous; not usually excessively bloody), weight loss, abdominal pain, anaemia and malaise. Perianal lesions and fistulae are common. Deep ulcers and fissures in the bowel wall produce a cobblestone appearance; inflammation occurs in all layers of the bowel wall with granulomas found in 50-60%. Patients tend to have recurrent relapses and although the mortality rate is variable, it appears to be at least twice that of the general population. Most deaths are associated with surgery. There is a slightly increased risk of carcinoma of the colon and cholangiocarcinoma.

Ref: Kumar & Clark. Clinical Medicine, 3rd Ed. W. B. Saunders. Ch. 4.

QUESTION 158

A. FALSE B. TRUE C. FALSE D. FALSE E. FALSE

Extra-gastrointestinal manifestations (including uveitis and episcleritis) occur in both diseases and may reflect the activity of the intestinal disease, but are more common in Crohn's disease. Both conditions show a peak in the 2nd-4th decade, but whilst Crohn's disease affects both sexes equally, ulcerative colitis (UC) affects more women than men. Histological differences in rectal or colonic biopsies distinguish the two conditions: inflammation is transmural and patchy in Crohn's but superficial and continuous in UC; granulomas are common in Crohn's but rare in UC; crypt abscesses and goblet cell depletion are mainly a feature of UC. Although classically a condition of the rectum and colon only, UC may produce inflammation of the terminal ileum: so called 'backwash ileitis'.

Ref: Kumar & Clark. Clinical Medicine, 3rd Ed. W. B. Saunders. Ch. 4.

QUESTION 159

A. TRUE B. TRUE C. TRUE D. TRUE E. TRUE

Malabsorption of specific substances occurs in many types of disease, for example, vitamin B12 in Crohn's disease. Other causes of small intestine malabsorption include coeliac disease, dermatitis herpetiformis, Whipple's disease, radiation, parasitic infection, tropical sprue (unknown but probably infective aetiology, possibly an enterotoxin producing coliform) and bacterial overgrowth (of E. coli and Bacteroides; found in structurally normal gut apart from occasional cases in the elderly). Intestinal resection is usually well tolerated but malabsorption may occur after resection of as little as 30% of the gut. Periodic acid-Schiff (PAS)-positive macrophages are a characteristic EM finding in the stunted villi of patients with Whipple's disease which may cause malabsorption.

Ref: Kumar & Clark. Clinical Medicine, 3rd Ed. W. B. Saunders. Ch. 4.

QUESTION 160

A. FALSE B. FALSE C. TRUE D. FALSE E. FALSE

Chylous ascitic fluid is characteristic of lymphatic obstruction for example by carcinoma. Intestinal TB usually results from re-activation of primary Mycobacterium tuberculosis infection. The ileocaecal area is most commonly affected. HIV infection is associated with an increased risk of tuberculosis infection. X-ray evidence of pulmonary TB is found in approximately 50% of patients. Other findings may include mesenteric thickening and lymph node enlargement on ultrasound examination, a palpable mass, other systemic manifestations of TB. Treatment (usually with rifampicin, isoniazid, pyrazinamide) should be continued for one year.

Ref: Kumar & Clark. Clinical Medicine, 3rd Ed. W. B. Saunders. Ch. 4.

QUESTION 161

A. FALSE B. FALSE C. FALSE D. FALSE E. FALSE

The oesophagus is a muscular tube with skeletal muscle in its upper third, smooth muscle in the lower third and both types in the middle third. Nerve supply is mainly vagal via oesophageal plexuses but also via sympathetic nerves. Primary peristalsis is a continuation of the swallowing reflex which starts in the pharynx when food enters the oesophagus. Secondary peristalsis results from direct stimulation by food etc. in the oesophageal lumen and is unrelated to swallowing. Tertiary non-peristaltic contractions, which are common in the elderly, are of uncertain function. In brain stem death spontaneous contractions disappear and provoked contractions show a low amplitude pattern. Activity may be decreased by atropine and SNP and increased by neostigmine.

Ref: Kumar & Clark. Clinical Medicine, 3rd Ed. W. B. Saunders. Ch. 4.

QUESTION 162

A. TRUE B. TRUE C. FALSE D. FALSE E. TRUE

Patients undergoing a barium meal may be given carbon dioxide producing granules or tablets with the barium in order to enhance accuracy of the study. In enteroclysis, large volumes of dilute barium are introduced via a tube through the duodenum; this is particularly good for visualising small bowel strictures. Intestinal obstruction usually produces dilated bowel loops and fluid levels seen on an erect plain abdominal film. Adverse reactions to radiological contrast usually follow intra-venous administration of iodine-containing substances (this may be due to high osmolality, immunological mechanisms and/or direct toxicity). Along with computed tomography (CT) and magnetic resonance imaging (MRI), endoscopic ultrasound can be used to assess tumour size and spread.

Ref: Kumar & Clark. Clinical Medicine, 3rd Ed. W. B. Saunders. Ch. 4.

QUESTION 163

A. TRUE B. TRUE C. TRUE D. TRUE E. TRUE

HIV infection has three main gastrointestinal manifestations: oesophageal symptoms, wasting and diarrhoea. Aetiology is diverse but includes all of the above.

Ref: Kumar & Clark. Clinical Medicine, 3rd Ed. W. B. Saunders. Ch. 4.

QUESTION 164

A. FALSE B. TRUE C. FALSE D. TRUE E. FALSE

Mouth lesions are common in people with AIDS. Conditions specifically associated with AIDS include Kaposi's sarcoma (perioral or often at the junction of hard and soft palate) and hairy leukoplakia (which is an indicator of poor prognosis). Geographic tongue affects 10% of the population and is of unknown aetiology. Stevens-Johnson syndrome is a severe form of erythema multiforme where bullae affect the oral mucosa and conjunctivae. Whilst candidiasis is a frequent problem in AIDS patients, it is a non-specific manifestation of immunosuppression.

Ref: Kumar & Clark. Clinical Medicine, 3rd Ed. W. B. Saunders. Ch. 4.

QUESTION 165

A. TRUE B. TRUE C. FALSE D. TRUE E. TRUE

The cells which produce gut hormones are derived from neural ectoderm (amine precursor uptake and decarboxylation: APUD cells). Many of the substances produced have similar structures and may be found in other tissues, particularly the brain. Their roles are not yet fully elucidated. VIP causes splanchnic vasodilation.

Ref: Kumar & Clark. Clinical Medicine, 3rd Ed. W. B. Saunders. Ch. 4.

QUESTION 166

A. TRUE B. TRUE C. FALSE D. FALSE E. FALSE

Colorectal carcinoma is rare in Africa and Asia probably for environmental rather than racial reasons. The aetiology is strongly linked with genetic inheritance; mutations on chromosome 5 are the cause of FAP but also have a part in sporadic colon cancer. No universal screening programme has yet been employed in the UK although faecal occult blood testing has been shown to reduce mortality. Colonoscopy is used in patients with risk factors such as a strong family history, ulcerative colitis and certain polyposis syndromes. Two thirds of tumours occur at the recto-sigmoid region. The mainstay of treatment is surgical, although adjuvant chemo- and radiotherapy are used to try and improve survival in Duke's B and C tumours.

Ref: Kumar & Clark. Clinical Medicine, 3rd Ed. W. B. Saunders. Ch. 4.

QUESTION 167

A. FALSE B. TRUE C. TRUE D. TRUE E. FALSE

IBS and non-ulcer dyspepsia are very common conditions embraced by the term 'functional bowel disease'. Pain (classically left iliac fossa), constipation and/or diarrhoea, distension and bloating are all common features. Inconsistent motility abnormalities can sometimes be demonstrated but do not always correlate with bouts of pain. A high-fibre diet, mebeverine (a spasmolytic), reassurance and even anti-depressants may all have a place in treatment. Diverticulae are common in the elderly and do not in themselves necessarily cause pain.

Ref: Kumar & Clark. Clinical Medicine, 3rd Ed. W. B. Saunders. Ch. 4.

QUESTION 168

A. TRUE B. FALSE C. FALSE D. FALSE E. FALSE

A hiatus hernia occurs when part of the stomach herniates through the diaphragm into the thorax. There are two main types. The stomach may push up beside the oesophagus ('para-oesophageal' or rolling). The sphincter stays below the diaphragm and remains competent. Surgery may be needed to alleviate pain. In the other type, the gastro-oesophageal junction may 'slide' up through the hiatus. The condition is common with many remaining asympto-matic. About 80% are 'sliding'. In most cases of reflux there is no hiatus hernia.

Ref: Kumar & Clark. Clinical Medicine, 3rd Ed. W. B. Saunders. Ch. 4.

QUESTION 169

A. FALSE B. TRUE C. TRUE D. TRUE E. TRUE

Constipation is a feature of many conditions including dietary deficiencies, immobility, myx-oedema, irritable bowel syndrome, hypercalcaemia and treatment with certain drugs (e.g. opi-ates, atropine, tricyclics). Diarrhoea is more common post-gastrectomy, but constipation may occur.

Ref: Kumar & Clark. Clinical Medicine, 3rd Ed. W. B. Saunders. Ch. 4.

QUESTION 170

A. TRUE B. FALSE C. FALSE D. TRUE E. FALSE

Dysphagia has a number of causes including neurological disease (e.g. bulbar palsy, myasthenia gravis, syringomyelia), pharyngeal pouch, achalasia, oesophagitis, systemic sclerosis and malig-nancy. Constant dysphagia and pain should make one suspicious of a malignant stricture. Barrett's oesophagus is a columnization of the lower oesophageal epithelium due to chronic reflux, which pre-disposes to development of adenocarcinoma. Tylosis (hyperkeratosis of palms and soles) is a familial condition which is associated with squamous cell carcinoma of the oesophagus.

Oesophageal carcinoma spreads predominantly by local invasion; at presentation 50% will have regional lymph node involvement.

Ref: Kumar & Clark. Clinical Medicine, 3rd Ed. W. B. Saunders. Ch. 4.

QUESTION   171

A. TRUE B. FALSE C. TRUE D. TRUE E. TRUE

Other associations include Barrett's oesophagus (columnar metaplasia of the oesophageal epithelium; a pre-malignant change), alcohol (predisposes to other mucosal tumours, e.g. bladder and colorectal), coeliac disease (classically lymphomas but may get any GI tumour) and Plummer-Vinson syndrome. Tylosis is an AD-inherited disease characterised by hyperkeratosis of palms and soles and high risk of oesophageal tumours.

QUESTION   172

A. FALSE B. TRUE C. FALSE D. TRUE E. TRUE

The clinical manifestations of iron deficiency result from tissue iron depletion. Epithelial tissues are most affected. The glossitis is usually painless and associated with atrophy of the papillae (vitamin B12 deficiency is associated with a painful glossitis). Nail changes include spoon-shaped deformity (koilonychia) and brittleness. Dysphagia and iron-deficiency anaemia are seen in the Plummer-Vinson syndrome (Patterson-Kelly-Brown syndrome). Dermatitis herpetiformis is associated with a gluten-sensitive enteropathy with features similar to coeliac disease: iron deficiency and anaemia may be seen. The condition responds to dapsone.

QUESTION   173

A. TRUE B. TRUE C. TRUE D. FALSE E. FALSE

The biochemical picture of pyloric stenosis (mimicked to some extent by bulimia) consists of metabolic alkalosis with respiratory compensation and dehydration.

QUESTION   174

A. TRUE B. TRUE C. TRUE D. FALSE E. TRUE

Dermatitis herpetiformis is a bullous skin disorder associated with gluten sensitive enteropathy (coeliac disease) and Vitamin K malabsorption.

Pseudoxanthoma elasticum is a disorder of elastin (AR or AD) and the fragile arterioles are prone to spontaneous minor bleeds. Other features of this condition include flexural 'xanthoma-like' lesions due to lax skin. Breaks in Bruch's membrane give typical retinal changes – angioid streaks; patients get premature atherosclerosis.

Acanthosis nigricans produces darkened, velvety thickened skin flexures and neck and multiple warty papillomata may be profuse. It is associated with carcinoma of the stomach (and insulin resistance).

Neurofibromatosis can affect any nerve and the neurofibromas may be found in both the small and large bowel.

QUESTION 175

A. FALSE B. FALSE C. TRUE D. TRUE E. FALSE

Smoking reduces the frequency of attacks of ulcerative colitis. Markers of disease activity in UC are peripheral arthropathy, pyoderma gangrenosum, erythema nodosum, apthous ulceration, uveitis and episcleritis. Ankylosing spondylitis, sacroiliitis and liver involvement (sclerosing cholangitis, chronic active hepatitis) usually do not respond to treatment of UC. Patients with UC have a colon cancer risk of ~10% at 15 years (early onset, whole colon involvement). Thus they should undergo colonoscopy and multiple biopsies at yearly intervals 7-8 years after diagnosis. Crypt abscesses are found in UC which is a disease characterised by inflammation of mucosa only (cf. Crohn's where the full thickness of the bowel wall is involved). Pseudopolyps are islands of relatively normal mucosal tissue isolated by ulceration of the surrounding mucosa. They are not pre-malignant.

Treatment: surgery for mega-colon, bleeding, perforation, >5 days symptoms not settling or evidence of mucosal dysplasia on biopsy.

QUESTION 176

A. FALSE B. FALSE C. TRUE D. TRUE E. FALSE

The liver receives its blood flow from the hepatic artery (25% of total blood flow but 50% of oxygen) and the portal vein (75% of total blood flow but only 50% of total oxygen supply). This constitutes 25% of the resting cardiac output. Riedel's lobe is an extension of the lateral portion of the right lobe which can occasionally be palpated in a normal abdomen. The right and left hepatic ducts join at the porta hepatis to form the common hepatic duct; the cystic and hepatic ducts form the common bile duct.

Ref: Kumar & Clark. Clinical Medicine, 3rd Ed. W. B. Saunders. Ch. 5.

QUESTION 177

A. TRUE B. FALSE C. FALSE D. TRUE E. FALSE

The liver performs many metabolic roles including breakdown of glycogen and hormones (e.g. vasopressin, aldosterone, oestrogens). Urea and VLDLs are examples of the liver's synthetic functions, which also include production of bile containing bilirubin, the product of red blood cell breakdown.

Ref: Kumar & Clark. Clinical Medicine, 3rd Ed. W. B. Saunders. Ch. 5.

QUESTION 178

A. TRUE B. TRUE C. FALSE D. FALSE E. FALSE

ALP is an enzyme found in the canalicular and sinusoidal membranes as well as many other tissues e.g. bone, intestine, placenta. Isoenzyme analysis differentiates between hepatic and other sources. Serum ALP is raised in cholestasis from any cause and in conditions where there is infiltration of the liver such as cirrhosis or metastatic disease, when jaundice is frequently absent. AST is a mitochondrial enzyme found in heart, muscle, kidney and brain as well as liver; high levels occur in acute myocardial infarction. Hyperglobulinaemia is a feature of chronic liver disease probably due to diminished antigen phagocytosis in the sinusoids. ALT is a cytosol enzyme which is more specific for the liver than AST. Elevation of gamma GT parallels that of ALP in cholestasis as they have a similar path of excretion.

Ref: Kumar & Clark. Clinical Medicine, 3rd Ed. W. B. Saunders. Ch. 5.

QUESTION 179

A. FALSE B. TRUE C. FALSE D. FALSE E. FALSE

Gilbert's syndrome is an asymptomatic condition of probable multifactorial aetiology which affects 2-5% of the population. Investigation shows a raised unconjugated bilirubin which rises with fasting and mild illness. A liver biopsy is not needed to confirm the diagnosis.

Ref: Kumar & Clark. Clinical Medicine, 3rd Ed. W. B. Saunders. Ch. 5.

QUESTION 180

A. TRUE B. TRUE C. TRUE D. TRUE E. TRUE

Haematological abnormalities associated with liver disease are common, and include: pancytopaenia secondary to hypersplenism; hypochromic anaemia because of chronic bleeding; macrocytosis which may be accompanied by target and spur cells (altered cell shape due to membrane abnormalities); aplastic anaemia occurs in up to 2% of patients with acute viral hepatitis.

Ref: Kumar & Clark. Clinical Medicine, 3rd Ed. W. B. Saunders. Ch. 5.

QUESTION 181

A. FALSE B. TRUE C. FALSE D. TRUE E. FALSE

High titres of antimitochondrial antibody (M2 is specific) are found in over 95% of patients with PBC, in which raised IgM is also a feature. AFP is normally produced by the fetal liver; significant elevation indicates hepatocellular carcinoma whereas slightly raised AFP is associated with hepatitis, chronic liver disease and teratomas. Along with other antibodies, kidney microsomal antibodies can be a feature of CAH.

Persistence of HbsAg following acute infection indicates chronic infection or carrier status. HbeAg is a marker for development of chronic liver disease.

Ref: Kumar & Clark. Clinical Medicine, 3rd Ed. W. B. Saunders. Ch. 5.

QUESTION 182

A. TRUE B. TRUE C. TRUE D. FALSE E. TRUE

Spider naevi and liver palms are usually associated with chronic liver disease but can occur in acute failure. Hypothermia, cerebral oedema, hypoglycaemia and hyperventilation may all occur particularly in fulminant hepatic failure of which viral hepatitis is the commonest cause.

Ref: Katz, Benumof & Kadis. Anesthesia and Uncommon Diseases. 3rd Ed. W. B. Saunders. Ch. 12.

QUESTION 183

A. FALSE B. TRUE C. TRUE D. TRUE E. TRUE

Many viruses can cause hepatitis. Transmitted by mosquito bites, a flavivirus causes Dengue fever; hepatitis is not a feature of this disease. Herpes simplex viruses, either 1 or 2, may cause hepatitis, particularly in immunocompromised patients. Ebola virus disease is a severe haemorrhagic, febrile illness in which hepatitis occurs. Delta virus is a defective RNA hepatotrophic virus which causes hepatitis only in the presence of hepatitis B infection; delta agent cannot act alone. This is a good example of a question which is open to individual interpretation. Sorry!!

Ref: Kumar & Clark. Clinical Medicine, 3rd Ed. W. B. Saunders. Ch. 1.

QUESTION 184

A. TRUE B. FALSE C. FALSE D. FALSE E. TRUE

Three types of non-A, non-B hepatitis (NANBH) have been described: C, D and E. The letter F is sometimes given to patients with fulminant hepatic failure (which can be caused by a number of different viruses) whilst hepatitis G refers to granulomatous hepatitis. NANBH is responsible for approximately 90% of post-transfusion hepatitis. A, C, D and E are all RNA viruses but hepatitis B is a DNA virus. Hepatitis E has no carrier status and does not progress to chronic liver disease; it is epidemic, particularly in developing countries and has a 1-2% mortality (up to 20% in pregnant women). Both hepatitis B and C are associated with development of liver cancer.

Ref: Kumar & Clark. Clinical Medicine, 3rd Ed. W. B. Saunders. Ch. 5.

QUESTION 185

A. TRUE B. FALSE C. TRUE D. TRUE E. FALSE

Viruses (Hepatitis B +/- D and others), autoimmune disease, drugs(e.g. methyldopa, isoniazid, ketoconazole), hereditary disorders (Wilson's disease, alpha 1-antitrypsin deficiency) and inflammatory bowel disease are all causes of chronic hepatitis. Methotrexate and haemachromatosis cause cirrhosis which is histologically different.

Ref: Kumar & Clark. Clinical Medicine, 3rd Ed. W. B. Saunders. Ch. 5.

QUESTION 186

A. FALSE B. FALSE C. FALSE D. TRUE E. TRUE

Hurler's syndrome is a mucopolysaccharoidosis inherited in an autosomal recessive fashion (inheritance of Hunter's syndrome, a similar disorder, is believed to be X-linked) which results in deposition of abnormal polysaccharides in numerous organs. Features include mental retardation, gargoyle facies, deafness, dwarfing, corneal clouding, musculoskeletal abnormalities and severe myocardial, coronary and valvular disease. The liver is frequently enlarged and disturbances in function are common.

Ref: Katz, Benumof & Kadis. Anesthesia and Uncommon Diseases. 3rd Ed. W. B. Saunders. Ch. 12.

QUESTION 187

A. FALSE B. FALSE C. TRUE D. TRUE E. FALSE

Liver transplantation is now an established treatment for a number of liver disease including primary biliary cirrhosis, chronic hepatitis B or C, alcoholic liver disease, metabolic disorders and acute fulminant hepatitis. Contraindications include sepsis, metastatic carcinoma, AIDS and patient psychological problems. Portal vein thrombosis is an example of a relative contraindication; these are mainly anatomical factors which would make surgery too difficult. Elective transplantation in low-risk patients has a 90% 1 year survival, and 5 year survival of up to 70-85%. Operative mortality is low, with most post-operative deaths occurring in the first 3 months. Lifelong immunosuppression is needed but is ineffective against ductopaenic rejection which needs retransplantation. Graft-versus-host disease is uncommon.

Ref: Kumar & Clark. Clinical Medicine, 3rd Ed. W. B. Saunders. Ch. 5.

QUESTION 188

A. TRUE B. TRUE C. FALSE D. FALSE E. FALSE

Portal hypertension is classified according to the site of obstruction: prehepatic (portal vein thrombosis), intrahepatic (e.g. cirrhosis, hepatitis, schistosomiasis) or posthepatic (e.g. Budd-Chiari, constrictive pericarditis). Portal-systemic anastomoses enlarge and may result in catastrophic haemorrhage. In cirrhotic patients, the circulation is hyperdynamic with peripheral and splanchnic dilatation; this is now thought to be due to endotoxaemia. Where portal vein thrombosis has occurred due to a congenital abnormality of the portal vein or neonatal sepsis, liver function is normal. Ascites develops because of increased lymph production and transudation of fluid into the peritoneal cavity; this transudate contains less than 11g/litre of protein. Injection sclerotherapy or banding is now the treatment of choice in prevention of recurrent variceal bleeding.

Ref: Kumar & Clark. Clinical Medicine, 3rd Ed. W. B. Saunders. Ch. 5.

QUESTION 189

A. FALSE B. TRUE C. FALSE D. TRUE E. FALSE

In ascites there is a reduction in effective, but not actual intravascular volume, due to peripheral vasodilatation. In Meig's syndrome an ovarian tumour is associated with ascites and pleural effusions. Dietary restriction of sodium and diuretics are the mainstay of treatment; fluid restriction is not thought necessary unless the patient is very hyponatraemic. Peritoneo-venous shunts are unsuitable for management of resistant ascites as they are prone to block. Spontaneous bacterial peritonitis is a serious complication of ascites with a high mortality; it is particularly common in patients with cirrhosis and ascites.

Ref: Kumar & Clark. Clinical Medicine, 3rd Ed. W. B. Saunders. Ch. 5.

QUESTION 190

A. TRUE B. TRUE C. FALSE D. TRUE E. TRUE

Portosystemic encephalopathy (PSE) is a chronic neuropsychiatric syndrome secondary to chronic liver disease (predominantly cirrhosis). Several factors may precipitate PSE in a patient with liver failure such as high dietary protein, gastrointestinal haemorrhage, constipation, narcotics, diuretic therapy, paracentesis and portosystemic shunting. The diagnosis is made on clinical information although other tests such as altered EEG or visual evoked responses and raised blood ammonia (if available) may be useful. Management is based around limiting protein intake and sterilising the bowel.

Ref: Kumar & Clark. Clinical Medicine, 3rd Ed. W. B. Saunders. Ch. 5.

QUESTION 191

A. TRUE B. TRUE C. FALSE D. FALSE E. FALSE

Cirrhosis may be 'primary' i.e. primary biliary cirrhosis (a disease of unknown, but possibly immunological aetiology) or 'secondary'. Secondary causes include gallstones, bile duct strictures, alcohol, haemachromatosis (an autosomal recessive inherited disease), Wilson's disease and alpha 1 antitrypsin deficiency. The oral contraceptive pill and renal tumours are associated with Budd-Chiari syndrome, where occlusion of the hepatic vein leads to hepatic congestion and ascites.

Caroli's disease is a rare condition where there is intrahepatic biliary dilatation resulting in recurrent cholangitis but not cirrhosis.

Ref: Kumar & Clark. Clinical Medicine, 3rd Ed. W. B. Saunders. Ch. 5.

QUESTION 192

A. TRUE B. FALSE C. TRUE D. FALSE E. TRUE

During pregnancy hepatic blood flow remains relatively constant despite alteration in plasma and blood volume. Liver size is unchanged. Plasma total protein concentration is reduced by dilution. Causes of jaundice include hepatitis (approximately 40% cases), hyperemesis gravidarum, pre-eclampsia, eclampsia, HELLP syndrome, cholestasis and acute fatty liver of pregnancy. In the latter histology shows microvesicles of fat in liver cells with little necrosis.

Ref: Kumar & Clark. Clinical Medicine, 3rd Ed. W. B. Saunders. Ch. 5.

QUESTION 193

A. FALSE B. FALSE C. TRUE D. TRUE E. FALSE

Reye's syndrome is a rare condition characterised by vomiting, depressed level of consciousness and hepatic failure. It occurs mainly in children but may also occur in adults. Jaundice is typically minimal or absent. It results in microvesicular fatty infiltration of the liver.

Ref: Kumar & Clark. Clinical Medicine, 3rd Ed. W. B. Saunders. Ch. 5.

QUESTION 194

A. TRUE B. TRUE C. FALSE D. FALSE E. TRUE

Carriers of hepatitis B and C have a high risk of developing hepatocellular carcinoma. Alcoholic cirrhosis, haemachromatosis, aflatoxin, androgenic steroids and the contraceptive pill have also been implicated to a greater or lesser extent. Schistosomiasis mansoni and japonicum produce granulomatous disease, fibrosis and inflammation of the liver.

Ref: Kumar & Clark. Clinical Medicine, 3rd Ed. W. B. Saunders. Ch. 5.

QUESTION 195

A. FALSE B. FALSE C. TRUE D. TRUE E. FALSE

The main pancreatic duct joins the common bile duct (CBD) before draining into the duodenum. The CBD is formed by union of the common hepatic and cystic ducts. 98% of the pancreas is taken up by exocrine cells. Enzyme secretion is stimulated by gut hormones e.g. secretin, cholecystokinin which act via cAMP and membrane phosphoinositides as second messengers. Serum amylase measurement is useful in acute disease but of no value in chronic disease.

Ref: Kumar & Clark. Clinical Medicine, 3rd Ed. W. B. Saunders. Ch. 5.

QUESTION 196

A. FALSE B. TRUE C. TRUE D. TRUE E. TRUE

Gallstones are present in 10-20% of the Western population but there is wide geographical variation. The majority are asymptomatic. Cholesterol stones develop in supersaturated bile i.e. where there is a relative lack of bile salts and phospholipid. Risk factors include acromegaly treated with octreotide and ileal resection or disease.

Ref: Kumar & Clark. Clinical Medicine, 3rd Ed. W. B. Saunders. Ch. 5.

QUESTION 197

A. TRUE B. TRUE C. TRUE D. TRUE E. TRUE

Other associations include malignancy (parotid tumours and lymphomas), cirrhosis, infections (mumps, bacterial parotitis), malabsorption states, Sjögren's syndrome, amyloidosis, drugs (iodides, thiouracil, lead), hyperlipidaemia and acromegaly.

QUESTION 198

A. FALSE B. FALSE C. TRUE D. TRUE E. FALSE

Hepatitis B is a DNA virus transmitted parenterally. HBsAg is seen in the serum 1-5 months after exposure (presence after 6 months implies carrier state and is seen in 5-10%). HBeAg is seen 6-12 weeks after exposure and implies high infectivity (persistence >12 weeks implies chronic infection). Anti-HBc implies previous exposure; anti-HBs alone is seen with vaccination. The glomerulonephritis associated with hepatitis B infection is membranous rather than minimal change.

QUESTION 199

A. FALSE B. TRUE C. TRUE D. FALSE E. FALSE

Clinical features of hepatic encephalopathy include inverted sleep-wake cycle, slurred speech, constructional apraxia, flap, fetor, brisk reflexes, increased tone and rigidity. It may be precipitated in patients with cirrhosis by infection, electrolyte imbalance, high protein intake (related to the release of ammonia) and some drugs. Blood ammonium levels are raised. The EEG is abnormal with slow delta waves and it never returns to normal (other causes of delta waves on the EEG include CO_2 retention, uraemia, B12 deficiency and hypoglycaemia). Treatment is with low protein diet, laxatives, purgatives and neomycin (debatable now) and drugs that may be of benefit are flumazenil (benzodiazepine antagonist) and bromocriptine.

QUESTION 200

A. TRUE B. FALSE C. FALSE D. FALSE E. FALSE

Hepatitis A is an RNA virus spread by the faeco-oral route and is nearly always a self-limiting illness – abrupt onset of high fever, short-lived elevation of transaminases and early appearance of IgM anti–HepA virus. Occasionally in adults the disease is more severe and can produce fulminant hepatic failure with high mortality (encephalopathy within 8 weeks of symptoms). Chronic liver disease and arthritis are features of hepatitis B and C.

FitzHugh-Curtis syndrome is due to chlamydia infection (fever, perihepatitis, shoulder-tip pain and friction rub over the liver, adnexal tenderness and occasionally endocarditis). Other chlamydial infections are NSU (C. trachomatis types D-K - Reiter's syndrome and pelvic inflammatory disease may follow), Lymphogranuloma venereum (LGV) (C. trachomatis types 1-3 - painful lymphadenopathy, proctitis, fistula to vagina or bladder) and Chlamydial pneumoniae (Psittacosis –C. psittaci or TWAR agent-C. pneumoniae). Treat with tetracycline (resistant to erythromycin).

QUESTION 201

A. FALSE B. TRUE C. FALSE D. TRUE E. FALSE

In pre-renal failure the kidney is trying to preserve sodium and water, and therefore, the urine will be concentrated. As such, fractional excretion of sodium [(Urinary Na x Plasma Creatinine) divided by (Plasma Na x Urinary Creatinine) x 100%] should be less than 1%. The urinary specific gravity will be > 1.020 and the urinary sodium will be less than 20 mmol/l. A urinary protein of greater than 150 mg/l suggests a diagnosis of microalbuminuria, seen in diabetic nephropathy, but not in pre-renal failure.

Ref: Kumar & Clark. Clinical Medicine, 3rd Ed. W. B. Saunders. Ch. 9.

QUESTION 202

A. TRUE B. TRUE C. TRUE D. TRUE E. TRUE

All of these conditions can give rise to an enlarged kidney.

Ref: Kumar & Clark. Clinical Medicine, 3rd Ed. W. B. Saunders. Ch. 9.

QUESTION 203

A. FALSE B. TRUE C. TRUE D. TRUE E. FALSE

Goodpasture's syndrome is mediated by an anti-glomerular basement membrane antibody, whilst aminoglycoside treatment leads to acute tubular necrosis.

Ref: Kumar & Clark. Clinical Medicine, 3rd Ed. W. B. Saunders. Ch. 9.

QUESTION 204

A. TRUE B. TRUE C. FALSE D. TRUE E. TRUE

Haematuria does not occur in diabetes unless associated with some other problem.

Ref: Kumar & Clark. Clinical Medicine, 3rd Ed. W. B. Saunders. Ch. 17.

QUESTION 205

A. TRUE B. TRUE C. TRUE D. FALSE E. TRUE

Minimal change glomerulonephritis can occur in diabetes mellitus but is not a direct complication of the diabetes. Treatment involves the use of steroids which will make the management of the diabetes more difficult. This demonstrates the importance of investigating diabetic patients with renal disease fully to ensure no other treatable conditions are missed.

Ref: Kumar & Clark. Clinical Medicine, 3rd Ed. W. B. Saunders. Ch. 17.

QUESTION 206

A. TRUE B. FALSE C. TRUE D. FALSE E. FALSE

Schistosoma haematobium infection leads to chronic inflammation of the bladder, urethra, and ureters, with the ultimate effect of an obstructive uropathy, rather than direct renal involvement. Staphlococcal infection does not ordinarily occur unless introduced during invasive procedures, whereas there can be post-streptococcal renal problems. Malaria can lead to Blackwater fever but this is a consequence of intra-vascular haemolysis, not direct renal disease.

Ref: Kumar & Clark. Clinical Medicine, 3rd Ed. W. B. Saunders. Chs 1, 8, 9.

QUESTION 207

A. TRUE B. TRUE C. TRUE D. FALSE E. TRUE

Hyperventilation may help in hyperkalaemia by driving potassium into the cells in response to the efflux of hydrogen ions caused by the respiratory alkalosis. In order for frusemide to be effective there still needs to be some renal function and response to a loop diuretic, which may have been lost in the acute renal insult, with a consequent loss of action. All the other measures work independently of the kidney. Secondly, frusemide, being nephrotoxic in its own right, may only serve to worsen the renal dysfunction.

Ref: Kumar & Clark. Clinical Medicine, 3rd Ed. W. B. Saunders. Ch. 9.

QUESTION 208

A. TRUE B. FALSE C. TRUE D. TRUE E. TRUE

Kanamycin (aminoglycoside), frusemide, amphotericin B, and cephaloridine are known to be nephrotoxic. Clarithromycin is a macrolide antibiotic of the same family as erythromycin.

Ref: Kumar & Clark. Clinical Medicine, 3rd Ed. W. B. Saunders. Ch. 9.

QUESTION   209

A. FALSE B. TRUE C. TRUE D. TRUE E. TRUE

Urea plasma concentration is defined as mass/volume and can therefore be raised by increased production or decreased plasma volume. Although acute renal failure may increase urea concentration, renal function is by definition impaired.

Ref: Kumar & Clark. Clinical Medicine, 3rd Ed. W. B. Saunders. Ch. 9.

QUESTION   210

A. TRUE B. TRUE C. TRUE D. FALSE E. TRUE

Liver failure will cause a disproportionately low urea due to its dysfunction rather than a raised creatinine. In situations such as the hepato–renal syndrome both the urea and creatinine levels are raised.

Ref: Kumar & Clark. Clinical Medicine, 3rd Ed. W. B. Saunders. Ch. 9.

QUESTION   211

A. TRUE B. TRUE C. TRUE D. TRUE E. TRUE

Chronic renal failure may lead to pericarditis, peripheral neuropathy, pruritus, secondary and tertiary parathyroidism. Primary hyperparathyroidism is when the excess PTH is inappropriate to the plasma calcium level (i.e. calcium is not low). Secondary hyperparathyroidism is when the raised PTH is appropriate (i.e. calcium is low). Tertiary hyperparathyroidism is a consequence of secondary hyperparathyroidism when a parathyroid adenoma results.

Ref: Kumar & Clark. Clinical Medicine, 3rd Ed. W. B. Saunders. Ch. 9.

QUESTION   212

A. TRUE B. TRUE C. TRUE D. FALSE E. TRUE

Pancreatitis and peritonitis are recognised complications of Continuous Ambulatory Peritoneal Dialysis (CAPD). In diabetic patients treated with CAPD insulin may be added to the dialysate bag (which contains glucose) in order to help control the blood glucose level. A transplanted kidney is positioned as a pelvic organ and as such is anastomosed to the iliac vessels.

Ref: Kumar & Clark. Clinical Medicine, 3rd Ed. W. B. Saunders. Ch. 9.

QUESTION 213

A. TRUE B. TRUE C. TRUE D. TRUE E. FALSE

The associated problems are well documented with their primary underlying renal disorder. APKD has an autosomal dominant manner of inheritance in the large majority of cases, with a single gene defect on the short arm of chromosome 16. Aniridia is a congenital absence of the iris of the eye. Berry aneurysms most commonly occur at the junction of the posterior communicating artery with the internal carotid.

Ref: Kumar & Clark. Clinical Medicine, 3rd Ed. W. B. Saunders. Ch. 9.

QUESTION 214

A. TRUE B. TRUE C. TRUE D. TRUE E. TRUE

Chlorpropamide increases the sensitivity of the renal tubules to Antidiuretic hormone (ADH), hence its theoretical use in nephrogenic diabetes insipidus. Excessive ADH, inappropriate ADH or the action of ADH-like substances will lead to a hyponatraemia with a normal extracellular volume, whereas in the hyponatraemia associated with diuretic use the patient loses water with the sodium and develops a decreased extracellular volume. In the case of heart failure the renal response to the decreased cardiac output is to conserve water, thereby causing a hyponatraemia with an increased extracellular volume.

Ref: Kumar & Clark. Clinical Medicine, 3rd Ed. W. B. Saunders. Ch. 9.

QUESTION 215

A. TRUE B. FALSE C. FALSE D. TRUE E. TRUE

Amiloride as a potassium sparing diuretic can cause hyperkalaemia. In Addison's disease there is loss of the mineralocorticoid effects leading to a raised potassium. Conn's syndrome (hyperaldosteronism) and carbenoxolone (an exogenous mineralocorticoid) will both lead to hypokalaemia due to increased loss of potassium via the sodium-potassium exchange pump in the distal convoluted tubule.

Ref: Kumar & Clark. Clinical Medicine, 3rd Ed. W. B. Saunders. Ch. 10.

QUESTION 216

A. TRUE B. FALSE C. TRUE D. FALSE E. TRUE

The effects of gravity on the distribution of blood flow are most marked in the standing position. The transmural pressure in the dependent veins increases and the dependent venous volume increases by ~500 ml. Cardiac filling pressure falls by several cmH$_2$O and stroke volume (and pulse pressure) declines. In healthy individuals the cardiopulmonary and carotid sinus reflexes restore the blood pressure; there is an increase in heart rate and cardiac contractility (sympathetic activity) with vasoconstriction of peripheral vascular beds, all within 1-2 min of standing. Capillary filtration in dependent tissues increases producing a 5-10% fall in plasma volume over the next hour. Salt and water excretion by the kidney diminishes due to a rise in serum renin, angiotensin II, vasopressin and aldosterone in combination with the reflex renal vasoconstriction.

QUESTION 217

A. TRUE B. TRUE C. FALSE D. FALSE E. TRUE

In mild-moderate renal failure, there is no intrinsic defect in the kidney's ability to excrete potassium and patients are able to maintain adequate potassium balance unless there is excessive intake. However, hypoaldosteronism impairs the renal potassium handling and contributes to hyperkalaemia. It is only when the GFR falls below 20ml/min (10-20% of normal) that this becomes a factor. Erythropoietin therapy is associated with a rise in serum potassium.

QUESTION 218

A. TRUE B. FALSE C. FALSE D. FALSE E. TRUE

The sensory supply to the bladder derives from both sympathetic and parasympathetic nervous systems. The vesical sphincter is innervated with sympathetic motor fibres while the bladder wall receives motor fibres from the parasympathetic system. Venous drainage is via the vesical plexus to the internal iliac vein, not the inferior mesenteric. The pubovesical and the lateral ligaments of the bladder are thickenings of the pelvic fascia.

QUESTION 219

A. TRUE B. TRUE C. TRUE D. TRUE E. FALSE

The calculated creatinine clearance is higher than the true GFR due to a small but significant active secretion of creatinine at the proximal tubule. This makes the creatinine clearance unreliable at low GFR. Bicarbonate resorption occurs in the proximal tubule due to the action of carbonic anhydrase. Defects result in tubular acidosis. Water deprivation tests the integrity of the distal tubule and collecting system rather than the proximal tubule.

QUESTION 220

A. FALSE B. TRUE C. TRUE D. FALSE E. FALSE

Bartter's syndrome (AR) usually presents as failure to thrive in childhood. There is hyperplasia of the juxtaglomerular apparatus and primary hyperreninaemia, resulting in hypokalaemic, hypochloraemic metabolic alkalosis but normal BP (unlike patients with Liddle's syndrome – hypertensive, pseudohyperaldosteronism). Urine prostaglandin, potassium and chloride excretion are elevated. Bartter's usually responds to diet, spionolactone, NSAIDs (PG synthetase inhibitors) and propranolol. Hypertension, if present, is sensitive to angiotensin II receptor antagonists (e.g. losartan).

QUESTION 221

A. FALSE B. TRUE C. TRUE D. FALSE E. TRUE

IgA nephropathy (Berger's disease) is the commonest primary glomerulonephritis. Presenting features include haematuria, proteinuria, nephrotic syndrome, rapidly progressive glomerulonephritis with renal failure and crescent formation and/or hypertension. It is associated with cirrhosis, gluten-sensitive enteropathy, dermatitis herpetiformis and Mycosis fungoides. Following transplantation, IgA deposits can occur in the transplanted kidney but rarely lead to recurrent disease. Only 20% go on to develop CRF over 20 years.

QUESTION 222

A. FALSE B. FALSE C. TRUE D. TRUE E. FALSE

Nephrotic syndrome is characterised by severe proteinuria that results in hypoalbuminaemia. Loss of transferrin results in hypochromic anaemia that is resistant to iron. Renal loss of immunoglobulins increases the susceptibility to infections. Decrease in plasma volume, loss of antithrombin III and increased levels of factors II, V, VII, VIII and X result in a procoagulant state (venous thromboses - e.g. renal vein). Serum cholesterol is raised due to increased synthesis of LDL apoprotein B. The decrease in plasma volume usually results in avid sodium retention.

QUESTION 223

A. TRUE B. FALSE C. TRUE D. TRUE E. FALSE

In patients with CRF, dementia may occur due to aluminium toxicity. Long-term haemodialysis is associated with an increased risk of hepatitis B and C infection (hepatitis E is transmitted by the faeco-oral route and is similar to hepatitis A in its clinical manifestations). Hypogonadism and infertility are common. Arthropathy may result from deposition of amyloid (failure to clear beta-2-microglobulin by haemodialysis). Patients with CRF have hyperuricaemia but this does not commonly result in acute gout.

QUESTION 224

A. FALSE B. FALSE C. FALSE D. TRUE E. FALSE

NSAIDs have a number of adverse effects on the kidney. By inhibiting prostaglandin synthesis they may precipitate acute ischaemic renal failure, sodium retention (leading to or exacerbating hypertension and heart failure), water retention (enhanced action of ADH and increased medullary tonicity) and hyporeninaemic hypoaldosteronism (causing hyperkalaemia). NSAIDs are associated with an acute allergic interstitial nephritis that can result in renal failure and proteinuria. Analgesic nephropathy results in papillary necrosis and chronic renal failure.

QUESTION 225

A. TRUE B. TRUE C. FALSE D. FALSE E. TRUE

Drugs that are recognised causes of acute interstitial nephritis include penicillin (and other beta-lactam antibiotics), sulphonamides, rifampicin, ethambutol, NSAIDs, diuretics (thiazides and loop diuretics), allopurinol, carbamazepine, methyldopa and cimetidine. Acute interstitial nephritis responds to stopping the drug and steroid therapy. Chronic interstitial nephritis is associated with lithium, phenacetin and cisplatinum.

QUESTION 226

A. TRUE B. FALSE C. FALSE D. TRUE E. TRUE

APKD is an autosomal dominant disorder (type 1 is linked to chr 16 while type 2 is as yet unlinked). Cysts derive from all parts of the nephron and are absent at birth. Clinically (and on ultrasound) cysts are evident from approx. age 30 onwards. Presentation is with loin pain, haematuria, hypertension, UTI, anaemia or polycythaemia. Associations include hepatic cysts (>50% and more common in females), pancreatic cysts (only 10%), saccular aneurysms (especially in the cerebral circulation), cardiac valve disease (aortic incompetence, mitral valve prolapse), colonic diverticular disease and herniae. Rarer associations include Peutz-Jegher's syndrome, myotonic dystrophy and hereditary spherocytosis.

QUESTION 227

A. FALSE B. TRUE C. FALSE D. TRUE E. FALSE

Renal osteodystrophy is associated with reduced phosphate excretion and hyperphosphataemia. This is treated with oral phosphate binders, dietary restriction of phosphate, oral calcium carbonate, aluminium hydroxide, etc. There is impaired 25-hydroxylation of cholecalciferol and as a result hypocalcaemia, elevated alkaline phosphatase and osteomalacia. There is secondary hyperparathyroidism with osteitis fibrosa cystica ('brown tumours' that are located in long bones, away from the joints: periarticular cysts are a feature of amyloid). Patients require calcium supplements as well as 1, 25-DHCC. Magnesium levels are typically raised as magnesium excretion is reduced. Radiographic changes include vascular calcification, 'rugger-jersey' spine and subperiosteal lesions.

QUESTION 228

A. TRUE B. FALSE C. TRUE D. FALSE E. TRUE

Bilateral renal enlargement is seen with polycystic kidney disease, medullary sponge disease, amyloidosis, acromegaly, acute interstitial nephritis, acute GN, acute tubular necrosis, acute urate nephropathy and radiation nephritis. Renal artery stenosis is associated with a shrunken kidney on the side of the lesion with compensatory hypertrophy of the contralateral kidney.

QUESTION 229

A. FALSE B. TRUE C. FALSE D. TRUE E. TRUE

Erythropoietin is a 165 aa glycoprotein synthesised by the peritubular cells in the kidney. Through specific cell-surface receptors it stimulates the proliferation and differentiation of erythroid lineage in the bone marrow and results in a gradual rise in red cell count and haemoglobin over weeks. Indications for use in renal failure include symptomatic anaemia (congestive cardiac failure, angina, etc.) requiring transfusions with an absolute Hb <8 g/dl. It is administered by subcutaneous injection. Side effects include 'flu-like' symptoms, headache, seizures, hypertension, thrombosis of shunts and fistulae (all due to a rapid rise in haematocrit) and hyperkalaemia.

QUESTION 230

A. FALSE B. FALSE C. TRUE D. TRUE E. FALSE

Increased doses of frusemide are usually required in renal failure, increasing the risk of oto-toxicity. Heparin and doxazosin do not require dose reduction. Digoxin and cimetidine are excreted by the kidney and require careful monitoring and reduced doses in CRF.

QUESTION 231

A. TRUE B. TRUE C. FALSE D. TRUE E. FALSE

Horner's syndrome is due to the disruption of sympathetic fibres to an eye. It results in enoph-thalmus, unilateral pupillary constriction, ptosis, nasal congestion and loss of sweating on the same side of the face. It can be caused by various lesions:

1. *Intracerbral lesions:* massive cerebral infarction, pontine glioma, lateral medullary syndrome, coning of the temporal lobe.
2. *Cervical cord lesions:* syringomyelia, cord tumours.
3. *T1 root lesions*: apical bronchial neoplasms, apical tuberculosis, cervical rib.
4. *Sympathetic chain in the neck*: cervical sympathectomy.

Ref: Kumar & Clark. Clinical Medicine, 3rd Ed. W. B. Saunders. Ch. 18.

QUESTION 232

A. TRUE B. FALSE C. FALSE D. FALSE E. FALSE

The Argyll–Robertson pupil is small, irregular and fixed to light, but constricts on conver-gence. It is a feature of neurosyphilis. Diabetes mellitus and aneurysms of the posterior communicating artery are associated with third nerve palsies which lead to dilated pupils. The Holmes–Adie pupil is usually a unilaterally dilated pupil with little reaction to light and incomplete constriction to convergence. It occurs mainly in females and is known as the myotonic pupil. In severe hypothermia the pupils are fixed and often dilated.

Ref: Kumar & Clark. Clinical Medicine, 3rd Ed. W. B. Saunders. Ch. 18.

QUESTION   233

A. TRUE   B. FALSE   C. TRUE   D. TRUE   E. TRUE

Papilloedema is caused by intracranial space occupying lesions, cerebral oedema, subarachnoid haemorrhage, benign intracranial hypertension, metabolic causes (CO_2 retention, chronic hypoxia, hypocalcaemia), malignant hypertension, optic neuritis, disc infiltration (i.e. leukaemia), ischaemic optic neuropathy and retinal venous obstruction (i.e. thrombosis).

Ref: Kumar & Clark. Clinical Medicine, 3rd Ed. W. B. Saunders. Ch. 18.

QUESTION   234

A. FALSE   B. TRUE   C. TRUE   D. TRUE   E. FALSE

The following structures pass through the cavernous sinus:

- Internal carotid artery
- Abducent nerve VI
- Oculomotor nerve III
- Trochlear nerve IV
- Ophthalmic division of trigeminal nerve Va
- Maxillary division of trigeminal nerve Vb

Ref: Kumar & Clark. Clinical Medicine, 3rd Ed. W. B. Saunders. Ch. 18.

QUESTION   235

A. FALSE   B. FALSE   C. FALSE   D. TRUE   E. TRUE

Damage to the facial nerve may occur in the pons, cerebellopontine angle, within the petrous temporal bone, and within the face. Causes of facial nerve palsy within the petrous temporal bone are Bell's palsy, trauma, infection of the middle ear, herpes zoster and tumours (e.g. glomus tumour). Sarcoidosis and mumps cause facial nerve palsies as the nerve passes through the parotid gland. Acoustic neuromas produce lesions at the cerebellopontine angle.

Ref: Kumar & Clark. Clinical Medicine, 3rd Ed. W. B. Saunders. Ch. 18.

QUESTION   236

A. FALSE   B. FALSE   C. FALSE   D. FALSE   E. FALSE

The glossopharyngeal nerve supplies the sensation of taste to the posterior two-thirds of the tongue. Lesions at the jugular foramen cause palsies of cranial nerves IX and X. Nystagmus occurs in lesions of the ocular or the vestibular systems and their connections. Eighth cranial nerve lesions cause a decrease of both air conduction and bone conduction.

Caloric testing with ice cold water causes nystagmus with the fast component to the opposite side whereas with warm water, the fast component occurs to the same side. In the presence of an eighth nerve lesion the response is decreased or absent.

Ref: Kumar & Clark. Clinical Medicine, 3rd Ed. W. B. Saunders. Ch. 18.

QUESTION 237

A. FALSE B. TRUE C. TRUE D. FALSE E. FALSE

In pseudobulbar palsy there are bilateral upper motor neurone lesions of the lower cranial nerves (IX - XII). The main causes are motor neurone disease, multiple sclerosis and cerebrovascular disease. Signs of pseudobulbar palsy are a spastic tongue, dysarthria, a gravelly voice and emotional lability. The gag and palatal reflexes are preserved. Muscle fasciculation is a lower motor neurone sign. Cog wheel rigidity occurs in Parkinson's disease.

Ref: Kumar & Clark. Clinical Medicine, 3rd Ed. W. B. Saunders. Ch. 18.

QUESTION 238

A. TRUE B. FALSE C. TRUE D. TRUE E. TRUE

Spastic paraparesis indicates bilateral damage to the corticospinal tracts. Causes include all the causes of spinal cord compression, multiple sclerosis, myelitis, motor neurone disease, subacute combined degeneration of the cord, syringomyelia, syphilis, hydrocephalus and multiple cerebral infarcts. Bilateral cerebral lesions may produce a similar picture.

Ref: Kumar & Clark. Clinical Medicine, 3rd Ed. W. B. Saunders. Ch. 18.

QUESTION 239

A. FALSE B. FALSE C. TRUE D. FALSE E. FALSE

Upper motor neurone lesions are characterised by, spastic increase in tone, drift of upper limb, exaggerated tendon reflexes, weakness, extensor planter response, loss of abdominal reflexes, no muscle wasting and normal electrical excitability of muscle.

Ref: Kumar & Clark. Clinical Medicine, 3rd Ed. W. B. Saunders. Ch. 18.

QUESTION 240

A. FALSE B. TRUE C. TRUE D. TRUE E. FALSE

The clinical features produced by diseases of the extrapyramidal system include:

1. The features of Parkinson's disease: resting tremor, cog-wheel rigidity, bradykinesia, festinant gait, scanning speech
2. Chorea, dystonia, hemiballismus

Nystagmus occurs in disorders of the ocular system, cerebellum and their connections. Dysdiadokinesis occurs with cerebellar lesions.

Ref: Kumar & Clark. Clinical Medicine, 3rd Ed. W. B. Saunders. Ch 18.

QUESTION 241

A. FALSE B. FALSE C. TRUE D. TRUE E. TRUE

Features of cord compression are radicular pain at the site of compression, spastic paraparesis or tetraparesis and sensory loss which rises to the level of compression. Sphincter disturbance is common. Root pain may be felt at the site of compression and may be worsened by coughing. Ipsilateral pyramidal signs in association with contralateral loss of pain and temperature sensation is known as the Brown-Sequard syndrome of hemisection of the cord.

Ref: Kumar & Clark. Clinical Medicine, 3rd Ed. W. B. Saunders. Ch. 18.

QUESTION 242

A. FALSE B. TRUE C. FALSE D. TRUE E. FALSE

The circle of Willis is supplied by two internal carotid arteries and by the basilar artery, which is formed by the union of the two vertebral arteries. The posterior cerebral arteries are formed from the basilar and posterior communicating arteries in the circle of Willis.

The posterior inferior cerebellar artery is the largest branch of the vertebral artery supplying the cerebellum, medulla oblongata and choroid plexus of the fourth ventricle. The anterior spinal artery is formed from a contributory branch of each vertebral artery.

Ref: Kumar & Clark. Clinical Medicine, 3rd Ed. W. B. Saunders. Ch. 18.

QUESTION 243

A. FALSE B. FALSE C. TRUE D. TRUE E. TRUE

The clinical features of transient ischaemic attacks arising from the posterior circulation (vertebrobasilar system) are diplopia, vertigo, vomiting, choking, dysarthria, ataxia, hemisensory loss, hemianopic visual loss, transient global amnesia, tetraparesis and loss of consciousness. Transient ischaemic attacks of the anterior circulation (carotid artery) cause hemiparesis, amaurosis fugax, aphasia, hemisensory loss, and hemianopic visual loss. Amaurosis fugax is often the first clinical sign of carotid stenosis.

Ref: Kumar & Clark. Clinical Medicine, 3rd Ed. W. B. Saunders. Ch. 18.

QUESTION 244

A. TRUE B. TRUE C. FALSE D. FALSE E. TRUE

The lateral medullary syndrome (Wallenberg's syndrome) is caused by thromboembolism of the posterior inferior cerebellar artery or the vertebral artery. There is sudden vertigo, vomiting, ipsilateral ataxia, facial numbness (V), diplopia (VI), nystagmus, Horner's syndrome, glossopharyngeal and vagus nerve lesions and contralateral (spinothalamic) loss of pain and temperature.

Ref: Kumar & Clark. Clinical Medicine, 3rd Ed. W. B. Saunders. Ch. 18.

QUESTION 245

A. FALSE B. FALSE C. FALSE D. TRUE E. TRUE

Berry aneuryms account for 70% of subarachnoid haemorrhages. Aneuryms of the posterior communicating artery may present with third nerve palsies. The CSF becomes xanthochromic several hours after subarachnoid haemorrhage. Lumbar puncture is not necessary if the diagnosis is made by CT and is contraindicated if raised intracranial pressure is suspected. Blood clot in the subarachnoid space can lead to obstruction of CSF flow and hydrocephalus.

Ref: Kumar & Clark. Clinical Medicine, 3rd Ed. W. B. Saunders. Ch. 18.

QUESTION 246

A. FALSE B. TRUE C. TRUE D. TRUE E. FALSE

Subdural haemorrhage occurs when blood accumulates in the subdural space following the rupture of a vein. It is almost always due to head trauma, which may be minor. The latent period between injury and symptoms may be weeks or months. Chronic subdural haematomas are common in the elderly and in patients with alcohol abuse. The level of consciousness often fluctuates. In the elderly some chronic subdural haematomas resolve spontaneously and can be monitored with serial CT scans.

Ref: Kumar & Clark. Clinical Medicine, 3rd Ed. W. B. Saunders. Ch. 18.

QUESTION 247

A. TRUE B. TRUE C. TRUE D. TRUE E. FALSE

Skull and paranasal sinus infection, dehydration, pregnancy and the oral contraceptive pill are aetiological factors in the development of dural venous thrombosis. It is also associated with central venous catheters inadvertently passed retrogradely up the internal jugular vein towards the jugular bulb. Lateral and sagittal sinus thrombosis is associated with raised intracranial pressure, headache, papilloedema and often epilepsy.

Ref: Kumar & Clark. Clinical Medicine, 3rd Ed. W. B. Saunders. Ch. 18.

QUESTION 248

A. TRUE B. TRUE C. FALSE D. FALSE E. TRUE

Partial (focal) seizures arise from abnormal electrical activity in an area of the brain. An acquired lesion (e.g. a tumour) is a cause of such activity. The onset of seizures in adult life has a 3% chance of being caused by a mass lesion. Jacksonian seizures originate in the motor cortex. They typically begin either in the corner of the mouth or in the thumb or index finger, spreading gradually to involve the limbs on the other side of the epileptic focus. Temporal lobe seizures (focal) are associated with disturbances of smell and feelings of familiarity. Tonic-clonic seizures are generalised seizures. 3 Hz spike and wave activity is pathognomonic of petit mal which is a generalised seizure and mainly a disorder of childhood. See reference for classification of types.

Ref: Kumar & Clark. Clinical Medicine, 3ʳᵈ Ed. W. B. Saunders. Ch. 18.

QUESTION 249

A. FALSE B. TRUE C. FALSE D. FALSE E. TRUE

Cataplexy is a sudden loss of tone in the lower limbs with preservation of consciousness precipitated by a sudden surprise or emotion. It may be accompanied by hypnagogic hallucinations (terrifying hallucinations on falling asleep), hypnopompic hallucinations (on waking) and sleep paralysis (a frightening inability to move whilst drowsy). The EEG is normal during these attacks. Treatment is with methylphenidate or other amphetamine-like drugs. Small doses of tricyclics may also help. It is related to narcolepsy.

Ref: Kumar & Clark. Clinical Medicine, 3ʳᵈ Ed. W. B. Saunders. Ch. 18.

QUESTION 250

A. TRUE B. FALSE C. TRUE D. TRUE E. FALSE

In Parkinson's disease, there is a poverty and slowing of movement (bradykinesia) and the gait is shuffling, festinant and associated with poor arm swinging. There is a characteristic resting tremor of 4-7 Hz that is decreased on movement. Stiffness of the limbs develop that is equal in opposing groups of muscles. When combined with tremor the increase in tone is broken up into a jerky resistance to passive movement i.e. cogwheel rigidity. The plantar responses are flexor. Intention tremor is a feature of cerebellar disease.

Ref: Kumar & Clark. Clinical Medicine, 3ʳᵈ Ed. W. B. Saunders. Ch. 18.

QUESTION 251

A. TRUE B. TRUE C. FALSE D. TRUE E. FALSE

Huntington's chorea is inherited as an autosomal dominant trait with full penetrance. A mutation has been identified on the short arm of chromosome 4. There is a reduction in neurotransmitters and the enzymes synthesizing acetylcholine and GABA in the striatum and the depletion of GABA, angiotensin converting enzyme and met-enkephalin in the substantia nigra. There is a relentless progression of chorea and dementia in middle life. Death usually occurs between 10 and 20 years after the onset. Tetrabenazine or sulpiride may be used to help control the chorea.

Ref: Kumar & Clark. Clinical Medicine, 3ʳᵈ Ed. W. B. Saunders. Ch. 18.

QUESTION 252

A. FALSE B. TRUE C. TRUE D. TRUE E. TRUE

This disorder is not inherited in a sex-linked manner, but it is three to four times more common in boys than girls. Coprolalia is present in one third of patients. Obsessive-compulsive symptoms occur frequently in patients with Gilles de la Tourette syndrome. Haloperidol is the most effective treatment.

Ref: Kumar & Clark. Clinical Medicine, 3rd Ed. W. B. Saunders. Ch. 18.
Gelder, Gath, Mayou & Cowen. Oxford Textbook of Psychiatry. 3rd Ed. Oxford University Press. Ch. 12.

QUESTION 253

A. FALSE B. FALSE C. TRUE D. TRUE E. TRUE

Multiple sclerosis is a demyelinating disease of the brain and spinal cord of unknown cause. There is a positive association between multiple sclerosis and antigens HLA-A3, B7 and DR2. Optic neuropathy causes blurred vision, scotomata and defects in colour vision. Visual evoked responses are abnormal. Brain stem demyelination manifests itself by the sudden onset of diplopia, vertigo and nystagmus. Diplopia in multiple sclerosis is caused by a number of different lesions; a sixth nerve lesion and internuclear ophthalmoplegia are two examples. A spastic paraparesis is caused by demyelination in the spinal cord. Peripheral nerve studies are normal. The appearance and pressure of cerebrospinal fluid is normal. There is a raised cell count (mainly mononuclear cells), raised total protein and oligoclonal bands of IgG within the CSF.

Ref: Kumar & Clark. Clinical Medicine, 3rd Ed. W. B. Saunders. Ch. 18.

QUESTION 254

A. FALSE B. TRUE C. FALSE D. FALSE E. TRUE

In bacterial meningitis the CSF becomes turbid in appearance, the mononuclear cell count rises from less than 5 per cubic mm to approx. 50 per cubic mm. Polymorphonuclear cells which are absent normally, increase to 200 - 300 per cubic mm. The protein count rises from 0.2 - 0.4 g per litre to 0.5 - 2.0 g per litre. The CSF glucose rises to a value greater than half the blood glucose. Pneumococci are gram positive intracellular diplococci. Mycobacterium tuberculosis are acid-fast bacilli that stain with Ziehl-Nielsen stain.

Ref: Kumar & Clark. Clinical Medicine, 3rd Ed. W. B. Saunders. Ch. 18.

QUESTION 255

A. TRUE B. FALSE C. TRUE D. FALSE E. FALSE

Neurological sequelae of herpes varicella zoster infection are, acute disseminated encephalomyelitis, shingles, residual neuralgia and the Ramsay Hunt syndrome (rare form of zoster on the tympanic membrane and external auditory canal often accompanied by a facial nerve palsy). Herpes varicella zoster is not oncogenic. Subacute sclerosing panencephalitis is a degenerative neurological disease which occurs following infection with either the measles or rubella virus. The aetiology of Reye's syndrome is unknown. It is an encephalitic illness of children associated with fatty infiltration of the liver and hypoglycaemia. It is said to be associated with aspirin therapy in children.

Ref: Kumar & Clark. Clinical Medicine, 3rd Ed. W. B. Saunders. Ch. 18.

QUESTION 256

A. TRUE B. TRUE C. FALSE D. TRUE E. TRUE

Tertiary syphilis may present in various forms:

1. Asymptomatic neurosyphilis; positive CSF serology without symptoms
2. Meningovascular syphilis; either subacute meningitis, an expanding intracranial gumma which causes epilepsy and focal deficits or paraparesis caused by spinal meningovasculitis
3. Tabes dorsalis; lightning pains, ataxia, neuropathic joints, ptosis, optic atrophy and the Argyll Robertson pupil (pupil fixed to light, but responds to accommodation)
4. General paralysis of the insane; progressive dementia, brisk reflexes, extensor plantar reflexes and tremor occur. Death follows within three years of onset.

Ref: Kumar & Clark. Clinical Medicine, 3rd Ed. W. B. Saunders. Ch. 18.

QUESTION 257

A. TRUE B. TRUE C. TRUE D. FALSE E. TRUE

Patients with HIV infection frequently develop neurological disease, which includes: acute meningitis, chronic meningitis, AIDS-dementia complex, encephalitis, CNS lymphoma, progressive multifocal leucoencephalopathy, acute HIV transverse myelitis, myelopathy secondary to viral infection, mononeuropathy, mononeuritis multiplex and polyneuropathy.

Ref: Kumar & Clark. Clinical Medicine, 3rd Ed. W. B. Saunders. Ch. 18.

QUESTION 258

A. TRUE B. TRUE C. FALSE D. TRUE E. TRUE

This disorder was described by Creutzfeld in 1920 and independently by Jakob in 1921. It is transmitted by proteinaceous infectious particles (prions). It causes a progressive dementia associated with cerebellar ataxia, spasticity and extrapyramidal signs. The incubation period is long, sometimes up to several years. Death occurs within two years from onset of symptoms.

Ref: Kumar & Clark. Clinical Medicine, 3rd Ed. W. B. Saunders. Ch. 18.
Gelder, Gath, Mayou & Cowen. Oxford Textbook of Psychiatry. 3rd Ed. Oxford University Press. Ch. 11.

QUESTION 259

A. FALSE B. TRUE C. TRUE D. TRUE E. TRUE

Metatstatic disease accounts for 25% of all intracranial tumours. The most frequently occurring primary lesions in decreasing order of frequency are: bronchus, breast, stomach, prostate, thyroid and kidney.

Ref: Kumar & Clark. Clinical Medicine, 3rd Ed. W. B. Saunders. Ch. 18.

QUESTION 260

A. TRUE B. FALSE C. TRUE D. FALSE E. FALSE

The triad of headache, vomiting and papilloedema in respect to a mass lesion imply that obstruction to CSF flow is occurring. This picture is produced early by lesions in the posterior fossa and as a later event by lesions above the tentorium. Herniation of the cerebellar tonsils through the foramen magnum compresses the medulla to cause impairment of consciousness, respiratory depression, bradycardia, decerebrate posturing and death. Herniation of the uncus of the temporal lobe compresses the third cranial nerve against the petroclinoid ligament and stretching it by downward displacement of the posterior communicating artery. False localising signs are false because they are not related to the site of the mass. The development of false localising signs indicates that brain shift is taking place and urgent surgical intervention may be necessary. Technetium brain scans have a high false negative rate.

Ref: Kumar & Clark. Clinical Medicine, 3rd Ed. W. B. Saunders. Ch. 18.

QUESTION 261

A. FALSE B. FALSE C. TRUE D. TRUE E. FALSE

Benign intracranial hypertension consists of marked papilloedema without other signs. Mass lesions are absent. Ventricular size is normal. Steroids have been implicated as a possible cause. Shunting or surgical decompression may be necessary. Thiazide diuretics reduce the intracranial pressure in this condition. Weight reduction is important. It is a condition occurring mainly in young obese women with menstrual irregularities.

Ref: Kumar & Clark. Clinical Medicine, 3rd Ed. W. B. Saunders. Ch. 18.

QUESTION 262

A. TRUE B. TRUE C. TRUE D. TRUE E. TRUE

There are several types of migraine:

1. Migraine with aura. Prodromal symptoms are usually visual and are related to ischaemia in the distribution of the intracranial artery i.e. scotomata with ophthalmic artery involvement and hemianopia with posterior cerebral artery involvement.

2. Migraine without aura.
3. Basilar migraine. The prodromal features are due to ischaemia of the posterior cerebral circulation. Circumoral tingling, numbness of the tongue, vertigo, diplopia, transient blindness, syncope, dysarthria, and ataxia.
4. Hemiplegic migraine. Classical migraine accompanied by hemiparesis which usually recovers in 24 hours.
5. Ophthalmoplegic migraine. Third nerve palsy occurring during a migraine attack.
6. Facioplegic migraine. Unilateral facial weakness occurring during a migraine attack.

QUESTION 263

A. FALSE B. TRUE C. TRUE D. TRUE E. FALSE

The clinical features include headache felt over the inflamed superficial temporal artery. Arterial pulsation is lost and becomes hard and tortuous. Pain in the face, jaw and mouth is caused by inflammation of the facial, maxillary and lingual branches of the external carotid artery. Pain is made worse on eating (jaw claudication). Visual loss due to inflammation of the ciliary and /or retinal artery occurs in 25% of untreated patients. Amaurosis fugax may precede visual loss. Polymyalgia rheumatica occurs in 50% of patients. Erythema nodosum is not associated with giant cell arteritis.

Ref: Kumar & Clark. Clinical Medicine, 3rd Ed. W. B. Saunders. Ch. 18.

QUESTION 264

A. TRUE B. TRUE C. TRUE D. TRUE E. TRUE

Occlusion of the anterior spinal artery causes an acute paraparesis or tetraplegia with dissociated sensory loss. Pain and temperature sensation are lost below the level, but proprioception, vibration sense, and the perception of light touch are retained. It is caused by any thrombotic or embolic vascular disease (e.g. endocarditis, hypotension, fat embolism, air embolism, decompression sickness, atheroma, diabetes mellitus, syphilis and polyarteritis nodosa). It also occurs in aneurysmal disease of the aorta and by compression by osteophytes in cervical spondylosis.

Ref: Kumar & Clark. Clinical Medicine, 3rd Ed. W. B. Saunders. Ch. 18.

QUESTION 265

A. TRUE B. FALSE C. FALSE D. FALSE E. TRUE

Syringomyelia is a condition in which fluid filled cavities (in continuity with the central canal) occur within the spinal canal. The syrinx gradually destroys the spinothalamic tract, anterior horn cells, and lateral corticospinal tracts. The vestibular system, trigeminal nuclei, sympathetic system and twelfth nerve nuclei may become affected. The signs produced by a syrinx in the cervical region are dissociated sensory loss (i.e. loss of pain and temperature, but not touch and proprioception), lower motor neurone signs in the upper limbs, wasting of the small muscles of the hand and a spastic paraparesis.

If the cavity extends into the brain stem (syringobulbia) there is atrophy of the tongue, nystagmus, Horner's syndrome, hearing loss and impairment of facial sensation. Bony abnormalities at the foramen magnum, spina bifida, Arnold-Chiari malformation or hydrocephalus are often seen in conjunction with syringomyelia.

Ref: Kumar & Clark. Clinical Medicine, 3rd Ed. W. B. Saunders. Ch. 18.

QUESTION 266

A. FALSE B. FALSE C. FALSE D. FALSE E. TRUE

In motor neurone disease there is progressive degeneration of motor neurones in the spinal cord, in the somatic motor nuclei of the cranial nerves and within the cortex. There are never sensory deficits, cerebellar or extrapyramidal signs. Ocular movements are not affected.

There are three patterns of motor neurone disease:

1. Progressive muscular atrophy. This is characterised by peripheral muscle wasting, fasciculation and weakness.
2. Amyotrophic lateral sclerosis. The picture is that of a spastic paraparesis or tetraparesis with lower motor neurone signs and fasciculation.
3. Progressive bulbar palsy. This is characterised by bulbar and pseudobulbar palsy i.e. a mixture of upper motor neurone and lower motor neurone signs in the lower cranial nerves.

Ref: Kumar & Clark. Clinical Medicine, 3rd Ed. W. B. Saunders. Ch. 18.

QUESTION 267

A. FALSE B. FALSE C. TRUE D. TRUE E. TRUE

Neurofibromatosis (von Recklinghausen's diseases), tuberose sclerosis (Bourneville's disease), Huntington's chorea, and von Hippel-Lindau syndrome (retinocerebellar angiomatosis) are all transmitted by autosomal dominant inheritance. Ataxia telangiectasia is a rare autosomal recessive disease where there is a progressive ataxic syndrome in association with immune defects. Sydenham's chorea usually occurs in children as a consequence of beta-haemolytic streptococcal infection.

Ref: Kumar & Clark. Clinical Medicine, 3rd Ed. W. B. Saunders. Ch. 18.

QUESTION 268

A. TRUE B. TRUE C. TRUE D. FALSE E. TRUE

Friedreich's ataxia is usually inherited in an autosomal recessive manner, although an autosomal dominant subset exists as well. It is characterised by degeneration of dorsal root ganglia, spinocerebellar tracts, corticospinal tracts and Purkinje cells of the cerebellum. Clinical manifestations are: ataxia, nystagmus, dysarthria, loss of proprioception, pescavus, kyphoscoliosis, cardiomyopathy and optic atrophy. Adenoma sebaceum is a feature of tuberose sclerosis.

Ref: Kumar & Clark. Clinical Medicine, 3rd Ed. W. B. Saunders. Ch. 18.

QUESTION 269

A. TRUE B. FALSE C. TRUE D. FALSE E. TRUE

The common sites of compression of the peripheral nerves are:

- Carpal tunnel – median nerve
- Cubital tunnel – ulnar nerve
- Spiral groove of humerus – radial nerve
- Supinator muscle – posterior interosseous nerve
- Inguinal ligament – lateral cutaneous nerve of thigh
- Neck of fibula – common peroneal nerve
- Flexor retinaculum – posterior tibial nerve

Ref: Kumar & Clark. Clinical Medicine, 3rd Ed. W. B. Saunders. Ch. 18.

QUESTION 270

A. FALSE B. TRUE C. FALSE D. TRUE E. TRUE

Autonomic neuropathy occurs in the following disorders: uraemia, diabetes, porphyria, amyloidosis and Guillain-Barré syndrome. Thyroid disease may cause a sensorimotor neuropathy. Alcohol abuse is not associated with autonomic neuropathy. The clinical features include postural hypotension, retention of urine, impotence, diarrhoea, diminished sweating, impaired pupillary responses and arrhythmias.

Ref: Kumar & Clark. Clinical Medicine, 3rd Ed. W. B. Saunders. Ch. 18.

QUESTION 271

A. FALSE B. TRUE C. TRUE D. TRUE E. TRUE

Drugs that have been reported to be associated with polyneuropathies are:
Phenytoin, chloramphenicol, procarbazine, isoniazid, dapsone, gold, amphotericin, nitrofurantoin, vincristine, chlorambucil, disulfiram, and cisplatin.

Ref: Kumar & Clark. Clinical Medicine, 3rd Ed. W. B. Saunders. Ch. 18.

QUESTION 272

A. FALSE B. TRUE C. FALSE D. TRUE E. TRUE

Wernicke-Korsakoff syndrome is an encephalopathy associated with alcohol abuse and other causes of thiamine (Vitamin B1) deficiency. It is comprised of a triad of ocular signs, ataxia and confusion. It is due to ischaemic damage to the brain stem and its connections. Untreated it may lead to an irreversible amnesic syndrome and residual brain stem signs. Features include:

- Ocular signs –nystagmus, strabismus
- Ataxia - broad-based gait, cerebellar signs and vestibular palsy (absent response to caloric stimulation)
- Confusion - apathy, confabulation, stupor and coma.
- Thiamine is the treatment of choice and should be given immediately.

Ref: Kumar & Clark. Clinical Medicine, 3rd Ed. W. B. Saunders. Ch. 18.

QUESTION 273

A. TRUE B. FALSE C. FALSE D. FALSE E. FALSE

Subacute combined degeneration of the spinal cord is caused by vitamin B12 deficiency. The signs are of distal sensory loss (posterior column), absent ankle jerks and extensor plantar reflexes. Optic atrophy and retinal haemorrhages may occur. Macrocytosis and megaloblastic changes occur in the bone marrow. Treatment with parenteral B12 reverses the peripheral nerve damage but has little effect on the central nervous system.

Ref: Kumar & Clark. Clinical Medicine, 3rd Ed. W. B. Saunders. Ch. 18.

QUESTION 274

A. TRUE B. FALSE C. TRUE D. TRUE E. FALSE

Polymyositis is characterised by inflammation of skeletal muscle with infiltration by mononuclear cells. Weakness is typically proximal. Investigations show a raised ESR, mild normochromic, normocytic anaemia and raised creatine phosphokinase. The electromyogram shows myopathic changes (short duration spiky polyphasic muscle action potentials with occasional spontaneous fibrillation).

Ref: Kumar & Clark. Clinical Medicine, 3rd Ed. W. B. Saunders. Ch. 18.

QUESTION 275

A. TRUE B. FALSE C. FALSE D. FALSE E. FALSE

This condition is characterised by weakness and fatiguability of muscles associated with IgG antibodies to acetylcholine receptor protein. The heart is not affected. Routine blood tests are normal. The ESR is not raised. Myasthenia gravis can be precipitated by infections, aminoglycosides and magnesium sulphate. Treatment with anticholinesterases commonly produces colic and diarrhoea. Thymectomy offers long term benefit. It improves the prognosis of those patients positive for receptor antibodies and in those who have had the disease for less than ten years. Small cell carcinoma of the bronchus is associated with the myasthenic (Eaton-Lambert) syndrome. The antibody concerned is different and affects acetyl choline release at the NMJ. Weakness improves with muscle contraction and activity unlike myasthenia gravis.

Ref: Kumar & Clark. Clinical Medicine, 3rd Ed. W. B. Saunders. Ch. 18.

QUESTION 276

A. FALSE B. TRUE C. TRUE D. TRUE E. TRUE

Duchenne muscular dystrophy is inherited as an X-linked recessive disorder. A defect has recently been localised to the Xp21 region of the X chromosome. Cardiomyopathy and kyphoscoliosis are common. In the paediatric population many cases of hyperkalaemia, rhabdomyolysis, malignant hyperthermia and acidodis have been reported in patients with biopsy proven Duchenne muscular dystrophy who were given suxamethonium. Gastric dilatation is common in the perioperative period and the prophylactic use of a nasogastric tube is recommended.

Ref: Kumar & Clark. Clinical Medicine, 3rd Ed. W. B. Saunders. Ch. 18.
Katz, Benumof & Kadis. Anesthesia and uncommon diseases. 3rd Ed. W. B. Saunders. Ch. 15.

QUESTION 277

A. FALSE B. FALSE C. TRUE D. FALSE E. FALSE

Dystophia myotonica is characterised by continued muscle contraction after the cessation of voluntary effort. The EMG shows continuous low-voltage activity with high-voltage fibrillation like potential bursts. Nerve conduction studies are normal. Clinical features include cataracts, frontal baldness, intellectual impairment, cardiomyopathy and cardiac conduction defects, hypogonadism, pituitary hypoplasia, glucose intolerance and low serum IgG. Dystrophia myotonia is a disorder of muscle function and is therefore not attenuated by regional local anaesthetic blockade or by competitive muscle relaxants. Anticholinesterases may exacerbate myotonia. Weakness after a heavy carbohydrate meal is a characteristic feature of hypokalaemic periodic paralysis.

Ref: Kumar & Clark. Clinical Medicine, 3rd Ed. W. B. Saunders. Ch. 18.

QUESTION 278

A. FALSE B. TRUE C. TRUE D. FALSE E. TRUE

Myaesthenia gravis is caused by antibody to the acetylcholine receptor on the postsynaptic membrane. Presenting features include ptosis - worse with upgaze, variable strabismus, facial weakness (myasthenic 'snarl' when the patient smiles), nasal weak voice, dysphagia (and sometimes painful swallowing); tendon reflexes are usually normal or increased. It is associated with autoimmune diseases: thyrotoxicosis (5%), hypothyroidism, rheumatoid arthritis, diabetes mellitus, polymyositis, SLE, pernicious anaemia, Sjîgren's syndrome, pemphigus and sarcoid.

Eaton-Lambert syndrome is caused by antibody to presynaptic calcium channels. It is associated with small cell lung carcinoma. Unlike myasthenia, patients exhibit post-exercise increase in power and tendon reflexes (post-tetanic potentiation). Cholinergic drugs have no effect. Treat with guanethidine (increases acetylcholine release from nerve terminals).

QUESTION 279

A. TRUE B. TRUE C. TRUE D. TRUE E. TRUE

Other causes of deterioration include pregnancy, thyrotoxicosis, sepsis, aminoglycosides, CNS depressants, D-penicillamine, hypokalaemia.

QUESTION 280

A. FALSE B. TRUE C. TRUE D. FALSE E. TRUE

The tensilon test is diagnostic for myasthenia gravis: pretreat the patient with atropine to prevent bradycardias and nausea, then test the effects of iv edrophonium and placebo (saline) on muscle power. The test is positive if edrophonium improves power. The false negative rate is approx. 10% due to muscle wasting.

AChR-Ab has approx. 90% sensitivity; approx. 70% in pure ocular myasthenia. False positives seen in first-degree relatives and rheumatoid arthritis patients on D-penicillamine. The EMG finding of post-tetanic inhibition suggests myasthenia while post-tetanic potentiation occurs with Eaton-Lambert syndrome. Creatine kinase is a muscle enzyme and not involved in the diagnosis of NMJ disease.

QUESTION 281

A. FALSE B. TRUE C. TRUE D. TRUE E. FALSE

Myotonic dystrophy has an autosomal dominant inheritance. Age of onset is typically 20-30 years. Clinical features include classical face (long, haggard appearance) and myotonia (tonic spasm of muscle) on percussion. Patients exhibit distal limb and shoulder girdle weakness. Other features include frontal balding, cataracts, cardiac conduction defects and dilated cardiomyopathy, end organ resistance to insulin (DM) and gonadotrophins (atrophy of testes or ovaries), type II respiratory failure (hypoventilation), low IQ.

Treatment: phenytoin, quinine and procainamide may reduce myotonia. Screen family with EMG and provide genetic counselling.

QUESTION 282

A. TRUE B. TRUE C. TRUE D. TRUE E. TRUE

Causes of peripheral neuropathy: (use the mnemonic 'DAM IT BICH ')

Drugs (vincristine, metronidazole, gold, isoniazid (B6 deficiency), phenytoin (folate deficiency), ethambutol, cisplatin, amiodarone);
Alcohol, amyloid;
Metabolic (DM, hypothyroid, CRF, porphyria - acute, intermittent and variegate);
Infection (diptheria, Guillain-Barré syndrome);
Tumour (Ca lung);
B vitamin deficiency (B1, B6, B12);

Idiopathic;
Connective tissue diseases (SLE, PAN) Charcot-Marie tooth;
Heavy metal (Pb/Hg) poisoning.

Painful peripheral neuropathy occurs with diabetic amyotrophy, ethanol, beriberi, drug toxicity (metronidazole), AIDS, Strachan syndrome (orogenital ulcers, sensory neuropathy, amblyopia).

QUESTION 283

A. FALSE B. FALSE C. FALSE D. FALSE E. TRUE

Ménière's disease presents with vertigo, tinnitus and deafness and is thought to be caused by idiopathic dilatation of the endolymph. Treat with prochlorperazine.
Vestibular neuronitis commonly follows a viral infection in younger patients and vascular disease in the elderly. Usually abrupt onset with severe nausea with any movement. May be followed by benign positional vertigo.

Central causes of acute vertigo include multiple sclerosis, brainstem infarct, cerebellar damage (CVA, trauma, etc.), drugs (phenytoin, alcohol). May be seen with Wernicke's encephalopathy.

QUESTION 284

A. FALSE B. TRUE C. TRUE D. FALSE E. FALSE

The pupil is dilated in IIIrd nerve palsy (compressive lesion), Holmes-Adie syndrome (myotonic pupil - often unilateral and poorly responsive to light; associated with reduced or absent ankle and knee reflexes), midbrain lesions, congenital syphilis, anticholinergic treatment (atropine), cocaine intoxication.
Causes of Horner's syndrome include Pancoast's tumour (apical lung carcinoma involving sympathetic chain), iatrogenic (sympathectomy), syringomyelia, lateral medullary syndrome, Shy-Drager syndrome (causes Parkinsonism with postural hypotension and atonic bladder). Other causes of small pupil include myotonic dystrophy, pontine lesions, acute iritis, opiates and organophosphates. The Argyll-Robertson pupil is seen in neurosyphilis - the pupil is unreactive to light but reacts to accommodation (a similar phenomenon may be seen in DM).

QUESTION 285

A. TRUE B. TRUE C. TRUE D. TRUE E. FALSE

Transient ischaemic attacks by definition leave no residual deficit. The cause is usually platelet thromboembolism but may be seen in hyperviscosity states (e.g. polycythaemia, sickle crises and myeloma). 30% of patients will have a completed stroke and of these about 30% will do so in the first 3 months. However, the commonest cause of death in these patients is acute myocardial infarction.

Antiplatelet drugs (aspirin or ticlopidine) reduce non-fatal MI or CVA and vascular mortality. Anticoagulation is advocated for patients with recurrent TIAs not controlled on antiplatelet therapy and patients with cardiac embolic source. Carotid endarterectomy is beneficial in patients with >70% stenosis of the internal carotid artery on the symptomatic side.

QUESTION 286

A. TRUE B. TRUE C. FALSE D. TRUE E. TRUE

Amantadine is a non-specific dopamine receptor antagonist; side-effects include an amphetamine-like effect which may result in insomnia. Benztropine/benzhexol are anticholinergic drugs that are used for relief of bradykinesia or tremor. Selegiline is a MAO-B (monoamine oxidase type B) inhibitor and trials show that it delays disability in patients with Parkinson's disease. L-DOPA is usually combined in preparations with a peripheral dopa-decarboxylase inhibitor (Madopar = L-dopa + benserazide; Sinemet = L-dopa + carbidopa) to reduce the side-effects. Dopamine is antagonised by phenothiazines such as chlorpromazine. Psychosis in patients with Parkinson's disease may respond to clozapine.

QUESTION 287

A. TRUE B. TRUE C. TRUE D. TRUE E. TRUE

Type I neurofibromatosis (von Recklinghausen's disease) is autosomal dominant (gene on Chr 17). Clinical manifestations include:

- Skin: Cafe au lait spots: more than 5, >1.5 cm diameter, axillary freckling, subcutaneous or dermal nodules;
- Pulmonary fibrosis and 'honeycomb' appearance on CXR. Rib notching from neurofibromata may also be seen on the CXR;
- Eyes: Lisch nodules in iris (melanocytic hamartomas), retinal white dots (astrocytic hamartomas) and exophthalmos;
- Sarcomatous change occurs in 5-15% of neurofibromata. Nerve compression;
- Other tumours: Gliomas, meningiomas, medulloblastomas, phaeochromocytoma and medullary carcinoma of thyroid.

QUESTION 288

A. TRUE B. FALSE C. FALSE D. TRUE E. FALSE

The commonest presentation of motor neurone disease is upper limb fasiculation and spastic gait (amyotrophic lateral sclerosis). 25% of patients have mainly lower motor neurone changes (progressive muscular atrophy) and carry a better prognosis. 25% present with progressive bulbar palsy and either flaccid, spastic or combined bulbar symptoms. Patients in this group usually die before their limbs are involved. There is no effective therapy (beta-IFN is used for selected patients with multiple sclerosis). Recently, riluzole (an 'anti-excitotoxic agent') has been reported to prolong tracheostomy-free survival in patients with amyotrophic lateral sclerosis, slow the deterioration in muscle strength and prolong survival. However, only 2 randomised trials have been reported and further data is awaited. There are usually no sensory symptoms (rarely subclinical involvement seen on nerve conduction studies) and it never affects extra-ocular movements (III, IV and VI).

QUESTION 289

A. TRUE B. TRUE C. TRUE D. TRUE E. TRUE

Other causes include: postural hypotension, carotid sinus hypersensitivity, cardiac dysrhythmia, micturition syncope, raised intracranial pressure (especially when coughing or sneezing), hyperventilation and anxiety, drug or alcohol ingestion

QUESTION 290

A. TRUE B. FALSE C. FALSE D. TRUE E. FALSE

Temporal lobe epilepsy is the commonest form of epilepsy following prolonged febrile convulsions. MRI scans on such patients show temporal lobe fibrosis which is thought to be the pathological epileptic focus. TLE is rare in childhood. Treatments: carbamazepine, vigabatrin or lamotrigine. Note in the classification of seizure types: 'Partial' = one hemisphere involved; 'General' = both hemispheres involved (e.g. tonic-clonic 'grand mal' seizures); 'Simple' = no impairment of consciousness (e.g. focal motor seizure). Partial seizures and simple seizures may secondarily generalise with both hemispheres becoming involved. TLE is a form of complex, partial seizure. Petit mal is a generalised seizure and not a complex partial seizure (like TLE).

QUESTION 291

A. FALSE B. TRUE C. TRUE D. FALSE E. FALSE

Other causes of intracranial calcification include craniopharyngioma, pineal, tuberose sclerosis, toxoplasmosis, CMV, TB, cystercicosis, berry aneurysm. Hyperparathyroidism causes basal ganglia calcification.

QUESTION 292

A. FALSE B. TRUE C. TRUE D. TRUE E. FALSE

The risk factors for developing intracranial aneurysms are increasing age and smoking. They are also seen in association with coarctation of the aorta, renal artery stenosis, Ehlers–Danlos syndrome, polyarteritis nodosa, Wegener's granulomatosis and infective endocarditis. 90% arise from the anterior communicating artery. Mycotic aneurysms from septic emboli tend to be peripheral (smaller vessels 'distal' in the vascular tree) and multiple.

QUESTION 293

A. TRUE B. FALSE C. TRUE D. TRUE E. TRUE

Lesions of the hypothalamus are seen with: tumour (craniopharyngioma, glioma), granulomata, histiocytosis X, radiation to pituitary or trauma. The nuclei of the hypothalamus are important in regulating appetite, sleep, body temperature and drinking and lesions may affect one or all of these homeostatic functions.

QUESTION 294

A. TRUE B. TRUE C. FALSE D. TRUE E. FALSE

After closed head injury with loss of consciousness, there is commonly a period of retrograde amnesia which shrinks with time. The duration of post-traumatic amnesia does not shrink with time. Other recognised sequelae include benign postural vertigo, 'punch-drunk' syndrome (dementia with extrapyramidal and long tract signs), chronic subdural and hydrocephalus.

QUESTION 295

A. TRUE B. FALSE C. TRUE D. FALSE E. TRUE

Other causes of raised total protein in the CSF include chronic ethanol intake, amyloid, diabetes mellitus, acoustic neuroma and saggital sinus thrombosis, but all are very rare.

Benign intracranial hypertension is commonly a disease of obese young women taking the oral contraceptive pill. Other drugs implicated are tetracyclines and hypervitaminosis A. Clinical features include papilloedema and headaches but no dilatation of the ventricles on CT scan of the brain. Treated by repeated lumbar puncture, diuretics and/or shunt.

QUESTION 296

A. TRUE B. TRUE C. FALSE D. TRUE E. TRUE

Primary hypothyroidism refers to failure (and atrophy) of the thyroid gland. Causes include autoimmune thyroid disease (associated with IDDM, Addison's disease or pernicious anaemia), Hashimoto's thyroiditis (years later), post-surgery or radioiodine therapy, drug-induced (especially amiodarone), dietary iodine-deficiency or congenital. Secondary hypothyroidism follows pituitary failure.

Clinical features of hypothyroidism (primary and secondary) include dry skin and hair, menorrhagia, muscle cramps, infertility, pericardial and pleural effusions, periorbital oedema, raised CPK, raised serum cholesterol, gout, delusions ('myxoedema madness'), bradycardia and slow-relaxing reflexes.

Features favouring secondary (pituitary) hypothyroidism are signs of hypopituitarism (hypopigmentation, etc.), normal cholesterol, TSH not elevated in spite of low free T4, no rise in TSH on infusion of TRH.

QUESTION 297

A. FALSE B. TRUE C. TRUE D. FALSE E. TRUE

Coma may be the presenting feature of hypothyroidism in the elderly and may be complicated by severe hypothermia. Other features include hyporeflexia, bradycardia and seizures. Precipitants include sepsis, acute MI, stroke, immobility or trauma.

After taking blood for T3, T4 and TSH (and excluding other causes of coma, e.g. hypogly-caemia, etc.) treatment should be started with iv T3 or T4; hydrocortisone should be given if pituitary hypothyroidism is suspected. Treat hypothermia and heart failure in the standard way. Survival ~80% with appropriate therapy.

Ref: Kumar & Clark. Clinical Medicine, 3rd Ed. W. B. Saunders. Ch. 16.

QUESTION 298

A. TRUE B. FALSE C. FALSE D. TRUE E. FALSE

Thyroid storm refers to severe hyperthyroidism and is a medical emergency. The initial treat-ment should be with propylthiouracil (PTU - 200 mg q 6h): this is better than carbimazole as it stops peripheral conversion of T4 to T3. This should be followed with IV iodide, 1 hour after PTU has been given. Steroids are usually given to try to prevent Addisonian crisis (which may be masked by the severe thyrotoxicosis); they also inhibit T4 release and peripheral conversion. Other measures include fluids, fanning, tepid sponging and full supportive treatment. Mortality is reported as 10%.

Causes of thyrotoxicosis: Graves' disease, toxic nodule, metastases of follicular carcinoma of the thyroid (can make T4), Hashimoto's (lymphocytic) thyroiditis (in the acute phase), acute viral thyroiditis, extrinsic compression of thyroid by mass, amiodarone and struma ovarii (TSH-secreting ovarian carcinoma).

Ref: Kumar & Clark. Clinical Medicine, 3rd Ed. W. B. Saunders. Ch. 16.

QUESTION 299

A. TRUE B. FALSE C. FALSE D. FALSE E. TRUE

de Quervain's thyroiditis is a transient thyrotoxic state characterised by a tender goitre, fever, malaise, neck pain and tachycardia. The F:M ration is 2:1. Giant cells are seen on biopsy and there is suppression of uptake on radioisotope (Tc-99) scans. The aetiology is probably viral (not bacterial).

Other types of thyroiditis:

1. *Hashimoto's* (F>>M, diffuse painless goitre full of lymphocytes on biopsy; associated with HLA DR5 and anti-thyroid antibodies; approx. 80% of patients will get hypothyroidism later);
2. *Riedel's* (fibrosis of thyroid; associated with other fibrosing diseases, e.g. retroperitoneal fibrosis, Peyronie's disease, sclerosing cholangitis; approx. 50% of patients will get hypothyroidism later);
3. *Post-partum thyroiditis* (F>M, similar to Hashimoto's with painless goitre, transient thyrotoxicosis ± transient hypothyroidism and lymphocytes in biopsy).

Ref: Kumar & Clark. Clinical Medicine, 3rd Ed. W. B. Saunders. Ch. 16.

QUESTION 300

A. FALSE B. TRUE C. TRUE D. TRUE E. TRUE

Thyroid eye disease is associated with specific autoantibodies that produce retro-orbital inflammation and lymphocytic infiltration of the extraocular muscles. Antibodies against the thyroid may also be present although the patient is not always biochemically or clinically hyperthyroid. Main impairment is in up and lateral gaze. Treatment: eyedrops, Fresnel prisms, retroorbital/systemic steroids, lateral tarsoraphy, muscle transposition, orbital decompression, cyclosporin, orbital radiotherapy and sometimes plasmapheresis.

In Graves' disease, T4 is responsible for lid lag and retraction, diarrhoea, linear growth acceleration in children and AF. Acropachy and proptosis are not related to the T4 levels. Other findings are hypercalciuria (not hypercalcaemia) and periosteal new bone formation.

Causes of uniocular proptosis: contralateral Horner's (i.e. a misdiagnosis), axial proptosis along the axis of the eyeball (optic nerve glioma, meningioma, Graves') *vs* non-axial (lymphoma, metastasis to orbit, pseudotumour oculi (seen with Riedel's thyroiditis), cavernous sinus pathology, Wegener's disease).

*Ref: **Kumar & Clark. Clinical Medicine, 3rd Ed. W. B. Saunders. Ch. 16.***

QUESTION 301

A. FALSE B. TRUE C. FALSE D. FALSE E. TRUE

Graves' disease in pregnancy is associated with fetal hyperthyroidism due to maternal antibodies crossing the placenta and causing (in essence) fetal Graves' disease. Fetal heart rate provides a direct biological assay of thyroid status. Neonates are hyperthyroid as the maternal antibody persists for up to 2 months and may need treatment with propylthiouracil. Signs include irritability, failure to thrive, weight loss, diarrhoea and eye signs. Thyroid function tests are difficult to interpret in neonates. Carbimazole is worse than propylthiouracil at causing neonatal goitre. Radioiodine cannot be used as it causes cretinism and goitre. Maternal T4 does not easily cross the placenta.

Side-effects of the anti-thyroid drugs (propylthiouracil and carbimazole): agranulocytosis (approx. 0.1% of patients), rash, fever, arthralgia, and jaundice.

*Ref: **Kumar & Clark. Clinical Medicine, 3rd Ed. W. B. Saunders. Ch. 16.***

QUESTION 302

A. TRUE B. TRUE C. TRUE D. TRUE E. TRUE

Primary adrenal failure is associated with hyperpigmentation (palmar creases and buccal mucosa of Caucasians). In patients where this is due to an autoimmune process, other autoimmune disorders such as vitiligo, diabetes mellitus and myasthenia gravis are more common. Common abnormalities on investigation include eosinophilia (mechanism unknown), low sodium, raised or normal potassium, raised urea, mild metabolic acidosis, hypocalcaemia or hypercalcaemia (seen in about 6%, mechanism uncertain). The ECG shows low voltage QRS complexes and T waves (the hyperkalaemia is usually too mild to produce any of the typical changes), prolongation of the PR interval and the corrected QT interval. The patients have an increase in ADH secretion (in response to the hypovolaemia produced by hypoadrenalism) and so exhibit a delay in the excretion of a free water load (this may used as a diagnostic test).

Patients with secondary adrenal failure usually exhibit pallor (due to pituitary failure). In these patients aldosterone is preserved so the electrolytes are less affected. However, the patients may still get hypovolaemia from diarrhoea and vomiting or diabetes insipidus (resulting in raised urea), and hyponatraemia due to SIADH or hypothyroidism.

Ref: Kumar & Clark. Clinical Medicine, 3rd Ed. W. B. Saunders. Ch. 16.

QUESTION 303

A. FALSE B. TRUE C. FALSE D. TRUE E. TRUE

Cushing's syndrome results in loss of the diurnal rhythm of cortisol secretion and produces a persistently elevated serum (and 24 hour urine) cortisol.

Adrenal tumours usually do not suppress with dexamethasone. Serum ACTH is undetectable. In Cushing's disease (i.e. adrenal hyperplasia due to excess pituitary ACTH secretion), there may be some suppression of the serum cortisol with high-dose dexamethasone but usually not to normal values. Serum ACTH is elevated but less than in ectopic ACTH production. Hypokalaemia suggests ectopic ACTH secretion (and is often associated with mild alkalosis). Only 10-30% of patients with ectopic ACTH secretion suppress with high-dose dexamethasone.

Metyrapone inhibits 11-beta-hydroxylase (a step in the synthesis of cortisol) and results in a loss in the negative feedback of cortisol on the pituitary. This produces a rise in ACTH secretion and a rise in urinary 17-oxogenic steroids (17-OGS). In pituitary Cushing's, metyrapone produces a large rise in urinary 17-OGS: in ectopic ACTH secretion or adrenal tumours, although serum cortisol levels fall, there is usually no increase in urinary 17-OGS.

Patients with depression and alcoholism may exhibit 'pseudo-Cushing's' - this is thought to be due to an increase in release of CRF by the hypothalamus. They will increase 24-hour urine cortisol, loss of diurnal secretion of cortisol; low-dose dexamethasone may fail to suppress the serum cortisol but this will almost invariably suppress with high-dose dexamethasone.

Ref: Kumar & Clark. Clinical Medicine, 3rd Ed. W. B. Saunders. Ch. 16.

QUESTION 304

A. TRUE B. FALSE C. FALSE D. FALSE E. TRUE

Any cause of Cushing's syndrome results in loss of the diurnal rhythm of cortisol secretion and produces a persistently elevated serum (and 24-hour urine) cortisol. Serum ACTH is undetectable with adrenal tumours; an exaggerated response to CRF administration is seen in pituitary-dependent Cushing's syndrome. Adrenal tumours usually do not suppress with dexamethasone (low or high dose).

Metyrapone inhibits 11-beta-hydroxylase (a step in the synthesis of cortisol) and results in a loss in the negative feedback of cortisol on the pituitary. This produces a rise in ACTH secretion and a rise in urinary 17-oxogenic steroids (17-OGS). It may be used in the diagnosis of Cushing's syndrome: in pituitary Cushing's, metyrapone produces a large rise in urinary 17-OGS while in ectopic ACTH secretion or adrenal tumours, although serum cortisol levels may fall, there is usually no change in urinary 17-OGS excretion. Prior to surgery, it is important to reduce cortisol levels to 300-400 nmol/l and metyrapone (or aminogluthemide) may be used.

QUESTION 305

A. TRUE B. TRUE C. FALSE D. FALSE E. TRUE

Adrenal tumours are incidental findings in about 1% of abdominal CT scans. If >6 cm in diameter, there is a 90% risk of malignancy; small tumours are usually benign. Most tumours are non-functional but patients should be screened to exclude Conn's syndrome, phaeochromocytoma or Cushing's (serum electrolytes, postural drop in blood pressure, urine catecholamines (and VMA or metanephrines)).

Multiple endocrine neoplasia type 1 (Werner's syndrome) is the association of parathyroid adenomas (90%), pituitary adenomas (60%) and pancreatic tumours (50%). Other features not in the definition include adrenal tumours (40%) and thyroid carcinoma (20%). The gene is found on chr 11 and the disorder exhibits dominant inheritance. Family members should be screened by a fasting serum calcium (raised in affected individuals).

QUESTION 306

A. FALSE B. TRUE C. TRUE D. TRUE E. TRUE

Multiple endocrine neoplasia type IIa (Sipple's syndrome) is the association of phaeochromocytoma (hypertension, often malignant, multiple, and extra-adrenal), medullary carcinoma of the thyroid (secretion of calcitonin causes flushing) and parathyroid hyperplasia (and occasionally gliomas or meningiomas).

Multiple endocrine neoplasia type III (= MEN IIb) has the same features as MEN type IIa but in addition is associated with a Marfanoid habitus, mucosal and intestinal neuromata; protruberent lips produce a characteristic facies. Hyperparathyroidism is relatively rare.

The gene for this (IIa and IIb) has been termed the ret locus and is located on chromosome 10.

QUESTION 307

A. TRUE B. FALSE C. TRUE D. FALSE E. FALSE

Renin is released from the juxtaglomerular apparatus in response to decrease in renal blood flow (e.g. pressure changes in the afferent arteriole, sympathetic tone within the renal arterioles), increased chloride (low Na) and osmotic changes in the distal tubule via macula densa and local prostaglandin synthesis. It converts angiotensinogen to angiotensin I; this is converted to angiotensin II by ACE (mainly in the lungs). Angiotensin II stimulates aldosterone release by the zona glomerulosa of the adrenal cortex; other effects include peripheral vasoconstriction and stimulation of thirst.

Increase in serum renin is seen in renal artery stenosis, congestive cardiac failure, hypovolaemia, hypotension, certain drugs (diuretics, ACE inhibitors, spironolactone) and Addison's disease. Serum renin is reduced by beta-blocker therapy, ANP or angiotensin II infusion. Hypertension may be associated with a low, normal or high renin.

QUESTION 308

A. FALSE B. FALSE C. FALSE D. TRUE E. FALSE

Congenital adrenal hyperplasia is most commonly due to 21-hydroxylase deficiency (90%); less commonly 11-hydroxylase or 3-beta-hydroxysteroid dehydrogenase deficiency. All are autosomal recessive, can cause male precocious puberty, have a low serum cortisol (and high ACTH) and have large adrenals on CT scanning. Clinical features depends on the enzyme defect:

*   *21-hydroxylase deficiency* produces vomiting, dehydration (salt-losing picture in over 70%: not HYPERtension), virilization in girls; boys display precocious puberty or ambiguous genitalia (increase in 17-hydroxyprogesterone)
*   *11-hydroxylase deficiency* produces raised 11-deoxycortisol (acts as a mineralocorticoid to produce hypertension and low potassium similar to Conn's syndrome) in addition to virilisation;
*   *incomplete masculinization* (hypospadias with cryptorchidism) is seen with 3-beta-hydrox ysteroid dehydrogenase deficiency.

Treat with glucocorticoids (and mineralocorticoids as necessary) aiming to normalize ACTH and 17-OH progesterone levels.

QUESTION 309   WITHDRAWN

A. FALSE B. TRUE C. TRUE D. TRUE E. FALSE

Causes of cataracts include hypoparathyroidism ('stellate' - punctate and radially distributed), DM (classical 'snowflake' cataract with IDDM), Wilson's disease ('sunflower' - does not usually impair vision), myotonic dystrophy ('scintillatory' cataract), steroid therapy, chronic uveitis, radiation damage, trauma, maternal rubella, ricketts, Marfan's syndrome, galactosaemia and Still's disease.

QUESTION 310

A. TRUE B. TRUE C. TRUE D. TRUE E. FALSE

Primary hyperparathyroidism most commonly presents as (or is diagnosed because of) asymptomatic hypercalcaemia: a normal PTH in the presence of hypercalcaemia is inappropriate and suggests hyperparathyroidism. Symptoms from hypercalcaemia may be non-specific (abdominal pains, constipation, depression), or result from renal calculi, pancreatitis, peptic ulcer (calcium causes gastrin release). Bone disease (cysts or fractures) may occur. Hypertension may occur and although initially due to hypercalcaemia, does not always respond to lowering the serum calcium level. Urinary calcium, cAMP and hydroxyproline excretion are all increased and there may be a mild hyperchloraemic metabolic acidosis.

Most commonly due to a single adenoma (90%). MEN type I produces parathyroid hyperplasia in association with pituitary adenoma and pancreatic islet cell tumours. In MEN type IIa and IIb, parathyroid tumours are associated with medullary thyroid carcinoma and phaeochromocytoma.

Cutaneous moniliasis, vitiligo and cataracts are features of HYPOparathyroidism

QUESTION 311

A. TRUE B. FALSE C. TRUE D. FALSE E. TRUE

Patients with acromegaly have hypercalciuria and renal stones (direct action of GH on renal tubules) but rarely have hypercalcaemia (only where acromegaly forms part of multiple endocrine neoplasia type I: parathyroid hyperplasia, pituitary and pancreatic tumours). There is an increased risk of colonic polyps which may be malignant. Excessive daytime drowsiness is seen as an enlargement of the tongue produces obstructive sleep apnoea. Other features include DM, osteoarthritis, carpal tunnel syndrome, hypertension, cardiomyopathy and skin tags. Biochemical abnormalities include raised serum phosphate, hyperglycaemia, raised triglycerides and prolactin.

Growth hormone secretion is stimulated by high protein meals and suppressed by glucose in normal individuals. In acromegaly, basal growth hormone levels are raised and these fail to suppress after a glucose load; other conditions where GH fails to suppress include poorly controlled diabetes mellitus, myxoedema, Cushing's syndrome and anorexia nervosa.

The major cause of morbidity and mortality in patients with acromegaly is cardiovascular (myocardial infarction).

QUESTION 312

A. TRUE B. FALSE C. TRUE D. FALSE E. FALSE

Nelson's syndrome is a rare condition that follows bilateral adrenalectomy. There is loss of the feedback inhibition by cortisol on the pituitary and an increase in secretion of ACTH and MSH (melanocyte stimulating hormone); the latter produces hyperpigmentation. Pituitary radiotherapy after adrenalectomy may prevent it. Pituitary enlargement may cause a bitemporal hemianopia.

Sheehan's syndrome is pituitary necrosis following post-partum haemorrhage and hypovolaemia. Symptoms are those of pan-hypopituitarism with loss of LH/FSH (loss of libido, amenorrhoea, impotence, etc.), TSH (hypothyroidism), ACTH (Addison's - recurrent hypoglycaemia), GH and prolactin.

QUESTION 313

A. TRUE B. FALSE C. TRUE D. TRUE E. TRUE

Appetite, sleep, body temperature and thirst are controlled by the hypothalamus and lesions may affect any of these functions. Lesions of the hypothalamus may be caused by tumour (e.g. craniopharyngioma, glioma), granuloma (TB, sarcoid), histiocytosis X, spread of radiation to pituitary and trauma. The hypothalamus produces dopamine which inhibits prolactin release from the pituitary: lesions of the hypothalamus will result in HYPERprolactinaemia.

QUESTION 314

A. FALSE B. TRUE C. FALSE D. TRUE E. FALSE

Gestational diabetes is associated with macrosomia and sudden fetal death, not cardiac defects or other fetal congenital abnormalities: the risk of sudden death is increased with poor diabetic control. It is usually seen in the second trimester and carries a higher risk of subsequent diabetes mellitus. Diagnosis usually requires an oral glucose tolerance test as the renal threshold for glucose is reduced in pregnancy (so glycosuria does not necessarily imply DM). The OGTT often returns to normal between pregnancies but diabetes recurs with subsequent pregnancies.

QUESTION 315

A. TRUE B. TRUE C. TRUE D. TRUE E. FALSE

Autoimmune Addison's may coexist with DM. Autonomic neuropathy produces the dumping syndrome with wide swings in blood glucose. Renal disease reduces insulin requirement and patients on chlorpropamide also get hypos.

QUESTION 316

A. TRUE B. TRUE C. TRUE D. TRUE E. FALSE

The pigmentation in Addison's disease is typically buccal (opposite the molars), on the flexor regions and in recent scars. Loss of body hair may also occur. Pigmentation also occurs in Cushing's syndrome, when purple striae may be seen. Pretibial myxoedema is a non-tender, non-pitting swelling on the anterior surface of the shin seen in Graves disease. Proximal myopathy may occur with both hypothyroidism and thyrotoxicosis. It also occurs with high dose steroids and Cushing's syndrome. Other endocrine causes include acromegaly and osteomalacia.

Ref: Kumar & Clark. Clinical Medicine, 3rd Ed. W. B. Saunders. Ch. 16.

QUESTION 317

A. FALSE B. TRUE C. FALSE D. FALSE E. TRUE

Glucocorticoid, mineralocorticoid and sex steroid production are all reduced in Addison's disease. Adrenal adenomas causing primary hyperaldosteronism (Conn's syndrome) usually present with hypokalaemia and hypertension. Primary hyperparathyroidism is the commonest endocrine abnormality in MEN(1). Pancreatic, pituitary and more rarely thyroid tumours may also be seen. Diabetes insipidus causes a failure of urine concentration, resulting in low urine osmolality and high plasma osmolality. Low urine osmolality with low plasma osmolality suggests an excess water load.

Ref: Kumar & Clark. Clinical Medicine, 3rd Ed. W. B. Saunders. Ch. 16.

QUESTION 318

A. TRUE B. FALSE C. TRUE D. TRUE E. FALSE

Thyroid crisis is a medical emergency with a mortality of 10-20%. Hypokalaemia, hypomagnesaemia and hypercalcaemia occur. Treatment consists of beta-blockers, steroids, antithyroid drugs and iodine. Beta-blockers antagonise the effects of thyroid hormones. Propranolol is the drug of choice as it also inhibits peripheral conversion of T4 to T3. A relative deficiency of steroids may be present (and glucocorticoids also inhibit peripheral T4 to T3 conversion). If patients are allergic to iodine, lithium can be used to block thyroid hormone release.

Ref: Oh. Intensive Care Manual. 4th Ed. Butterworth Heinemann. Ch. 52.

QUESTION 319

A. FALSE B. TRUE C. TRUE D. FALSE E. FALSE

Primary hyperparathyroidism is usually caused by single adenomas (80%). Excess parathyroid hormone is secreted and leads to hypercalcaemia and hypophosphataemia. The hypercalcaemia reduces the concentrating ability of the renal tubules (a form of nephrogenic diabetes insipidus). The hydrocortisone suppression test suppresses hypercalcaemia to normal or near normal levels in sarcoidosis, vitamin D mediated hypercalcaemia and some malignancies. Chvostek's sign occurs in hypocalcaemia and may be seen following parathyroidectomy.

Ref: Kumar & Clark. Clinical Medicine, 3rd Ed. W. B. Saunders. Ch. 16.

QUESTION 320

A. TRUE B. FALSE C. TRUE D. TRUE E. FALSE

The adrenals have an outer cortex with three zones (reticularis, fasciculata and glomerulosa) which produce steroids and an inner medulla producing catecholamines. The steroids are grouped in three classes: glucocorticoids, mineralocorticoids and androgens. Aldosterone is the main mineralocorticoid, and secretion is controlled by the renin/angiotensin system. Glucocorticoid secretion is under hypothalamo/pituitary control via ACTH. Cushing's disease is caused by increased circulating ACTH from pituitary hyperplasia or tumour. Congenital adrenal hyperplasia is an autosomal recessive condition caused by deficiency in an enzyme in the cortisol synthetic pathway.

Ref: Kumar & Clark. Clinical Medicine, 3rd Ed. W. B. Saunders. Ch. 16.

QUESTION 321

A. TRUE B. FALSE C. TRUE D. TRUE E. TRUE

Cushing's syndrome may be due to a primary excess of glucocorticoids (with suppression of ACTH) or a secondary excess caused by increased circulating ACTH from the pituitary (Cushing's disease) or other tumour (e.g. bronchial carcinoma or carcinoid). Pseudo-Cushing's syndrome can be caused by alcohol excess. There are many signs including plethora, thin skin, bruising, purple striae, hypertension and proximal myopathy. Impaired glucose tolerance or frank diabetes mellitus are common.

Ref: Kumar & Clark. Clinical Medicine, 3rd Ed. W. B. Saunders. Ch. 16.

QUESTION 322

A. FALSE B. FALSE C. TRUE D. TRUE E. FALSE

GH secretion from the anterior pituitary is stimulated by growth hormone releasing hormone from the hypothalamus. It causes the hepatic production of insulin like growth factor. GH release is mainly nocturnal, especially during REM sleep, but may also be stimulated by Bovril, exercise, clonidine, arginine and insulin. Excess is usually due to a growth hormone secreting pituitary tumour.

Ref: Kumar & Clark. Clinical Medicine, 3rd Ed. W. B. Saunders. Ch. 16.

QUESTION 323

A. TRUE B. TRUE C. TRUE D. TRUE E. TRUE

Acromegaly is usually due to a growth hormone secreting pituitary tumour. These are often large, and lateral skull X-ray is abnormal in 90%. Untreated acromegaly results in increased mortality from hypertension, heart failure, and coronary artery disease. Treatment may be surgical (trans-sphenoidal or trans-frontal approach), radiotherapy or medical (octreotide or bromocriptine).

Ref: Kumar & Clark. Clinical Medicine, 3rd Ed. W. B. Saunders. Ch. 16.

QUESTION 324

A. FALSE B. FALSE C. FALSE D. FALSE E. TRUE

Multiple pituitary hormone deficiencies may occur due to compression by a large tumour. GH and the gonadotrophins are usually affected first. TSH and ACTH are affected late. Hyperprolactinaemia may occur because of the loss of inhibitory control by dopamine. Bitemporal hemianopias or upper temporal quadrantanopias are the commonest visual field defects. Sheehan's syndrome is caused by pituitary infarction following PPH. Kallmann's is a syndrome of isolated gonadotrophin deficiency. Nelson's syndrome may occur after adrenalectomy and consists of an ACTH secreting pituitary tumour causing local effects and pigmentation.

Ref: Kumar & Clark. Clinical Medicine, 3rd Ed. W. B. Saunders. Ch. 16.

QUESTION 325

A. TRUE B. TRUE C. TRUE D. FALSE E. FALSE

Polyarteritis nodosa is initially non-specific though is later characterised by renal impairment, hypertension, polyneuropathy, lung disease, arrhythmias and heart failure. Rheumatoid arthritis also causes vasculitis but is not commonly associated with hypertension. Congenital adrenal hyperplasia leads to cortisol deficiency and, more rarely, aldosterone deficiency. It may present early with adrenal failure. Hypertension is not a feature.

Ref: Kumar & Clark. Clinical Medicine, 3rd Ed. W. B. Saunders. Chs 8 and 16.

QUESTION 326

A. FALSE B. TRUE C. FALSE D. TRUE E. FALSE

90% of phaeochromocytomas arise in the adrenal, and 90% are benign. Urinary 5HIAA is used in the diagnosis of carcinoid syndrome (urinary VMA for phaeochromocytoma). MIBG scanning is useful for localising extra-adrenal tumours. Treatment should start with alpha blockade, followed by beta blockade if necessary.

Ref: Kumar & Clark. Clinical Medicine, 3rd Ed. W. B. Saunders. Ch. 16.

QUESTION 327

A. TRUE B. TRUE C. FALSE D. TRUE E. FALSE

20-70% of patients receiving long term lithium therapy have some degree of nephrogenic diabetes insipidus. Amphotericin B may also cause it (though resolution after starting the liposomal counterpart has been described). Nicotine increases secretion of ADH. Central diabetes insipidus may occur after head injury or brain death.

Ref: Oh. Intensive Care Manual. 4th Ed. Butterworth Heinemann. Ch. 51.

QUESTION 328

A. TRUE B. FALSE C. TRUE D. FALSE E. TRUE

Both autonomic and somatic neuropathies of many different types may complicate diabetes mellitus. Particularly important are vagal neuropathies resulting initially in resting tachycardia and loss of sinus arrhythmia., but later causing denervation (when the heart resembles one post-transplant). Renal lesions (one of which is the Kimmelstein–Wilson lesion) lead initially to microalbuminuria. This is defined as the renal loss of albumin greater than normal but too small to be detected by dipsticks.

Ref: Kumar & Clark. Clinical Medicine, 3rd Ed. W. B. Saunders. Ch. 17.

QUESTION 329

A. FALSE B. TRUE C. TRUE D. FALSE E. FALSE

Hyperglycaemic emergencies may be precipitated by thiazide diuretics, steroids or an inter-current illness. Gastric stasis occurs commonly in DKA. Cerebral oedema may be caused by the rapid correction of hyperosmolality and is more common in children and young adults. DKA is an absolute indication for long term insulin treatment. It has a lower mortality (1-10%) than HONK (40-70%).

Ref: Kumar & Clark. Clinical Medicine, 3rd Ed. W. B. Saunders. Ch. 17.
Oh. Intensive Care Manual. 4th Ed. Butterworth Heinemann. Ch. 50.

QUESTION 330

A. TRUE B. TRUE C. FALSE D. TRUE E. TRUE

Ketoconazole and fluconazole may precipitate acute adrenal insufficiency, which inhibit steroid synthesis. A tetracosactrin test (ACTH stimulation test) can be performed immediately provided there is no undue delay in corticosteroid administration. Fludrocortisone is unnecessary acutely as high dose hydrocortisone provides sufficient mineralocorticoid activity. It should be introduced later.

Ref: Kumar & Clark. Clinical Medicine, 3rd Ed. W. B. Saunders. Ch. 16.
Oh. Intensive Care Manual. 4th Ed. Butterworth Heinemann. Ch. 53.

QUESTION 331

A. TRUE B. FALSE C. TRUE D. TRUE E. FALSE

The porphyrias are a group of disorders of haem synthesis. Acute intermittent porphyria (AIP) is characterised by an inherited deficiency of porphobilinogen deaminase. In the latent phase of AIP, the activity of this enzyme may be used to aid the diagnosis . Due to a negative feed-back loop involving the end product (haem), 5 amino laevulinate (ALA) synthase activity is increased leading to an increase in ALA and porphobilinogen (PBG) which are excreted in the urine. As the enzyme defect in AIP is early in the metabolic chain there is no increase in faecal metabolites. Although the condition is inherited as a Mendelian dominant it is more common in women. Skin lesions do not occur in AIP. They only occur in situation were there is excessive production of porphyrins.

Ref: Zilva JF, Pannall PR & Mayne PD. Clinical Chemistry in Diagnosis and Treatment.

QUESTION 332

A. FALSE B. FALSE C. TRUE D. TRUE E. FALSE

The porphyrias are a group of diseases characterised by overproduction and excretion of porphyrins; porphyrins are intermediate compounds produced during haem synthesis.

Each disease form results from a specific enzyme defect, porphobilinogen deaminase in the case of AIP. There is no protoporphyrin in the urine as this compound appears downstream in the pathway from the abnormal enzyme. Urine from these patients goes red-brown on standing; Ehrlich's aldehyde is part of a different bedside test and is performed by mixing equal volumes of urine and reagent. The result is a pink colouration which persists if 2 volumes of chloroform are added. Abdominal pain, vomiting, polyneuropathy, hypertension and neuropsychiatric disorders may all be presenting features. Photosensitivity occurs in variegate porphyria, hereditary coproporphyria and porphyria cutanea tarda, but is not a feature of AIP.

Ref: Kumar & Clark. Clinical Medicine, 3rd Ed. W. B. Saunders. Ch. 17.

QUESTION 333

A. FALSE B. TRUE C. TRUE D. TRUE E. FALSE

Nicotinic acid is synthesised from niacin (found in plants, fish, offal or synthesised from tryptophan) and can be converted to nicotinamide (part of NAD and NADP). The latter two act as hydrogen acceptors in oxidative reactions and thus in electron transport. Cholecalciferol requires hydroxylation at the 1- and 25-position to generate the active 1, 25-dihydroxycholecalciferol, the active form of Vitamin D. Folic acid is metabolised to tetrahydrofolate which serves as an intermediate carrier of hydroxymethyl, formyl and methyl groups, necessary for purine and pyramidine biosynthesis. Many antimetabolite and immunosuppressive drugs (e.g. methotrexate) depend on inhibition of these reactions. Pyridoxal phosphate (B6) is involved in amino acid metabolism. Thiamine is involved in the glycolytic pathway and the pentose phosphate shunt.

QUESTION 334

A. TRUE B. FALSE C. TRUE D. TRUE E. TRUE

Features of zinc deficiency include acrodermatitis enteropathica, alopecia, poor wound healing, impaired taste sensation and photophobia. Vitamin C deficiency (not Vitamin A) results in scurvy - fatigue, weakness, arthralgia, gingivitis, poor wound healing, purpura, subperiosteal haemorrhages. Vitamin A deficiency is associated with night-blindness, Bitot's spots and hyperkeratosis. Clinical manifestations of iron deficiency include anaemia, koilonychia, atrophic glossitis, angular stomatitis, candidiasis and pica. Niacin deficiency results in pellagra - diarrhoea, dermatitis and dementia. Other features include glossitis and Casal's necklace (dermatitis in the exposed area around the neck). Copper deficiency results in hypochromic, microcytic anaemia and disordered keratinisation.

QUESTION 335

A. TRUE B. TRUE C. TRUE D. TRUE E. FALSE

Gluconeogenesis can take place from lactate, glycerol (from triglyceride metabolism) and amino acids. 90% occurs in the liver in the initial stages, but as the body continues in a state of starvation, other organs can contribute; the kidney may later produce up to 50% of the body requirement of glucose. Lipolysis releases triglycerides which are broken down to glycerol and free fatty acids. These are metabolised to acetyl CoA and diverted to ketone body production as acetyl CoA cannot directly be used for gluconeogenesis.

QUESTION 336

A. TRUE B. TRUE C. TRUE D. FALSE E. FALSE

Lactic acidosis results from accumulation of lactic acid sufficient to cause changes in blood pH. Normal concentrations are 0.6-1.2 mmol/l but this may rise to 10 mmol/l after severe physical exercise, rapidly returning to normal on stopping exertion. The causes are divided into Type A - precipitated by any cause of severe tissue hypoxia (e.g. haemorrhagic shock or MI with severe LVF), and Type B - no features of tissue hypoperfusion except as a late event, and is due to disturbed metabolism of lactate (e.g. liver disease, uraemia, debilitated patients, diabetics given metformin, some leukaemias, etc.). The natural isomer is L-lactate and the body is unable to metabolise the D-isomer. Rarely, alterations in gut flora in patients can result in absorption and accumulation of this isomer and acidosis (clinically - confusion, ataxia, nystagmus, stupor; treated with iv bicarbonate, thiamine and antibiotics to alter gut flora).

Ref: Kumar & Clark. Clinical Medicine, 3rd Ed. W. B. Saunders. Ch. 10.

QUESTION 337

A. TRUE B. TRUE C. TRUE D. FALSE E. FALSE

A protein meal stimulates both insulin and glucagon secretion; the glucagon prevents the hypoglycaemia that would result from the increased insulin levels if there were no carbohydrate with the protein. Somatostatin infusion inhibits both insulin and glucagon secretion and produces hypoglycaemia, suggesting that glucagon is essential for the liver to release glucose. In addition, cortisol and growth hormone are required for normal glucose efflux from the liver. ILGF-I and ILGF-II are peptides that appear to function primarily as growth factors rather than influencing glucose uptake by tissues. ILGF-I is synthesised by the liver in response to growth hormone (not insulin). Beta-oxidation of free fatty acids to form acetyl CoA and ketone bodies provides the energy required for gluconeogenesis in starvation. This is inhibited by insulin.

QUESTION 338

A. TRUE B. FALSE C. TRUE D. FALSE E. FALSE

Hyperuricaemia may be caused by increased uric acid production or decreased excretion: Increased production: HGPRT deficiency (Lesch-Nyhan syndrome - choreoathetosis, self-mutilation, mental deficiency, gout), glucose-6-phosphatase deficiency, hereditary fructose intolerance, myelo- and lymphoproliferative diseases, chronic haemolytic anaemias, Gaucher's disease, severe psoriasis; Decreased excretion: renal failure, nephrogenic DI (reduced GFR), hypertension, hypothyroidism, Bartter's syndrome, sarcoidosis, drugs (low-dose salicylates, pyrazinamide, ethambutol).

HYPOuricaemia may be due to decreased production or increased excretion:

Decreased production: xanthine oxidase deficiency, severe liver disease, acute intermittent por-phyria, allopurinol therapy.

Increased excretion: Fanconi's syndrome, Wilson's disease, myeloma kidney, cystinosis, galac-tosaemia, hyperparathyroidism, uricosuric drugs (high-dose aspirin, NSAIDs, probenecid).

QUESTION 339

A. TRUE B. FALSE C. TRUE D. TRUE E. TRUE

The main drugs that precipitate attacks of AIP are:

Barbiturates
Alcohol
Etomidate
Phenytoin
Pentazocine
Corticosteroids
Imipramine
Tolbutamide

Anticholinergics, anticholinesterases, relaxants, droperidol, opioids, nitrous oxide, volatile agents, and propofol are all considered to be safe drugs.

Ref: Stoelting & Dierdorf. Anaesthesia and Co-Existing Disease. 3rd Ed. Churchill Livingstone.

QUESTION 340

A. FALSE B. TRUE C. TRUE D. FALSE E. FALSE

TPN is associated with hyperglycaemia which may need treatment with exogenous insulin. Hypoglycaemia may occur if the feed is stopped while there are elevated circulating levels of endogenous insulin. The metabolic acidosis that occurs is hyperchloraemia due to the liberation of HCl during the metabolism of amino acids present in the TPN solution. Central vein thrombosis is a recognised complication along with catheter related sepsis. The common elec-trolyte abnormalities are hypokalaemia, hypocalcaemia, hypomagnesaemia and hypophos-phataemia.

Ref: Stoelting & Dierdorf. Anaesthesia and Co-Existing Disease. 3rd Ed. Churchill Livingstone.

QUESTION 341

A. FALSE B. TRUE C. TRUE D. TRUE E. FALSE

Coagulation involves a series of enzymic reactions that lead to the conversion of soluble plasma fibrinogen to a fibrin clot. All the factors in the coagulation cascade are either enzyme precursors (Factors XII, XI, X, IX and thrombin) or cofactors (V, VIII). Fibrinogen is the exception as it is the subunit of fibrin. Fibrin does not occur in normal circulating blood. Factor V is a cofactor in the conversion of prothrombin to thrombin by activated factor X. Factor VIII is a complex protein with both coagulant (VIII:C) and platelet adhesion properties (VIII:vWF). Factor VIII and calcium ion are cofactors in association with activated factor IX that activates factor X. Plasminogen is part of the naturally occurring fibrinolytic system. It is an inactive plasma protein that is converted to plasmin by plasminogen activators derived from plasma, blood cells or tissues. Thromboplastin is derived from animal brain extract and is added to blood in the measurement of the prothrombin time.

Ref: Kumar & Clark. Clinical Medicine, 3rd Ed. W. B. Saunders. Ch. 6.

QUESTION 342

A. FALSE B. TRUE C. FALSE D. FALSE E. FALSE

Compounds found in normal circulating blood are either cofactors in the clotting cascade or enzymic precursors. Fibrinogen is the precursor of fibrin which is responsible for initial clot formation after it has been split by thrombin (the activated enzyme derived from prothrombin). Plasmin is part of the fibrinolytic pathway and is formed from plasminogen which circulates as an inactive plasma protein. Plasminogen is activated by activators derived from the plasma, blood cells or tissues. Plasmin is a serine protease that breaks down both fibrinogen and fibrin into fragments known as FDP's. It may also breakdown factors V and VIII. D-Dimers are the breakdown product of cross linked fibrin and represent a single intermolecular cross link between the gamma chains of two fibrin monomers. This cross link does not occur in fibrinogen and so D-Dimers are more specific for fibrin degradation than FDP's. Factor Xa is the activated form of factor X. It is a vitamin K dependent glycoprotein coagulation factor produced by the liver. It can be activated by both the intrinsic and extrinsic pathway.

Ref: Kumar & Clark. Clinical Medicine, 3rd Ed. W. B. Saunders. Ch. 6.

QUESTION 343

A. FALSE B. FALSE C. TRUE D. TRUE E. TRUE

The bleeding time is a measure of platelet plug formation in vivo. It is performed by making two 1mm deep, 1cm long incisions in the forearm with a blood pressure cuff inflated to 40 mmHg. The normal bleeding time is between 3 and 10 minutes. It is used to assess capillary function, platelet number/function and the ability of platelets to adhere to the vessel wall and form a plug. It is useful in the investigation of a spontaneous bruising and bleeding tendency. ITP is associated with low platelet numbers and prolongation of the bleeding time. In von Willebrand's disease there is a qualitative platelet defect due to deficiency of factor VIII:vWF which plays a role in platelet adhesion to damaged subendothelium as well as stabilizing factor VIII:C in plasma. Renal failure is associated with abnormal platelet function in the presence of normal numbers. Desmopressin may improve platelet function and shorten the bleeding time. Haemophilia is a deficiency of factor VIII or IX. Sickle cell disease is an abnormality of the beta globin chain with the substitution of valine to glutamine in position 6. The bleeding time is not affected in either condition.

Ref: Kumar & Clark. Clinical Medicine, 3rd Ed. W. B. Saunders. Ch. 6.

QUESTION 344

A. FALSE B. TRUE C. FALSE D. TRUE E. FALSE

The prothrombin time screens the extrinsic pathway of the coagulation system. It is performed by adding calcium and tissue thromboplastin to a sample of citrated platelet poor plasma and measuring the time required for fibrin clot formation. It is most sensitive to deficiencies in the vitamin K dependent clotting factors (II, VII, IX and X). It is also sensitive to deficiencies in factor 5. PTT is used to monitor warfarin therapy. It is insensitive to fibrinogen deficiency and not affected by heparin. The prothrombin time is elevated in liver disease and vitamin K deficiency (reduced synthesis of clotting factors), intravascular coagulation (consumption), congenital factor II,V,VII,X deficiency, warfarin therapy and after massive transfusion. It is normal in both haemophilia and von Willebrand's disease where the PTTK is elevated in association with reduced factor VIII levels. Vitamin C is involved in the hydroxylation of proline to hydroxyproline, necessary in the formation of collagen. Deficiency leads to scurvy with associated parafollicular haemorrhages and spontaneous bruising. There is capillary fragility and normal clotting factor levels.

Ref: Kumar & Clark. Clinical Medicine, 3rd Ed. W. B. Saunders. Ch. 6.

QUESTION 345

A. TRUE B. TRUE C. TRUE D. FALSE E. FALSE

The activated partial thromboplastin time APTT is assessed by mixing patients plasma with phospholipid, an activator substance and calcium. The normal is 30-50 seconds depending on the exact methodology. This test screens the intrinsic pathway and adequacy of all coagulation factors except factor XIII and VII. It may not detect mild clotting defects associated with factor levels of 25-40% of normal. It appears to be the best test to monitor heparin therapy. The APTT is elevated in the following situations:

- Deficiency of any individual coagulation factor (note this includes vitamin K-dependent factors) except factors XIII,VII
- Non specific inhibitors - lupus anticoagulant
- Specific inhibitors of clotting factors - i.e. anti-factor VIII antibodies
- Haemophilia A and B
- DIC
- Heparin and Warfarin therapy

The PTT may or may not be abnormal in von Willebrand's disease depending on the level of VIII:C. Factor VIII:vWF is responsible for stabilizing VIII:C in plasma. It is coded for on chromosome 12. The gene for factor VIII:C is on the X chromosome. Type III von Willebrand's disease is recessively inherited and associated with barely detectable levels of vWF and hence VIII:C. This form of the disease has clinical features resembling haemophilia A.

Ref: Kumar & Clark. Clinical Medicine, 3rd Ed. W. B. Saunders. Ch. 6.

QUESTION 346

A. FALSE B. FALSE C. TRUE D. FALSE E. FALSE

Stroke is a rare presenting feature of DIC and is more commonly seen in TTP (thrombotic thrombocytopenic purpura). The causes of DIC are legion. Treatment should be aimed at the underlying cause (sepsis-meningococcus, Gram negative septicaemia, Staphylococcal septicaemia, malignancy- mucin-secreting adenocarcinoma, prostate cancer, promyelocytic leukaemia, liver failure, obstetric disaster - abruptio placentiae, amniotic fluid embolism, eclampsia, etc.).

Treatment: supportive - heparin may be useful in promyelocytic leukaemia, meningococcaemia, TTP and where thrombosis is potentially life-threatening (large leg DVT, pulmonary embolism, peripheral gangrene). Other measures include replacement of clotting factors (FFP and purified antithrombin III), e-aminocaproic acid or aprotinin (+ heparin) for life-threatening bleeding.

Ref: Kumar & Clark. Clinical Medicine, 3rd Ed. W. B. Saunders. Ch. 6.

QUESTION 347

A. TRUE B. FALSE C. TRUE D. FALSE E. TRUE

The causes of thrombocytopenia may be divided into those with increased platelet consumption, decreased platelet production or abnormal platelet distribution (hypersplenism).

Increased platelet consumption: idiopathic thrombocytopenic purpura (ITP), drug-induced (quinine, sulphonamides, heparin, gold compounds, D-penicillamine), SLE, lymphoproliferative disease, HIV-associated, post-transfusion purpura, DIC, septicaemia, TTP, haemolytic uraemic syndrome;

Decreased platelet production: marrow hypoplasia (chemotherapy, chloramphenicol, phenytoin, gold compounds, idiopathic aplastic anaemia, TAR (thrombocytopenia with absent radii), malignant invasion of bone marrow (leukaemia, carcinoma (breast, lung, renal, stomach, prostate) and myelofibrosis), dysmyelopoietic syndromes (folate, B12 deficiency, myelodysplastic syndromes); viral infection causing selective reduction in megakaryocytes.

Hypersplenism: Any cause of splenomegaly (e.g. liver disease, lymphoproliferative disease, tropical splenomegaly, etc.). This results in sequestration.

Dilutional loss associated with massive transfusion of stored blood.

Ref: Kumar & Clark. Clinical Medicine, 3rd Ed. W. B. Saunders. Ch. 6.

QUESTION 348

A. FALSE B. TRUE C. FALSE D. TRUE E. TRUE

The bleeding time reflects platelets and endothelial/vascular function and is prolonged when either of these is abnormal, e.g. von Willebrand's disease, Bernard-Soulier syndrome (absence of platelet glycoprotein Ib receptor for vWF), Glanzman's thrombasthenia (lack of platelet glycoprotein IIb/IIIa), uraemia, aspirin, liver disease, scurvy, Ehlers-Danlos syndrome, etc. Christmas disease is an X-linked disorder due to factor IX deficiency. This results in prolongation of the APTT, but not the bleeding time.

DDAVP stimulates the immediate release of factor VIII:C and von Willebrand factor (vWF) from endothelial cell stores and avoids the risks of factor transfusions. However, repeat doses are only fully effective when given about 48 hours later. It has no effect on factor IX:C levels. Osler-Weber-Rendu (hereditary haemorrhagic telangiectasia) is associated with abnormally fragile blood vessels (telangiectasia), which are prone to bleed. Alcoholic liver disease results in reduced synthesis of factors II, III, IX and X (low levels of protein C, S, antithrombin III), defective clearance of tissue plasminogen activator, dysfibrinogenaemia and thrombocytopenia. The liver is responsible for the synthesis of all coagulation factors except factor VIII.

Ref: Kumar & Clark. Clinical Medicine, 3rd Ed. W. B. Saunders. Chs 5 and 6.

QUESTION 349

A. FALSE B. TRUE C. TRUE D. TRUE E. FALSE

The bleeding time reflects platelets and endothelial/vascular function and is prolonged when either of these is abnormal, e.g. von Willebrand's disease, Bernard-Soulier syndrome (absence of platelet glycoprotein Ib receptor for vWF), Glanzman's thrombasthenia (lack of platelet glycoprotein IIb/IIIa), uraemia, aspirin, liver disease, thrombocytopenia (of any cause), scurvy, Ehlers-Danlos syndrome, etc. Platelet function is normal in the haemophilias.

Ref: Kumar & Clark. Clinical Medicine, 3rd Ed. W. B. Saunders. Ch. 6.

QUESTION 350

A. TRUE B. TRUE C. TRUE D. FALSE E. TRUE

The characteristic findings in DIC are a prolonged prothrombin, activated partial thromboplastin and thrombin times. Fibrinogen levels are decreased in association with the presence of fibrin and fibrinogen degradation products due to the activity of plasmin on both fibrin and fibrinogen. D-Dimer is present and represents the degradation of cross-linked fibrin into fragments that contain one intermolecular cross-link between two fibrin monomers. This cross linkage occurs in fibrin and not fibrinogen and so this test is specific for fibrin degradation unlike FDP's. D-Dimer assay can distinguish fibrin degradation products in DIC from fibrinogen degradation products in primary fibrinogenolysis. However it is not specific for DIC and the definitive diagnosis must depend on other tests including platelet counts and serum fibrinogen levels. Fibrinogen is synthesized in the liver and has a half life of 4 days. Thrombin cleaves fibrinogen to form insoluble fibrin monomers which polymerise to form a clot. Fibrinogen is an acute phase protein which may be raised in inflammatory states, pregnancy and patients taking the OCP. Factor V and VIII levels may be severely decreased in DIC but are not used for diagnostic purposes due to time and technical complexity.

Ref: Kumar & Clark. Clinical Medicine, 3rd Ed. W. B. Saunders. Ch. 6.

QUESTION 351

A. FALSE B. TRUE C. FALSE D. TRUE E. FALSE

In autoimmune thrombocytopenic purpura sensitized platelets are removed by the reticuloendothelial system. Acute AITP is seen in children and often follows a viral infection. Chronic AITP is characteristically seen in adult females and is usually idiopathic. It may occur in association with other autoimmune diseases (SLE, thyroid disease, haemolytic anaemia) and in patients with CLL or after viral infections (including HIV). Platelet antibodies are detectable in only 60-70% of patients.

Patients present with bruising, epistaxis and menorrhagia with major bleeding only occurring with severe thrombocytopenia. Splenomegaly is rare. FBC shows low platelets but the clotting profile is normal. In children remission is normal but steroids and immunoglobulins may have a role in the acute phase of the disease. Adults may not respond to steroids and may relapse. Splenectomy may be required (90% response rate). This is avoided in children due to the risk of severe pneumococcal infection. Refractory patients may require immunosuppressives. Immunoglobulin infusions block the Fc receptor in the spleen leading to a rapid but transient rise in platelet counts. Transfused platelets do not survive any longer than a patients own platelets. They may be of help in life-threatening bleeding.

Ref: Kumar & Clark. Clinical Medicine, 3rd Ed. W. B. Saunders. Ch. 6.

QUESTION 352

A. FALSE B. TRUE C. TRUE D. FALSE E. FALSE

Haemophilia A is inherited as an X-linked recessive condition. The gene in huge and constitutes 0.1% of the X chromosome. The gene for factor VIII:vWF is on chromosome 12. It affects approximately 1 in 10,000 males and there is no family history in about one third of cases representing sporadic new mutations. All patients have normal vWF levels. Females are asymptomatic carriers unless homozygous for the defective gene. Clinical features depend on the level of factor VIII:C:-

<1% - frequent spontaneous bleeds
<5% - severe bleeding following injury and occasional spontaneous bleeds
>5% - milder disease with post-traumatic bleeding only

The APTT is prolonged in haemophilia in patients with factor VIII levels below 50%. The prothrombin time is normal as this test does not measure factor VIII activity. Bleeding time is also normal as there is no platelet dysfunction. Clot retraction is a measure of platelet function.

For major surgery factor VIII levels should be raised to 100% preoperatively and maintained above 50% until healing has occurred. Factor VIII has a half life of 12 hours and must be given twice daily to maintain adequate levels. Recombinant factor VIII is now available. DDAVP may be used to increase factor VIII levels transiently in mild disease. It avoids the problems of blood products. It stimulates the release of factor VIII from endothelial cell storage sites which become depleted and therefore limit its use. 10% of severe haemophiliacs develop factor VIII autoantibodies. Anticipated factor VIII concentrations following injection are therefore not achieved. Very high doses may be needed.

Ref: Kumar & Clark. Clinical Medicine, 3rd Ed. W. B. Saunders. Ch. 6.

QUESTION 353

A. TRUE B. TRUE C. FALSE D. TRUE E. FALSE

The intrinsic pathway of the clotting cascade depends on factors XII, XI, IX, VIII, X, V, II and I. It is assessed by the APTT. Platelet function is not affected and so the platelet count and bleeding times are normal. The prothrombin time tests the function of the extrinsic pathway and is dependent on factors VII, X, V, II (prothrombin) and I (fibrinogen). The clot retraction test is a qualitative measure that evaluates the function of the platelet contractile mechanism.

Ref: Kumar & Clark. Clinical Medicine, 3rd Ed. W. B. Saunders. Ch. 6.

QUESTION 354

A. FALSE B. FALSE C. FALSE D. TRUE E. TRUE

Haemophilia is an X-linked disorder resulting from a deficiency of factor VIII or IX (Christmas disease). The severity of bleeding disorder reflects the level of factor. Aspirin inhibits platelet function and is contraindicated in patients with haemophilia. Haematomas usually do not require decompression and may be managed by bed-rest and factor replacement. A Factor VIII level of 30% is enough to control a haemarthrosis, but for surgery it is usual to aim for 100% in the preoperative phase and maintain a level of 50% for 10-14 days thereafter. DDAVP produces a rise in Factor VIII and avoids the risks of intravenous factor. It can be used in mild haemophiliacs. It stimulates the immediate release of Factor VIII:C and von Willebrand factor (vWF) from endothelial cell stores but repeat doses are only fully effective when given about 48 hours later when stores of factor VIII are regenerated. Compared to Factor VIII, a larger volume of Factor IX diffuses into the extravascular tissues and the half-life of infused Factor IX is longer than that of Factor VIII (24 versus 12 hours).

Ref: Kumar & Clark. Clinical Medicine, 3rd Ed. W. B. Saunders. Ch. 6.

QUESTION 355

A. FALSE B. FALSE C. FALSE D. TRUE E. TRUE

Vitamin K is needed for the gamma-carboxylation of glutamic acid residues on factors II, VII, IX and X as well as protein C and S. Without it these factors cannot bind calcium and form complexes with PF-3 to carry out their normal function. Vitamin K deficiency is associated with inadequate stores (haemorrhagic disease of the new-born), malabsorption due to cholestasis and oral anticoagulants which are vitamin K antagonists. Scurvy is associated with capillary fragility due to defective collagen production. Haemophilia B is a genetic absence or reduced level of factor IX. Although low levels of factor IX are also associated with a deficiency of vitamin K, in haemophilia B they are not correctable by the administration of vitamin K. Heparin works by potentiating the activity of anti-thrombin III.

Ref: Kumar & Clark. Clinical Medicine, 3rd Ed. W. B. Saunders. Ch. 6.

QUESTION 356

A. TRUE B. TRUE C. TRUE D. FALSE E. FALSE

About 10% of normal red cell precursors die within the confines of the bone marrow. This is called ineffective erythropoiesis. This is substantially increased in anaemias such as thalassaemia major where there is imbalanced globin chain production and the megaloblastic anaemias due to Vitamin B12 or folate deficiency which is essential for normal DNA synthesis. Pernicious anaemia is the commonest form of B12 deficiency. There is atrophy of the gastric mucosa with failure of intrinsic factor production leading to Vitamin B12 malabsorption. Folate deficiency may be nutritional or associated with excess utilization, malabsorption and antifolate drug therapy (phenytoin, primodone, methotrexate, pyrimethamine, trimethoprim). Sideroblastic anaemias are inherited or acquired disorders with refractory anaemia and ring sideroblasts in the marrow with hypochromic cells in the blood film. There is a variable defect in red cell maturation with intramedullary destruction of precursors and a considerable degree of ineffective erythropoiesis. Fanconi's anaemia is a form of aplastic anaemia associated with the congenital absence of radii. Aplastic anaemia is anaemia due to marrow failure where there is the absence of red cell precursors and so erythropoiesis is absent rather than ineffective.

Ref: Kumar & Clark. Clinical Medicine, 3rd Ed. W. B. Saunders. Ch. 6.

QUESTION 357

A. TRUE B. FALSE C. TRUE D. TRUE E. TRUE

The Coombs' test is also known as the direct antiglobulin test and detects autoantibodies on the surface of the patients red cells. Washed red cells are tested directly with a antihuman globulin reagent. Agglutination occurs if the red cells are coated with IgG antibodies. It is positive in:

- Autoimmune haemolytic anaemia
- Haemolytic disease of the new-born
- Alloimmune reactions to recently transfused cells
- Drug induced haemolytic anaemia - methyl-dopa, cephalosporins, penicillin, levodopa, quinidine, methadone.

CLL is associated with an autoimmune haemolytic anaemia that is normally Coombs' positive. Thalassaemia is an inherited haemolytic anaemia due to a haemoglobinopathy and not an autoantibody. 1% of patients on methyl-dopa develop haemolytic anaemia but 15% develop a positive Coombs' test (direct anti-globulin test).

Note that in the Indirect Coombs' test, patients serum is incubated with reagent red cells to detect antibodies in the serum against red cells. After unbound antibody is washed off, the cells are incubated with antihuman globulin which will cause agglutination if the cells have been coated by patient serum antibodies. This forms the basis of antibody detection in cross-matching of blood.

Ref: Detmer. Pocket Guide to Diagnostic Tests. Lange.

QUESTION 358

A. TRUE B. TRUE C. TRUE D. FALSE E. TRUE

Folates are found in foods in the reduced dihydrofolate or tetrahydrofolate forms with methyl, formyl or methylene groups attached to the pteridine part of the molecule. Dietary folate is converted to methyltetrahydrofolate in plasma and transported into cells. Vitamin B12 converts methyltetrahydrofolate into tetrahydrofolate. This acts as a coenzyme in the transfer of single carbon units for amino acid metabolism and DNA synthesis (deoxyuridine to deoxythymidine).

The following drugs may precipitate folate deficiency:

- *Dihydrofolate reductase inhibitors* – methotrexate, pyrimethamine, trimethoprim
- *Anticonvulsants* – phenytoin, primidone
- *Others* – nitrofurantoin, triamterene, pentamidine

Ref: Oxford Textbook of Medicine, 3rd Ed. Oxford University Press. Ch. 22.4.6.

QUESTION 359

A. TRUE B. TRUE C. TRUE D. FALSE E. FALSE

Cold haemolysis is seen in a number of conditions including lymphomas, infectious mononucleosis, mycoplasma pneumonia and paroxysmal cold haemoglobinuria (Donath-Landsteiner antibody). It is generally associated with an IgM antibody and the Direct Coombs' test is positive.

Coombs' test identifies RBC coated with immunoglobulin (Ig) and C'. Coombs' positive haemolysis frequently occurs secondary to an underlying disease (SLE, chronic lymphocytic leukaemia, Hodgkin's lymphoma or ovarian teratoma) or drug reaction (methyldopa, hydralazine, penicillin, insulin, quinine, isoniazid, sulphonamide, sulphonyl ureas and rifampicin).

Primaquine causes haemolysis in patients with G6PD deficiency (other drugs causing this are: dapsone, sulphonamides, Vitamin K (water-soluble preparation), probenecid, quinine and chloramphenicol). This is not antibody-mediated and is Coombs' negative.

Many forms of haemolytic anaemia are associated with splenomegaly in particular the haemoglobinopathies and pyruvate kinase deficiency.

Serum haptoglobins are reduced in haemolytic anaemia. They are synthesized in the liver and bind free haemoglobin following haemolysis. They are acute phase proteins and are increased in infection, malignancy and other inflammatory diseases.

Ref: Kumar & Clark. Clinical Medicine, 3rd Ed. W. B. Saunders. Ch. 6.
Detmer. Pocket Guide to Diagnostic Tests. Lange.

QUESTION 360

A. TRUE B. FALSE C. FALSE D. TRUE E. TRUE

Macrocytosis in the absence of megaloblastic changes may occur in the following conditions:

Pregnancy
New-born children
Alcohol excess
Liver disease
Reticulocytosis
Hypothyroidism
Aplastic and sideroblastic anaemia

Alcoholics may develop a megaloblastic anaemia due to the toxic effects of alcohol on ery-thropoiesis and a deficiency of folate in the diet. Methotrexate is a dihydrofolate reductase inhibitor and produces megaloblastic changes. Gluten-sensitive enteropathy (coeliac disease) is associated with both B12 and folate deficiency due to malabsorption and megaloblastosis.

Ref: Kumar & Clark. Clinical Medicine, 3rd Ed. W. B. Saunders. Ch. 6.

QUESTION 361

A. TRUE B. FALSE C. TRUE D. TRUE E. TRUE

Sickle cell disease is associated with aseptic necrosis of the femoral heads. In Thalassaemia states skeletal changes include maxillary hypertrophy, skull changes (extramedullary haematopoiesis) and osteomyelitis. Haemophilia causes chronic osteoarthritis. Sub-periosteal haemorrhages are seen in scurvy (Vitamin C deficiency). G-6-PDH deficiency is an inherited disorder associat-ed with haemolysis following an oxidant shock. There are no X-ray changes in the skeleton.

Ref: Kumar & Clark. Clinical Medicine, 3rd Ed. W. B. Saunders. Ch. 6.

QUESTION 362

A. FALSE B. TRUE C. TRUE D. TRUE E. TRUE

Sickle cell disease results from a point mutation that substitutes valine for glutamine in the beta-globin chain. Factors that promote sickling include hypoxia, acidosis, increase in serum osmolality, fever and sluggish blood flow. Sickling may result in either occlusion in the microvasculature (resulting in infarction of the tissues) or haemolysis of the sickle RBC.

Complications include renal failure, bone necrosis, infections, ulcers and hand-foot syndrome in children. Polyuria and nocturia are due to the decreased concentrating ability of renal tubules. Patients are susceptible to infections. In particular strep pneumoniae which can cause a fatal meningitis or pneumonia and salmonella which can lead to osteomyelitis in necrotic bone.

QUESTION 363

A. TRUE B. TRUE C. TRUE D. TRUE E. FALSE

In patients with sickle cell disease the main precipitants of sickling are:

- Infection
- Dehydration
- Cold
- Acidosis
- Hypoxia

In many cases the cause is unknown. HbS precipitates inside the red cell damaging the membrane increasing the likelihood of rupture and haemolytic anaemia. Tactoids of sickled cells increase the viscosity of the blood leading to stasis and potentially an infarctive crisis when vascular occlusion occurs. The portal circulation with a low PO_2 is at unique risk of occlusion.

Suxamethonium does not precipitate sickling. There is no evidence that either a single or combination of anaesthetic drugs is better for patients with sickle cell disease. Patients may occasionally have decreased levels of plasma cholinesterase activity.

Ref: Stoelting & Dierdorf. Anaesthesia and Co-Existing Disease. 3rd Ed. Churchill Livingstone. Ch. 24.

QUESTION 364

A. TRUE B. FALSE C. FALSE D. TRUE E. TRUE

Sickle cell trait is the heterozygous form of sickle cell disease with only one chromosome carrying the abnormal gene. The incidence in African Americans is about 8-10%. Most patients are asymptomatic or have occasional haematuria. The blood count and film are usually normal and typically there is HbA of about 60% and HbS about 40%. The diagnosis is made on the basis of a positive sickle test and Hb electrophoresis. It appears that sickle cell trait actually protects against Plasmodium falciparum malaria. Sickle cell trait may occur in association with other Hb chain abnormalities. HbSC disease is similar to HbSS disease but is associated with severe retinopathy and increased likelihood of thrombotic episodes. Anaesthesia in patients with sickle trait should still be carried out with care in order to avoid hypoxia which may still precipitate sickling.

Ref: Stoelting & Dierdorf. Anaesthesia and Co-Existing Disease. 3rd Ed. Churchill Livingstone Ch. 24.
Kumar & Clark. Clinical Medicine, 3rd Ed. W. B. Saunders. Ch. 6.

QUESTION 365

A. FALSE B. FALSE C. FALSE D. FALSE E. FALSE

Sickle cell disease occurs in patients with either HbSS or HbSC disease. HbS is the substitution of valine for glutamic acid at position 6 of the BETA chain of the globin molecule. Lysine is substituted for glutamic acid at the same location to produce HbC. The clinical course of patients with HbSC disease is similar to that of homozygous HbS disease. In addition to this there is an increased risk of thrombotic episodes that may be life threatening as well as a recognised retinopathy. Sickle cell disease occurs mainly in Africa. However it is also found in India, the Middle East and parts of southern Europe. The disease does not manifest itself in the first 6 months of life due to presence of HbF which is composed of two alpha and two gamma chains.

Ref: Stoelting & Dierdorf. Anaesthesia and Co-Existing Disease. 3rd Ed. Churchill Livingstone Ch. 24.
Kumar & Clark. Clinical Medicine, 3rd Ed. W. B. Saunders. Ch. 6.

QUESTION 366

A. TRUE B. TRUE C. TRUE D. FALSE E. TRUE

Reticulocytosis occurs with any type of haemolytic anaemia or loss of blood provided that the marrow is functional and there is no Fe/Folate or B12 deficiency. Other markers of increased red cell breakdown include:

- Elevated serum unconjugated bilirubin
- Excess urinary urobilinogen from bilirubin breakdown in the gut
- Reduced plasma haptoglobins that bind free Hb
- Raised LDH

- Intravascular haemolysis is suggested by raised levels of plasma Hb, haemosiderinuria, very low or absent haptoglobins and methaemalbuminemia (positive Schumm's test)

Ref: Kumar & Clark. Clinical Medicine, 3rd Ed. W. B. Saunders. Ch. 6.

QUESTION 367

A. FALSE B. TRUE C. TRUE D. TRUE E. FALSE

G-6-PDH deficiency is the most common of the inherited red cell enzyme disorders. The gene is on the X chromosome and is recessive. Up to 10% of black males in the USA are affected. Female carriers have a degree of protection against malaria. It affects people around the world but in particular Africa, around the Mediterranean, the Middle East and South East Asia. Drugs that form peroxides by their interaction with haemoglobin can trigger haemolysis. G-6-PDH is essential for the production of NADPH which inactivates these peroxides. Haemolysis may be induced by any oxidant shock.

Drugs implicated in haemolysis in these patients include:

Analgesics – aspirin, phenacetin
Antimalarials – primaquine, pyrimethamine, quinine, chloroquine
Antibacterials – sulphonamides, dapsone, nitrofurantoin, chloramphenicol
Others – Vitamin K, quinidine, probenicid, methylene blue, nalidixic acid, Vitamin C

Other triggers include:

Infection
Ingestion of fava beans – (contain vicine and convicine which produce free radicals in the course of their autoxidation)

There is considerable variation in the response to drugs. Drugs used in anaesthesia have not been implicated in haemolysis.

Ref: Stoelting & Dierdorf. Anaesthesia and Co-Existing Disease. 3ʳᵈ Ed. Churchill Livingstone Ch. 24.
Kumar & Clark. Clinical Medicine, 3ʳᵈ Ed. W. B. Saunders. Ch. 6.

QUESTION 368

A. FALSE B. FALSE C. TRUE D. TRUE E. FALSE

Pyruvate kinase deficiency is the most common of the enzyme defects in the anaerobic glycolytic pathway of red cells, and the second most common red cell metabolism defect after G-6-PDH deficiency. It is inherited as an autosomal recessive unlike G-6-PDH which is sex-linked. The enzyme deficiency leads to rigid red cells that are highly permeable to potassium and susceptible to rupture. Homozygotes have enzyme levels of 5-20% and haemolysis may be precipitated by infection and pregnancy. The blood film shows a reticulocytosis with distorted cells. Blood transfusions are often necessary and splenectomy may improve the patients clinical condition by reducing the rate of red cell destruction but not haemolysis. Pigment gall stones are common due to chronic haemolysis. Patients are often anaemic with Hb levels of 5-10 g/dL. However levels of 2, 3DPG in the red cells are raised due to the enzyme defect. Symptoms are therefore mild. Although the red cells are more permeable to potassium, the administration of suxamethonium has not been associated with hyperkalaemia.

Ref: Stoelting & Dierdorf. Anaesthesia and Co-Existing Disease. 3ʳᵈ Ed. Churchill Livingstone Ch. 24.
Kumar & Clark. Clinical Medicine, 3ʳᵈ Ed. W. B. Saunders. Ch. 6.

QUESTION 369

A. TRUE B. FALSE C. FALSE D. TRUE E. FALSE

The level of serum ferritin reflects body stores of iron more accurately than saturation of the serum iron binding capacity. Normal values are 30-300 mcg/l in males and 15-200 mcg/l in females.

MCH (mean cell haemoglobin) and MCHC (mean cell haemoglobin concentration) are indices of microcytosis rather than iron deficiency and are also low in conditions such as thalassaemia, sideroblastic anaemia and anaemia of chronic disease.

Free erythrocyte protoporphyrin represents porphyrin rings with no iron to make into haem – also seen in lead poisoning, sideroblastic anaemia and erythropoietic protoporphyria.

The characteristic features of iron deficiency anaemia are:

- Microcytosis (MCV < 80fl) and hypchromia (MCH <27pg)
- Anisocytosis (variation in size), Poikilocytosis (variation in shape)
- Low serum iron
- Raised serum iron binding capacity
- Low transferrin saturation (serum iron divided by iron binding capacity)
- Low serum ferritin (<15 mcg/l)
- Raised erythrocyte protoporphyrin

Ref: Kumar & Clark. Clinical Medicine, 3rd Ed. W. B. Saunders. Ch. 6.
Detmer. Pocket Guide to Diagnostic Tests. Lange.

QUESTION   370

A. TRUE B. TRUE C. TRUE D. TRUE E. TRUE

The following are diagnostic features on a blood film:

- Basophilic stippling – seen in beta–thalassaemia and lead poisoning;
- Target cells – liver disease, sickle cell disease and thalassaemia; low numbers in iron deficiency;
- Heinz bodies – denatured Hb seen in G-6-PDH deficiency;
- Howell-Jolly bodies – RNA remnants seen in HYPOsplenism;
- Cabot's rings – RNA/DNA remnants in thalassaemia and B12 deficiency;
- Pappenheimer bodies – granules of siderocytes: seen in lead poisoning, carcinomatosis and post splenectomy;
- Parasitic inclusions (malaria, babesiosis);
- Spherocytes – hereditary spherocytosis, immune haemolytic anaemia (IgG mediated), hypersplenism;
- Schistiocytes (fragmented red cells) – valve disease and prosthesis, microangiopathic disorders (DIC, TTP, HUS).

Causes of macrocytosis – alcohol, coeliac (folate/B12), hypothyroidism, pregnancy, phenytoin, AZT, azathioprine, myelodysplasia and PNH.

Ref: Epstein RJ. Medicine for Examinations. 3rd Ed. Churchill Livingstone. Ch. 5.

QUESTION 371

A. FALSE B. TRUE C. FALSE D. TRUE E. TRUE

Thrombocytosis (an elevated platelet count) is commonly seen as a response to acute or chronic illness (reactive thrombocytosis – platelet counts 500–1,000 (109/l), e.g. with malignancies or chronic inflammation (rheumatoid arthritis). Other causes include iron deficiency   and splenectomy. In myeloproliferative diseases, there may be autonomous production, e.g. chronic myeloid leukaemia (not CLL), polycythaemia rubra vera and essential thrombocytosis; in these conditions this may be associated with abnormal platelet function. (CLL causes an autoimmune thrombocytopenia.)
Iron overload can be divided into primary (as in haemochromatosis) or secondary. Causes of acquired iron overload include ineffective erythropoiesis (e.g. thalassaemia, sickle cell disease, sideroblastic anaemia, etc. where iron overload is due to increased dietary absorption as well as blood transfusion). Minor degrees of iron overload are also seen in alcoholic liver disease and porphyria cutanea tarda. For haemochromatosis, therapeutic venesection is an effective treatment; others require parenternal iron chelation therapy (desferrioxamine).

Aplastic anaemia is characterised by peripheral blood pancytopenia due to bone marrow failure. About half are idiopathic. The commonest cause is drug/toxin-induced – chloramphenicol, sulphonamides, anticonvulsants, chlorpropamide, propylthiouracil, carbimazole, phenothiazines, aspirin, gold compounds, D-penicillamine, carbon tetrachloride, benzene, DDT and radiation. Other causes include infection (e.g. hepatitis C, parvovirus, tuberculosis, rarely CMV or EBV). Fanconi's anaemia is a congenital disorder with hypoplastic kidneys, hypoplastic thumb and radii, microcephaly and mental retardation. Down's syndrome carries an increased risk of acute myeloid leukaemia, not aplastic anaemia.

Erythrocytosis has been associated with renal cysts, hydronephrosis, nephrotic syndrome, diffuse renal parenchymal disease and Bartter's syndrome and is seen in up to 15% of renal transplant recipients. Other causes of secondary erythrocytosis include smoking, chronic pulmonary disease, cyanotic heart disease, Pickwickian syndrome, high altitude, adrenal cortical hypersecretion and occasionally with exogenous androgen therapy.

QUESTION 372

A. TRUE B. FALSE C. TRUE D. TRUE E. TRUE

Hypercoagulable states may be divided into congenital or acquired defects.

Congenital: deficiency of antithrombin III, protein S or C (Factor V-Leiden mutation). Antithrombin III neutralises factors IXa, Xa, XIa and XIIa and thrombin. Levels are reduced in women taking the OCP and in patients with liver disease or on heparin. Low levels are associated with a heparin resistance hypercoagulable state. FFP contains ATIII and is a useful source when acute correction is needed. Protein C neutralises Va and VIIIa and binds thrombin. It also stimulates fibrinolysis. Deficiency is associated with recurrent thromboembolic disease including MI, CVA and PE's. It is not detectable on routine screening coagulation tests. Protein S is a co-factor for activated protein C.

Acquired: Malignancy (migratory thrombophlebitis), myeloproliferative disorders, paroxysmal nocturnal haemoglobinuria (PNH), SLE (anti-phospholipid syndrome), pregnancy, oestrogen therapy, postoperative, nephrotic syndrome (acquired antithrombin III deficiency), hyperlipidaemia and homocystinuria.

Glanzman's syndrome is a platelet defect (absence of platelet glycoprotein Ib receptor for vWF) and is associated with bleeding rather than thromboses.

QUESTION 373

A. FALSE B. TRUE C. TRUE D. TRUE E. FALSE

Coombs' test identifies red cells coated with immunoglobulin and/or complement. Causes of Coombs'-positive haemolysis include drugs (penicillin, insulin, quinine, isoniazid, sulphonamide, sulphonyl ureas, rifampicin, D-penicillamine, gold compounds), SLE, rheumatoid arthritis, CLL, Hodgkin's lymphoma and ovarian teratoma. Primaquine produces haemolysis by promoting oxidative crisis within the RBC of patients with G-6-PDH deficiency - this is not antibody mediated and Coombs' test is negative. Other potentially oxidative drugs include dapsone, sulphonamides, Vitamin K (water-soluble preparation), probenecid, quinine and chloramphenicol.

QUESTION 374

A. TRUE B. FALSE C. FALSE D. TRUE E. TRUE

Beta thalassaemia is due to the defective production of haemoglobin beta chains. There is an excess of alpha chains that precipitate in erythroblasts and red cells causing ineffective erythropoiesis. There is a single beta chain locus on chromosome 11 (NB there are two alpha chain loci on each chromosome) and most of the defects are point mutations unlike alpha thalassaemia in which there are gene deletions. Beta thalassaemia minor represents the carrier state (trait) in which there is only mild or no anaemia. The red cells are hypochromic and microcytic (low MCV/MCH) and may be confused with iron deficiency. Serum iron, ferritin and iron stores are however normal. Electrophoresis shows increased HbA2 and often HbF. It occurs commonly around the Mediterranean and an area stretching through to South East Asia. Beta thalassaemia trait can occur in association with HbS (also a beta chain disease). This is known as sickle cell beta-thalassaemia and clinically resembles full blown HbSS disease.

Ref: Kumar & Clark. Clinical Medicine, 3rd Ed. W. B. Saunders. Ch. 6.

QUESTION 375

A. TRUE B. TRUE C. FALSE D. FALSE E. TRUE

There are 2 alpha chain genes on each chromosome 16. Unlike beta thalassaemia, alpha thalassaemia is caused by gene deletions. If all 4 genes are deleted there are no alpha chains and only Hb Barts is present. This is not compatible with life and results in still born infants with hydrops fetalis. If 3 genes are deleted, patients are moderately anaemic and may have splenomegaly and gall stones. Patients are not usually transfusion dependent and have HbA,

Hb Barts and HbH (beta★4). Microcytosis is the characteristic feature of alpha thalassaemia trait. HbA2 and HbF levels are normal in alpha thalassaemia states. These are increased in beta thalassaemia.

Ref: Kumar & Clark. Clinical Medicine, 3rd Ed. W. B. Saunders. Ch. 6.

QUESTION 376

A. TRUE B. FALSE C. FALSE D. TRUE E. FALSE

Body fluids designated high risk for transmission of HIV are blood, vaginal secretions, breast milk, amniotic fluid, pericardial fluid, pleural fluid, semen, synovial fluid, cerebrospinal fluid, and peritoneal fluid.

Faeces, nasal secretions, sputum, saliva, sweat, urine and vomit are not considered to present a significant risk for transmission of HIV.

Ref: HIV and other blood borne viruses - guidance for anaesthetists. Association of Anaesthetists of Great Britain and Ireland. Ch. 3.

QUESTION 377

A. TRUE B. FALSE C. TRUE D. FALSE E. FALSE

The carboxypenicillins (carbenicillin and ticarcillin) and ureidopenicillins (azlocillin and piperacillin) are active against *Pseudomonas* infections.

Phenoxymethylpenicillin, the broad spectrum penicillins (ampicillin, amoxycillin, co-amoxi-clav and pivampicillin) and the penicillinase-resistant penicillins (cloxacillin, flucloxacillin and temocillin) are inactive against *Pseudomonas*.

Ref: Kumar & Clark. Clinical Medicine, 3rd Ed. W. B. Saunders. Ch. 1.
British National Formulary.

QUESTION 378

A. FALSE B. FALSE C. TRUE D. TRUE E. TRUE

Cloxacillin is not inactivated by penicillinase. Temocillin is a new penicillin with activity against penicillinase producing gram negative bacteria (except *Pseudomonas*). It is not active against gram positive bacteria. Ticarcillin with clavulinic acid (Timentin) is active against penicillinase producing bacteria. Piperacillin with the beta lactamase inhibitor tazobactam (Tazocin) is active against beta lactamase producing bacteria. Norfloxacin (a 4-Quinolone) is not a penicillin derivative.

Ref: Kumar & Clark. Clinical Medicine, 3rd Ed. W. B. Saunders. Ch. 1.
British National Formulary.

QUESTION 379

A. TRUE B. TRUE C. FALSE D. TRUE E. FALSE

The orally active cephalosporins are cephalexin, cephradine, cefadroxil, cefaclor, cefuroxime axetil (an ester of cefuroxime), cefixime, ceftibuten and cefpodoxime proxetil. Note that is not cefuroxime itself that is active orally. It is an ester of the parent drug that is active orally. It has the same spectrum of activity as the parent compound.

Ref: Kumar & Clark. Clinical Medicine, 3rd Ed. W. B. Saunders. Ch. 1.

QUESTION 380

A. TRUE B. FALSE C. FALSE D. FALSE E. FALSE

Vancomycin a glycopeptide is produced by *Streptomyces orientalis*. Vancomycin inhibits cell wall synthesis and thus is bactericidal. It is used to treat endocarditis, "line" sepsis caused by gram positive bacteria and pseudomembranous colitis.

Rapid infusion causes severe hypotension, wheezing, dyspnoea, urticaria, pruritus, flushing of the upper body (red man syndrome) and muscle spasm of the back and chest.

Ref: Kumar & Clark. Clinical Medicine, 3rd Ed. W. B. Saunders. Ch. 1.

QUESTION 381

A. FALSE B. FALSE C. FALSE D. TRUE E. TRUE

Erythromycin and azithromycin are both macrolide antibiotics. They inhibit protein synthesis and are thus bacteriostatic. Azithromycin has less activity against gram positive organisms than erythromycin, but has a broader spectrum of activity against gram negative organisms, Mycobacteria and Toxoplasma. Azithromycin has enhanced tissue and intracellular penetration and longer half-life that allows once daily dosing. Macrolide antibiotics are not active against Pseudomonas species.

Ref: Kumar & Clark. Clinical Medicine, 3rd Ed. W. B. Saunders. Ch. 1.

QUESTION 382

A. FALSE B. TRUE C. FALSE D. FALSE E. TRUE

Beta-lactam antibiotics inhibit bacterial cell wall synthesis and are bactericidal in action. Aztreonam is currently the only monocyclic beta lactam antibiotic. It's spectrum of activity is limited to aerobic gram negative bacilli i.e. *pseudomonas, neisseria* and *haemophilus*.

Imipenem is a carbapenem. Imipenem is active against gram positive and gram negative organisms including *Pseudomonas* and anaerobes. However it is partially inactivated in the kidney and is therefore combined with cilastin a specific enzyme inhibitor which blocks its renal metabolism. Meropenem is similar to imipenem, but is stable to the renal enzyme which inactivates imipenem.

QUESTION 383

A. TRUE B. TRUE C. TRUE D. TRUE E. FALSE

Ciprofloxacin a 4-fluoroquinolone, is active against gram negative bacteria (including pseudomonas) and some gram positive bacteria. It is the drug of first choice in travellers diarrhoea. Current therapy for eradication of *Helicobacter pylori* consists of a proton pump inhibitor e.g. Omeprazole 40 mg daily and clarithromycin 500 mg bd (or any other macrolide) plus either amoxycillin 500 mg tds or metronidazole 400mg tds for one week. This produces eradication in up to 90% of patients. Various eradication regimens exists.

Ref: Kumar & Clark. Clinical Medicine, 3rd Ed. W. B. Saunders. Ch. 1.

QUESTION 384

A. TRUE B. TRUE C. FALSE D. FALSE E. FALSE

Ganciclovir a guanine analogue is used to treat cytomegalovirus retinitis and colitis in patients with HIV. Its major complication is myelosuppression.

Acyclovir, famciclovir and valaciclovir are active against herpes viruses, especially when started at the onset of infection (the latter two are pro-drugs).

Idoxuridine is only effective if applied topically at the onset of infection with herpes viruses. It is too toxic for systemic use.

Ritonavir is a protease inhibitor. It is used in combination with nucleoside inhibitors (e.g. zidovudine, lamivudine, didanosine, stavudine and zalcitabine) in advanced HIV infection.

Tribavarin is used in severe respiratory syncitial virus bronchiolitis in children. When given during the first week of Lassa fever, it reduces the mortality from 50% to 5%.

Ref: Kumar & Clark. Clinical Medicine, 3rd Ed. W. B. Saunders. Ch. 1.
British National Formulary.

QUESTION 385

A. FALSE B. FALSE C. TRUE D. TRUE E. FALSE

Polyene antifungal drugs (amphotericin and nystatin) are not absorbed from the gastointestinal tract and are used to treat oral and intestinal candidiasis. Amphotericin is prepared in various lipid formulations for systemic use. Amphotericin is nephrotoxic.

Griseofulvin is given orally for fungal infections in the skin, nails, scalp and hair when topical therapy has failed. It is selectively concentrated in keratin. It is not effective when applied topically.

Concomitant administration of terfenadine and imidazole antifungal drugs (miconazole, ketoconazole and clotrimazole) is associated with ventricular arrhythmias. Ketoconazole is hepatotoxic. Fluconazole is used to treat local and systemic infections with candida and cryptococcus.

Ref: Kumar & Clark. Clinical Medicine, 3rd Ed. W. B. Saunders. Ch. 1.
British National Formulary.

QUESTION   386

A. FALSE   B. TRUE   C. TRUE   D. FALSE   E. TRUE

Clinical conditions associated with toxins produced by Staphylococcus aureus are:

- Staphylococcal food poisoning; enterotoxins A, B, C, D and E;
- Toxic shock syndrome; toxic shock syndrome toxin-1(TSST-1). Blood cultures are negative and anti-TSST-1 antibodies are present in serum;
- Scalded skin syndrome; exfolatin;
- Cellulitis, pneumonia, lung abscesses, endocarditis, pericarditis, meningitis, brain abscesses and osteomyelitis are due to local invasion of staphylococcus.

Ref: Kumar & Clark. Clinical Medicine, 3rd Ed. W. B. Saunders. Ch. 1.

QUESTION   387

A. TRUE   B. TRUE   C. TRUE   D. TRUE   E. FALSE

Patients with prosthetic heart valve lesions should be given prophylactic antibiotics when undergoing the following procedures:

- *Dental procedures:* extractions, scaling and surgery involving the gingival tissues;
- *Genitourinary surgery;*
- *Obstetric and gynaecological procedures:* vaginal delivery, cervical dilatation and curettage of the uterus and the insertion or removal of intrauterine contraceptive devices;
- *Gastrointestinal procedures:* endoscopy, colonoscopy, sigmoidoscopy, proctoscopy and barium enema;
- *Procedures on the upper airway:* tonsillectomy and adenoidectomy. Fibreoptic bronchoscopy rarely causes bacteraemia and prophylactic antibiotics are not indicated.

Ref: Kumar & Clark. Clinical Medicine, 3rd Ed. W. B. Saunders. Ch. 1.
Report of a Working Party of the British Society for Antimicrobial Chemotherapy. Lancet, 1982, 1323 – 1326.

QUESTION 388

A. FALSE B. FALSE C. TRUE D. TRUE E. TRUE

Usual pathogens associated with hospital acquired urinary tract infections are *Escherichia coli, Klebsiella, Proteus, Serratia, Pseudomonas* and other gram negative bacteria.

Ref: Kumar & Clark. Clinical Medicine, 3rd Ed. W. B. Saunders. Ch. 1.

QUESTION 389

A. FALSE B. FALSE C. TRUE D. FALSE E. TRUE

Modes of action of anti microbial agents:

1. *Inhibition of bacterial cell wall synthesis:* penicillins cephalosporins, monobactams, carbapenems and glycopeptides (vancomycin and teicoplanin).
2. *Damage to cell membrane:* Some antibiotics bind to the cell wall, resulting in the loss of the semipermeable properties of the membrane. Substances then pass out through the cell wall and death occurs. Polypeptide antibiotics (e.g. polymixins) act in this manner.
3. *Inhibition of protein synthesis by inhibiting ribosomal function:* chloramphenicol, tetracyclines, aminoglycosides, macrolides, fusidic acid and clindamycin.
4. *Inhibition of DNA synthesis:* nalidixic acid, quinolones, nitroimidazoles (e.g. metronidazole) and rifampicin.
5. *Inhibition of folate synthesis:* sulphonamides and trimethoprim.

Ref: Kumar & Clark. Clinical Medicine, 3rd Ed. W. B. Saunders. Ch. 1.

QUESTION 390

A. FALSE B. FALSE C. FALSE D. TRUE E. TRUE

Patients with heart valve lesions, septal defects, patent ductus arteriosus or prosthetic valves require antibacterial prophylaxis for dental surgery.

Patients who have had a splenectomy should also be given antibiotic prophylaxis to prevent pneumococcal sepsis.

Ref: Kumar & Clark. Clinical Medicine, 3rd Ed. W. B. Saunders. Ch. 1.
Report of the Working Party of the British Society for Antimicrobial Chemotherapy. Lancet. 1982. 2. 1323 - 1326.

QUESTION 391

A. TRUE B. FALSE C. FALSE D. TRUE E. TRUE

HIV positive patients are susceptible to a wide range of infections. The major protozoal and fungal pathogens are:

- Protozoa: *Pneumocystis carinii, Toxoplasma gondii, Cryptosporidium parvum, Isospora belli* and *Microspora spp.*
- Fungi: *Candida* spp., *Cryptococcus neoformans, Histoplasma capsulatum* and *Coccidiodes immitis.*

Pneumocystis carinii most commonly causes pneumonia. *Toxoplasma gondii* most commonly causes encephalitis and cerebral abscesses. *Cryptosporidium parvum* and Microsporidia spp. cause diarrhoea.
Cryptococcus neoformans most commonly causes meningitis, although it can cause pneumonia and disseminated infection. *Candida* spp. frequently infect the oropharynx.

Ref: Kumar & Clark. Clinical Medicine, 3rd Ed. W. B. Saunders. Ch. 1.

QUESTION 392

A. FALSE B. FALSE C. FALSE D. TRUE E. TRUE

Nalidixic acid and tetracycline exacerbate renal failure and should not be given to patients with kidney disease.
Chloramphenicol causes bone marrow suppression.
Fusidic acid is hepatotoxic.
Erythromycin produces cholestatic jaundice.

Ref: Kumar & Clark. Clinical Medicine, 3rd Ed. W. B. Saunders. Ch. 1.

QUESTION 393

A. FALSE B. TRUE C. FALSE D. FALSE E. TRUE

Enterococci are gram positive diplococci, non haemolytic, Lancefield group D streptococci. They are resistant to cephalosporins, but sensitive to ampicillin and amoxycillin. They are common causes of abdominal wound, urinary tract, biliary tract infections and endocarditis.

Ref: Kumar & Clark. Clinical Medicine, 3rd Ed. W. B. Saunders. Chs 1 and 11.

QUESTION 394

A. FALSE B. FALSE C. FALSE D. TRUE E. TRUE

Tuberculosis results from infection with Mycobacterium spp. It is spread by droplet infection. It is a granulomatous disease with central caseating necrosis. The primary infection usually involves the lungs. The primary infection usually heals leaving some surviving tubercle bacilli. Reactivation may occur in the event of a lowering of host resistance e.g. HIV infection. Therefore in adults TB usually results from reactivation of old disease.

The current recommended regimen by the Joint Tuberculosis Committee of the British Thoracic Society is:

- 2 months: isoniazid, rifampicin, and pyrazinamide. Ethambutol is added if resistance is likely.
- For a further 4 months; isoniazid and rifampicin.
- Second line drugs for resistant organisms are azithromycin, clarithromycin, ciprofloxacin and ofloxacin.

Ref: Kumar & Clark. Clinical Medicine, 3rd Ed. W. B. Saunders. Ch. 1.
British National Formulary.

QUESTION 395

A. FALSE B. FALSE C. TRUE D. FALSE E. FALSE

Sterilization implies the killing of all organisms including spores.
Disinfection removes or kills most organisms, but not spores.
Decontamination is the physical removal of infected material and can be achieved by thorough washing and scrubbing.

Methods of sterilization are:

1. Moist heat under pressure; e.g. 122° C for 30 min at 101.3 kPa, 126° C for 10 min at 135 kPa and 134° C for 3 min at 202.6 kPa.
2. Low pressure, low steam; 74° C at 37 kPa with formaldehyde vapour.
3. Dry heating; 150-170° C for 20-30 min.
4. Formaldehyde cabinets.
5. Ethylene or propylene oxide chamber.
6. Gamma irradiation.

Boiling objects for 5 minutes and immersion in disinfectant solutions are methods of disinfection.

Ref: Davey, Moyle & Ward. Ward's Anaesthetic Equipment. 3rd Ed. W. B. Saunders. Ch. 20.

QUESTION 396

A. FALSE B. TRUE C. FALSE D. TRUE E. TRUE

HIV is an RNA virus of the lentivirus family. It is called a retrovirus as it encodes the enzyme reverse transcriptase (an RNA-dependent DNA-polymerase) which allows DNA to be transcribed from the viral RNA within the infected cell. CD4 is a surface glycoprotein (gp) which binds to gp120 on the surface of the HIV particle. CD4 is also present on macrophages, Langerhans cells and dendritic cells of blood/lymph nodes. These cells act as reservoirs for virus and their immune responses (antigen presentation and T cell activation) are also impaired. Other cells such as microglial cells and colonic epithelial cells can also be infected but less efficiently. Anti-HIV antibodies usually appear 6-12 weeks after initial infection. HIV can be cultured from peripheral blood lymphocytes of asymptomatic individuals infected with the virus even before the anti-HIV titres rise. However, the levels of infective virus are generally low and the p24 antigen is not detectable by ELISA. Persistence of the p24 antigen is highly suggestive of higher disease burden and more rapid disease progression

QUESTION 397

A. TRUE B. FALSE C. TRUE D. TRUE E. FALSE

The commonest manifestation of seroconversion following HIV infection is a mononucleosis-like syndrome. Other recognised syndromes include aseptic meningoencephalitis, encephalopathy, myelopathy and peripheral neuropathy. In many individuals, seroconversion is subclinical. Following the acute infection (stage I), individuals are usually asymptomatic for 3-4 years (stage II) before developing persistent generalised lymphadenopathy (non-tender; stage III). Patients developing other disease are classified as stage IV. Predictors of progression to AIDS include: clinical features (fever, weight loss, oral hairy leukoplakia) and laboratory investigations (anaemia, reduced haematocrit, fall in CD4 count, raised ESR, rise in p24 antigen). The drug of choice for pneumocystis is cotrimoxazole. Pentamidine may be used in patients intolerant to cotrimoxazole.

QUESTION 398

A. FALSE B. TRUE C. TRUE D. TRUE E. TRUE

Metronidazole is associated with a painful neuropathy, altered taste and disulfiram-type reactions with alcohol.

Ciprofloxacin is associated with theophylline toxicity (as is erythromycin and cyclosporin), arthralgias in children, photosensitivity, abnormal LFTs, psychosis and crystalluria.

Amphotericin B produces fever, rigors, vomiting, renal failure, hypokalaemia, hypomagnesaemia and renal tubular acidosis and anaemia.

Tetracyclines are associated with benign intracranial hypertension, photosensitivity (esp. demeclocycline), vertigo (minocycline), diarrhoea, oesophagitis, moniliasis and hepatotoxicity.

Imipenem is associated with lowered seizure threshold and seizures in non–epileptic patients (as are high-dose ticarcillin or piperacillin, fluconazole and fluoroquinolones).

QUESTION 399

A. TRUE B. TRUE C. TRUE D. TRUE E. FALSE

Kaposi's sarcoma is commonly seen in homosexual patients with AIDS and faeco-oral contact seems to predispose for this. It is occasionally seen in intravenous drug users with AIDS but rarely occurs in haemophiliacs with AIDS. Kaposi's lesions on the palate are strongly associated with intrathoracic Kaposi's sarcoma. There is recent evidence that a novel Herpes virus (HHV-8) may be involved in the pathogenesis of Kaposi's sarcoma. A reduced gas transfer (TLCO) is sensitive but not specific.

Mycobacterial infections are rare until the CD4 count falls below $0.06 \times 10^9/l$. Approx. 50% of HIV-positive individuals develop this infection before they die. The presentation is non-specific; hepatomegaly and anaemia are the most common findings. Treatment is not curative and is required for life (e.g. rifampicin, ethambutol, clarithromycin). Prophylaxis is with ansamycin (rifabutin).

CMV causes pneumonitis in immunosuppressed individuals but rarely occurs without other pathogens in HIV. Treatment is with Ganciclovir but is rarely very effective.

QUESTION 400

A. FALSE B. FALSE C. TRUE D. TRUE E. TRUE

Vertical transmission of HIV occurs in approx. 15% of HIV-positive pregnancies. Note: the anti-HIV antibody is an IgG isotype and can cross the placenta. Thus all new-borns from HIV-positive mothers will be positive for the antibody - though not necessarily infected with the virus. No developmental abnormalities have been associated with transplacental passage of virus. However, in developing countries, there is a detrimental effect on pregnancy through maternal ill health. There is some evidence that vaginal delivery carries a higher risk of transmission of HIV than Caesarean section and in one study, first-born twins were at higher risk than their sibling. There is no increased risk of HIV transmission in subsequent pregnancies. HIV can be cultured from breast milk and can be transmitted to new-borns via this route. Zidovudine therapy for the mother before and during delivery and to the new-born infant for 6 weeks reduces the risk of perinatal transmission of infection from 26% to 8%.

QUESTION 401

A. TRUE B. TRUE C. TRUE D. FALSE E. FALSE

Glandular fever-like syndrome is produced by infection with EBV, CMV, toxoplasma, HHV-6 and HIV. EBV produces the classical picture with pharyngitis, palatine petechiae, tender cervical lymphadenopathy, splenomegaly, lymphocytosis and mildly deranged LFTs. CMV produces marked fever. Pharyngitis is typically absent; lymphadenopathy and lymphocytosis are less frequent. Granulomatous hepatitis and hepatomegaly are usual. Toxoplasmosis is commonly subclinical and produces non-tender 'rubbery' lymphadenopathy which may persist for up to a year. Unlike EBV or CMV it is not associated with an ampicillin rash. HHV-6 in adults produces a non-specific viral syndrome and is associated with atypical lymphocytosis. Primary HIV infection is associated with prominent rash, fever, pharyngitis and adenopathy. It is often accompanied by oral or genital ulcers. Lymphocytosis and abnormal LFTs are unusual.

Parvovirus B19 produces erythema infectiosum in children. In adults with sickle cell or spherocytosis it may precipitate an aplastic crisis. In women it is associated with a rubella-like syndrome and polyarthralgia. Coxsackie A is usually a subclinical infection but may be complicated by aseptic meningitis, acute haemorrhagic conjunctivitis, 'hand-foot-mouth' disease or herpangina.

QUESTION 402

A. FALSE B. TRUE C. FALSE D. TRUE E. TRUE

Legionnaire's disease is caused by *Legionella pneumophila* and occasionally *L. micdadei*. The organism thrives in water-containing reservoirs; there is no documented person-to-person spread. Clinical features include high fever, gastrointestinal upset, headache and encephalopathy. LFTs are abnormal and patients develop hyponatraemia, hypophosphataemia and renal failure.

Diagnosis is by direct fluorescence on pleural fluid or lung biopsy or silver stain on sputum or retrospectively by serology (takes 2 weeks). Pontiac fever is a self-limiting tracheobronchitis caused by the same organism. Treatment: erythromycin +/- rifampicin for 2 weeks.

QUESTION 403

A. TRUE B. TRUE C. TRUE D. FALSE E. FALSE

Chlamydia trachomatis is hyperendemic in some parts of the world and is the commonest avoidable cause of blindness world-wide (keratitis). In neonates it can produce a severe pneumonia. C. psittaci is the cause of psittacosis, an atypical pneumonia in individuals exposed to birds (e.g. pigeons). It can rarely cause a myocarditis and endocarditis. Diagnosis is by serology. C. pneumonia (also known as the TWAR agent) is a common cause of pneumonia in Finland. It produces an atypical pneumonia (similar to psittacosis) but is a prolonged illness with prominent pharyngitis and laryngitis. The organism is resistant to erythromycin (unlike C. psittaci) and treatment is with tetracycline. Radiological features are non-specific with patchy shadows in the lung fields; lobar consolidation is rare.

QUESTION 404

A. TRUE B. TRUE C. FALSE D. TRUE E. FALSE

Other relative contraindications include practising homosexuals and individuals who feel they require an HIV test.

QUESTION 405

A. TRUE B. FALSE C. TRUE D. TRUE E. TRUE

Infective agents known to be transmitted by blood include:

* *Viruses*: hepatitis A, B and C, delta agent, CMV, parvovirus B19, HTLV 1 and HTLV 2, EBV, herpes simplex, HIV-1 and HIV-2;
* *Parasites*: trypanosomes, toxoplasma, filaria and leishmania.

QUESTION 406

A. TRUE B. FALSE C. TRUE D. TRUE E. FALSE

Monoamine oxidase A metabolises intraneuronal noradrenaline and 5-hydroxytryptamine. Monoamine B metabolises dopamine. Isocarboxazid, phenelzine and tranylcypromine irreversibly inhibit the intracellular enzymes monoamine oxidase A and B. Moclobemide is a reversible inhibitor of monoamine oxidase A. Selegiline inhibits monoamine oxidase B and is used in the treatment of Parkinson's Disease.

Ref: Kumar & Clark. Clinical Medicine, 3rd Ed. W. B. Saunders. Chs 18 and 19.

QUESTION 407

A. FALSE B. TRUE C. FALSE D. TRUE E. TRUE

Fluoxetine, paroxetine and sertraline selectively inhibit the reuptake of serotonin (SSRIs). SSRIs are less sedative, less cardiotoxic and safer in overdose than tricyclic antidepressants. Nortriptyline is a tricyclic antidepressant. Venlafaxine is a new antidepressant which inhibits the reuptake of serotonin and noradrenaline.

Ref: British National Formulary. No 34. BMA & RPS. Ch. 4.

QUESTION 408

A. TRUE B. FALSE C. TRUE D. FALSE E. TRUE

Donepezil is a reversible inhibitor of anticholinesterase and is used in the treatment of mild to moderately severe Alzheimer's dementia. No dose adjustment is required for patients with renal or mild-moderate hepatic impairment. It has a vagotonic effect on the heart and should be used with caution in patients with sick sinus syndrome or other supraventricular conduction abnormalities. It should be used with care in patients at risk of peptic ulcer disease, asthma and obstructive airways disease. Its side effects are: diarrhoea, muscle cramps, fatigue, nausea, vomiting, insomnia, dizziness, syncope, bradycardia, heartblock, convulsions, bladder outflow obstruction and minor increases in muscle creatine kinase.

Ref: British National Formulary. No 34. BMA & RPS. Ch. 4.

QUESTION 409

A. TRUE B. TRUE C. FALSE D. TRUE E. TRUE

Electroconvulsive therapy is effective in the treatment of depressive psychosis, puerperal pyschosis, mania, acute catatonic states, schizoaffective disorders and acute schizophrenia with predominantly positive symptoms (such as delusions and thought disorder).

Ref: Gelder, Gath, Mayou & Cowen. Oxford Textbook of Psychiatry. 3rd Ed. Oxford University Press. Ch. 17.

QUESTION 410

A. FALSE B. FALSE C. TRUE D. FALSE E. TRUE

During ECT activation of the parasympathetic nervous system (i.e. bradycardia and hypotension) initially occurs, followed by a sympathetic response (tachycardia and hypertension). Arrhythmias during the parasympathetic phase include asystole, premature ventricular contraction or ventricular escape beats. The most frequent arrhythmias during the sympathetic phase are sinus tachycardia, ventricular tachycardia and premature ventricular contractions. There is little evidence that atropine in usual dosages prevents the vagal arrhythmias of ECT and the current advice of the Royal College of Psychiatrists (1995) is that atropine should not be given routinely.

The cerebral effects of ECT are increases in cerebral blood flow (up to 200%), cerebral oxygen consumption and intracranial pressure.
The neuroendocrine response to ECT are increases in ACTH, cortisol, noradrenaline, adrenaline and prolactin.

ECT is associated with a mortality of 3-5 per 100,000 treatments. Most deaths are caused by ventricular fibrillation or myocardial infarction.

Refs: Gelder, Gath, Mayou & Cowen. Oxford Textbook of Psychiatry. 3rd Ed. Oxford University Press. Ch. 17.
Miller. Anesthesia. 4th Ed. Churchill Livingstone. Ch. 70.

QUESTION   411

A. FALSE   B. TRUE   C. TRUE   D. TRUE   E. FALSE

The characteristic pathological features of Alzheimer's disease are:

- Global neuronal reduction particularly of the frontal, parietal and temporal cortex
- Neurofibrillary tangles composed of paired helical filaments
- Argentophil plaques composed mainly of amyloid protein
- Granulovacuolar degeneration
- Reduction of neurochemicals including the enzyme choline acetyltransferase, acetyl choline, noradrenaline, 5-hydroxytryptamine, glutamate and somatostatin.
- Lewy bodies are pathognomonic of Lewy body dementia a progressive dementing illness clinically distinguished from Alzheimer's disease by its fluctuating course and the occurrence of psychotic symptoms.

Ref: Kumar & Clark. Clinical Medicine, 3rd Ed. W. B. Saunders. Ch. 19.

QUESTION   412

A. FALSE   B. FALSE   C. FALSE   D. TRUE   E. TRUE

Depressive symptoms are the most common psychiatric manifestation of Cushing's disease and hyperparathyroidism.

Phaeochromocytomas are associated with episodic attacks of anxiety which may precipitate the symptoms of flushing, palpitations, sweating, tremulousness and headaches.

Addison's disease produces symptoms of withdrawal, apathy, fatigue, memory disturbance which may be misdiagnosed as dementia. Addisonian crises are accompanied by the features of an acute organic syndrome.

Insulinomas causes recurrent attacks of aggressive and uninhibited behaviour.

Ref: Kumar & Clark. Clinical Medicine, 3rd Ed. W. B. Saunders. Ch. 19.
Gelder, Gath, Mayou & Cowen. Oxford Textbook of Psychiatry. 3rd Ed. Oxford University Press. Ch. 12.

QUESTION   413

A. FALSE B. TRUE C. FALSE D. FALSE E. FALSE

Factors associated with a poor outcome in schizophrenia is associated with an insidious onset, male sex, negative symptoms that persist after resolution of positive symptoms and a family history of schizophrenia.

Ref: Kumar & Clark. Clinical Medicine, 3rd Ed. W. B. Saunders. Ch. 19.

QUESTION   414

A. FALSE B. FALSE C. TRUE D. TRUE E. FALSE

Delirium tremens is the most serious alcohol withdrawal state with a mortality of up to 10% because it often complicates other medical emergencies. It is associated with visual and auditory hallucinations, restlessness, tremor, agitation and disorientation which are worse at night. Vestibular disturbances are frequent and felt by the patient as rotation of the room or movement of the floor.

Treatment is with fluids, adequate sedation, prevention of hypoglycaemia, hypokalaemia, hypomagnesaemia, parenteral B vitamins and anticonvulsants for withdrawal convulsions. Coexisting infections markedly increase the mortality and must be treated. Disulfiram is contraindicated in delirium tremens.

Ref: Kumar & Clark. Clinical Medicine, 3rd Ed. W. B. Saunders. Ch. 19.
Gelder, Gath, Mayou & Cowen. Oxford Textbook of Psychiatry. 3rd Ed. Oxford University Press. Ch. 14.

QUESTION   415

A. TRUE B. TRUE C. TRUE D. TRUE E. FALSE

The psychiatric complications of alcohol abuse are delirium tremens, alcoholic hallucinations, pathological jealousy (Othello syndrome), Korsakoff's psychosis and depression. Cotard's syndrome is a severe depressive illness associated with nihilistic delusions.

Ref: Kumar & Clark. Clinical Medicine, 3rd Ed. W. B. Saunders. Ch. 19.

QUESTION   416

A. TRUE B. FALSE C. TRUE D. TRUE E. FALSE

In bulimia nervosa, patients characteristically have episodes of uncontrolled excessive eating. Patients attempt to avoid the fattening effects of periodic bingeing by vomiting, abusing laxatives and drug misuse (diuretics, thyroid extracts and anorectics).

The clinical features include hypochloraemic, hypokalaemic metabolic alkalosis, swollen salivary glands and eroded dental enamel as a result of vomiting.

Menstrual irregularity is common but amenorrhoea is rare and is usually a feature of anorexia nervosa. Severe weight loss is also a feature of anorexia nervosa.

Ref: Kumar & Clark. Clinical Medicine, 3rd Ed. W. B. Saunders. Ch. 19.

QUESTION 417

A. TRUE B. TRUE C. TRUE D. TRUE E. TRUE

All of the above are associated with an increased risk of suicide in depressed patients.

Ref: Kumar & Clark. Clinical Medicine, 3rd Ed. W. B. Saunders. Ch. 19.

QUESTION 418

A. FALSE B. TRUE C. FALSE D. FALSE E. FALSE

Puerperal psychosis occurs once in every 500-1,000 births. Over 80% occur within the first two weeks following delivery. Electroconvulsive therapy is very rapidly effective and enables the mother to resume the care of her baby quickly. Most patients make a full recovery. After subsequent childbirth the recurrence rate for depressive illness is approximately 15-20%.

Ref: Kumar & Clark. Clinical Medicine, 3rd Ed. W. B. Saunders. Ch. 19.
Gelder, Gath, Mayou & Cowen. Oxford Textbook of Psychiatry. 3rd Ed. Oxford University Press. Ch. 12.

QUESTION 419

A. FALSE B. TRUE C. TRUE D. TRUE E. FALSE

Reserpine and methyldopa may produce symptoms of depression.

Ref: Kumar & Clark. Clinical Medicine, 3rd Ed. W. B. Saunders. Ch. 19.

QUESTION 420

A. FALSE B. FALSE C. TRUE D. FALSE E. FALSE

Moclobemide binds reversibly to monoamine oxidase A (MAO-A) forming a compound which has a half-life of two hours. Full MAO activity is restored within 24 hours of stopping moclobemide. It is known as a RIMA (reversible inhibitor of monamine oxidase).

Foods containing tyramine should avoided in patients taking MAOI's. These are:

- all cheeses except cream, cottage and ricotta cheeses
- red wine, sherry, beer and liquors

- pickled or smoked fish
- brewer's yeast products
- broad bean pods
- beef or chicken liver
- fermented sausage (bologna, pepperoni and salami)
- foodstuffs past their sell by date (pheasant, venison, non-fresh dairy products)

A greater dose of tyramine is required to produce a pressor response with moclobemide, because MAO-B present in the gut wall and liver is still available to metabolise much of the tyramine ingested.

MAOI's are non specific in action and can interact with other drugs as a result of their inhibition of other enzymes. The hypoglycaemic action of sulphonylureas is potentiated. Adrenaline is metabolised by catechol-O-methyltransferase.

Ref: Gelder, Gath, Mayou & Cowen. Oxford Textbook of Psychiatry. 3rd Ed. Oxford University Press. Ch. 17.

QUESTION 421

A. TRUE B. FALSE C. TRUE D. TRUE E. TRUE

Hyponatraemia due to inappropriate secretion of antidiuretic hormone has been associated with all types of antidepressants and carbamazepine. It is not a feature of antipyschotic drugs.

Ref: British National Formulary. No 34. BMA and RPS. Ch. 4.

QUESTION 422

A. TRUE B. FALSE C. TRUE D. FALSE E. FALSE

The most serious effects of overdose of ecstasy are: delirium, coma, convulsions, ventricular arrhythmias, hyperpyrexia, rhabdomyolysis, acute renal failure, acute hepatitis, disseminated intravascular coagulation, adult respiratory distress syndrome, hyperreflexia, hypotension and intracerebral haemorrhage.

Ref: Kumar & Clark. Clinical Medicine, 3rd Ed. W. B. Saunders. Ch. 19.

QUESTION 423

A. TRUE B. TRUE C. FALSE D. TRUE E. FALSE

Depression is common in bulimia nervosa and may require treatment with antidepressants.

Ref: Kumar & Clark. Clinical Medicine, 3rd Ed. W. B. Saunders. Ch. 19.
Gelder, Gath, Mayou & Cowen. Oxford Textbook of Psychiatry. 3rd Ed. Oxford University Press. Ch. 12.

QUESTION 424

A. FALSE B. TRUE C. TRUE D. FALSE E. TRUE

Characteristics of hysteria are:

1. They occur in the absence of physical disease.
2. They are produced unconsciously.
3. They are not caused by overactivity of the sympathetic nervous system.
4. They often reflect a patient's ideas about illness.
5. The symptoms usually confer some advantage on the patient (secondary gain).

Most patients of recent onset recover quickly. Drug treatments have no part to play unless the symptoms are secondary to a depressive illness or anxiety neurosis requiring treatment.

Ref: Kumar & Clark. Clinical Medicine, 3rd Ed. W. B. Saunders. Ch. 19.

QUESTION 425

A. TRUE B. FALSE C. TRUE D. FALSE E. FALSE

Toxic symptoms begin to occur when serum lithium levels exceed 1.5 mmol/l. These are drowsiness, blurred vision, tremor, ataxia, dysarthria, polyuria, polydipsia (due to inhibition of the antidiuretic hormone sensitive adenylate cyclase in the distal tube of Henlé), metallic taste, nausea, vomiting, diarrhoea, hypothyroidism and leucocytosis.

Ref: Kumar & Clark. Clinical Medicine, 3rd Ed. W. B. Saunders. Ch. 19.

QUESTION 426

A. FALSE B. FALSE C. FALSE D. TRUE E. FALSE

ECT is the treatment of choice for puerperal psychosis. It is beneficial in patients with severe depression resistant to medical therapy, depression accompanied by dehydration or weight loss, drug-resistant mania, depression with suicidal ideation, delusions or psychotic symptoms. Contraindications include patients unfit for general anaesthesia, known ischaemic heart disease or stroke, or raised intracranial pressure. In young adults, prominent anxiety symptoms are usually associated with a poor outcome with ECT; in the elderly, agitation and anxiety predict a good outcome.

QUESTION 427

A. TRUE B. TRUE C. TRUE D. TRUE E. FALSE

Acutely, cocaine produces a stimulated euphoric feeling in the user. Other features include irritability, acute anxiety, paranoid ideation, hypertension, tachycardia, cardiac dysrhythmias, dilated pupils (responsive to light), dry mouth, aggression, hallucination (typically formication – tactile sensations on the skin), increased deep-tendon reflexes and respiratory arrest in overdose. Chronic use, in addition, produces impaired concentration, erectile and ejaculatory dysfunction, hypersomnia, psychotic symptoms (persecutory delusions, ideas of reference, etc.), nasal septal perforation from snorting, endocarditis from intravenous use and seizures from overdose.

QUESTION 428

A. FALSE B. FALSE C. TRUE D. TRUE E. FALSE

Remember to distinguish between side effects of a drug (i.e. with long-term use) from toxic effects due to overdose. Common side effects of lithium (with levels <1.0 mmol/l) include nausea, fine tremor, polyuria (nephrogenic DI), polydipsia, weight gain, leucocytosis, and metallic taste in mouth. Rarer side effects include goitre, hypothyroidism (biochemical abnormalities may occur without symptoms), hypokalaemia and exacerbation of psoriasis. Toxic effects of lithium (i.e. levels >1.3 mmol/l) include blurred vision, ataxia, dysarthria, anorexia, coarse tremor, vomiting, muscle weakness, hyperreflexia, oliguria, seizures, syncope, coma and death. Toxicity may be precipitated by ACE inhibitors, thiazides, NSAIDs, metronidazole, SSRI antidepressants and diltiazem (even with normal levels).

QUESTION 429

A. TRUE B. TRUE C. TRUE D. TRUE E. TRUE

Extrapyramidal syndromes are common with the high-potency neuroleptic agents. These includes acute dystonic reactions (torticollis, opisthotonos and oculogyric crises - treat with benztropine or procyclidine), neuroleptic-induced catatonia (mutism, withdrawal, rigidity, waxy flexibility - responds to stopping the neuroleptic and sometimes to amantadine), akathisia (motor restlessness), tardive dyskinesia (fasciculation of the tongue, facial and tongue hyperkinesias, chewing, grimacing, choreoathetoic movements - if diagnosed early may be reversible, but become irreversible with time), drug-induced Parkinsonism (responds to standard therapy for Parkinson's disease, which can then be tailed off). Other side effects include neuroleptic-malignant syndrome, anticholinergic effects, orthostatic hypotension, ventricular arrhythmias, cholestatic jaundice, lens and corneal pigmentation (chlorpromazine, thioradizine) and blurred vision.

QUESTION 430

A. TRUE B. FALSE C. TRUE D. TRUE E. FALSE

The neuroleptic-malignant syndrome is a potentially life-threatening complication of neuroleptic therapy and occurs in 1-2% of treated patients. It is characterised by hyperthermia, muscular rigidity, autonomic instability and fluctuating conscious level. Serum CK and WCC are elevated. The full blown syndrome occurs over 24-48 hours after a period of gradual muscular rigidity. Treatment involves stopping the neuroleptic, supportive measures (cooling, rehydration, renal, respiratory and cardiac support), and drug therapy (dantrolene, diazepam and other muscle relaxants; also dopamine agonists like bromocriptine, amantadine and L-dopa). Neuroleptics may be reintroduced cautiously after recovery: the recurrence rate is 10-30%.

QUESTION 431

A. TRUE   B. FALSE   C. FALSE   D. TRUE   E. FALSE

In a pure paracetamol overdose patients are normally fully conscious on admission. A decreased level of consciousness suggests another substance has been taken. A paracetamol level above 200 mg/l at 4 hours suggests treatment is indicated. Alcoholics and those taking enzyme-inducing drugs should be treated at half this level. Even after an overdose that causes severe hepatic damage long term sequelae don't develop, and normal therapeutic doses of parac-etamol can be taken.

Ref: Kumar & Clark. Clinical Medicine, 3rd Ed. W. B. Saunders. Ch. 14.

QUESTION 432

A. FALSE   B. TRUE   C. TRUE   D. TRUE   E. TRUE

Subacute combined degeneration of the cord is due to Vitamin B12 deficiency. Vitamin B1 deficiency occurs in chronic alcoholism and may cause Wernicke-Korsakoff syndrome or beri-beri. Beri-beri may present with cardiac failure and should be distinguished from alcoholic cardiomyopathy. Macrocytosis is caused by a direct toxic effect on the bone marrow or by folate deficiency.

Ref: Kumar & Clark. Clinical Medicine, 3rd Ed. W. B. Saunders.

QUESTION 433

A. TRUE   B. TRUE   C. TRUE   D. FALSE   E. TRUE

Penicillamine is useful in treating lead poisoning. Desferrioxamine is used to treat iron poisoning.

Ref: Oh. Intensive Care Manual. 4th Ed. Butterworth Heinemann. Ch. 77.

QUESTION 434

A. TRUE   B. TRUE   C. TRUE   D. TRUE   E. TRUE

Many anticholinergic effects may be seen after tricyclic overdose. After theophylline overdose, the elimination half-life will be decreased from approximately 10 to approximately 5 hours by repeated doses of activated charcoal. Charcoal haemoperfusion may be useful if seizures or malignant arrhythmias are occurring or if there is pre-existing hepatic or heart disease. Ethanol competitively inhibits the metabolism of methanol and is used to treat methanol over-dose. Atropine may be used to control parasympathetic overactivity occurring when organophosphates inhibit cholinesterase.

Ref: Oh. Intensive Care Manual. 4th Ed. Butterworth Heinemann. Ch. 77.

QUESTION 435

A. TRUE B. TRUE C. TRUE D. TRUE E. TRUE

Poisoning with lithium may occur in patients on long term therapy if a diuretic is administered. Patients with lithium levels greater than 3.5–4.0 mmol/l usually need haemodialysis. Digoxin overdose may be treated with the Fab fragments of digoxin specific antibodies. Cyanide prevents cellular respiration by inhibiting cytochrome oxidase, leading to a metabolic acidosis.

Ref: Kumar & Clark. Clinical Medicine, 3rd Ed. W. B. Saunders. Ch. 14.
Oh. Intensive Care Manual. 4th Ed. Butterworth Heinemann. Chs 72 and 77.

QUESTION 436

A. TRUE B. FALSE C. TRUE D. TRUE E. TRUE

CO affinity for haemoglobin is 240 times that of oxygen. It makes pulse oximetry readings tend to 100%. Poisoning may present with a decreased level of consciousness or coma, and toxicity is synergistic with cyanide.

Ref: Oh. Intensive Care Manual. 4th Ed. Butterworth Heinemann. Chs 72 and 77.
Davey, Moyle & Ward. Ward's Anaesthetic Equipment. 3rd Ed. W. B. Saunders. Ch. 16.

QUESTION 437

A. TRUE B. FALSE C. FALSE D. FALSE E. TRUE

Activated charcoal maintains a drug concentration gradient between mucosal blood and the gut lumen, so is useful even for drugs without significant enterohepatic circulation. It increases non-renal elimination of phenobarbitone, salicylate, diazepam, digoxin, theophylline and carbamazepine (amongst others). It is ineffective for cyanide, pesticides and elemental metals. Death following charcoal aspiration has been reported.

Ref: Oh. Intensive Care Manual. 4th Ed. Butterworth Heinemann. Ch. 77.

QUESTION 438

A. TRUE B. TRUE C. TRUE D. FALSE E. TRUE

Methanol is non-toxic. Acidosis and blindness occur due to its metabolism to formaldehyde and formate. Amanita phalloides poisoning is worse if mushrooms are eaten raw. Paraquat causes pulmonary oedema followed by pulmonary fibrosis. This is worsened by high oxygen concentrations.

Ref: Kumar & Clark. Clinical Medicine, 3rd Ed. W. B. Saunders. Ch. 14.
Oh. Intensive Care Manual. 4th Ed. Butterworth Heinemann. Ch. 77.

QUESTION 439

A. TRUE B. TRUE C. FALSE D. TRUE E. TRUE

Tricyclic overdose may cause a decreased level of consciousness, increased tone, hyperreflexia and extensor plantars. Pupils may be fixed and dilated. Urinary retention occurs. Sinus tachycardia or other arrhythmias (including ventricular arrhythmias) may occur. Increasing arterial pH to greater than 7.45 (using bicarbonate or hyperventilation) reduces free drug availability.

Ref: Kumar & Clark. Clinical Medicine, 3rd Ed. W. B. Saunders. Ch. 14.
Oh. Intensive Care Manual. 4th Ed. Butterworth Heinemann. Ch. 77.

QUESTION 440

A. TRUE B. FALSE C. FALSE D. FALSE E. TRUE

Salicylic acid or aspirin overdose causes a range of symptoms including tinnitus, hyperpyrexia, renal failure, respiratory failure, coma and death. Gastric emptying is slowed down, hence the advice 'Its never too late to aspirate for salicylate'. It causes respiratory alkalosis and a metabolic acidosis. The pKa of the drug (50% ionization) is 4.1. Renal excretion can be enhanced by increasing oral/iv fluid intake to induce a diuresis. Acids dissociate in alkaline urine therefore alkalinisation of the urine to a pH greater than 7 leads to an increase in the ionized proportion within the renal tubules. Since only uncharged molecules can traverse the lipid membranes of the tubular cells to be reabsorbed, salicylic acid remains 'trapped' in the urine and excretion is enhanced. Forced alkaline diuresis is normally reserved for plasma salicylate levels greater than 4.3 mmol/l.

QUESTION 441

A. FALSE B. FALSE C. TRUE D. FALSE E. FALSE

Immunoglobulin G (IgG) is the most abundant immunoglobulin in the serum. It is monomer composed of 2 heavy and 2 light chains with a molecular weight of 150,000 Daltons. It is the antibody of the secondary immune response and has in general a high affinity. It crosses the placenta freely and is the only antibody to do so in significant quantities. This has both therapeutic and pathological consequences. Each molecule has 2 antigen binding sites. There are 4 subclasses of IgG. IgG1 and IgG3 are mainly produced in response to protein antigens such as tetanus toxin and viruses. IgG2 and IgG4 are produced in response to polysaccharide antigen such as the pneumococcus or haemophilus. The natural haemagglutinins anti-A and anti-B are IgM antibodies.

Ref: Kumar & Clark. Clinical Medicine, 3rd Ed. W. B. Saunders. Ch. 2.

QUESTION 442

A. FALSE B. FALSE C. TRUE D. FALSE E. TRUE

IgM is a pentameric molecule mainly confined to the intravascular pool. The 5 chains containing 10 antigen binding sites are held together by J chains. It does not cross the placenta and is not normally produced until after birth. Antigen specific IgM is therefore a good marker of intrauterine infection. It is the antibody of the primary immune response and forms the natural anti-A and anti-B haemagglutinins. Haemolytic disease of the new-born is caused by anti-D IgG antibodies.

Ref: Kumar & Clark. Clinical Medicine, 3rd Ed. W. B. Saunders. Chs 2 and 6.

QUESTION 443

A. TRUE B. TRUE C. FALSE D. TRUE E. TRUE

IgA occurs in both serum and secretions. It is monomeric in serum but dimeric in secretions with two molecules being complexed by a J chain. Secretory IgA only occurs in secretions and is the association of IgA with a secretory component (a poly FC receptor). IgA itself appears as 2 subclasses A1 and A2. IgA1 predominates in serum but both occur in equal amounts in secretions. IgA does not cross the placenta or bind to mast cells. It is responsible for mucosal immunity and may be important in binding enterotoxins such as cholera, preventing the attachment of enteroviruses and preventing invasion by bacteria.

Ref: Kumar & Clark. Clinical Medicine, 3rd Ed. W. B. Saunders. Ch. 2.

QUESTION 444

A. TRUE B. TRUE C. TRUE D. TRUE E. TRUE

The acute phase proteins are a group of proteins that are synthesized in response to trauma, infection, necrosis, malignancy or other events in which there is inflammation. They appear to have a role in the immunopathological process and in the non-specific defence mechanism. The main acute phase proteins are C-reactive protein, serum amyloid protein, fibrinogen, haptoglobin, caeruloplasmin, alpha-1-antitrypsin and components of the complement system. CRP is used clinically as a marker of disease activity.

Ref: Kumar & Clark. Clinical Medicine, 3rd Ed. W. B. Saunders. Ch. 2.

QUESTION 445

A. FALSE B. FALSE C. TRUE D. TRUE E. TRUE

The human lymphocyte antigens form part of the Major Histocompatibility Complex (MHC) and are a series of closely linked genetic loci on the short arm of chromosome 6. The loci are highly polymorphic and exhibit co-dominance. There is wide inter-racial variation with the haplotype A1B8 being found mainly in Caucasians. The genes code for a series of cell-surface glycoproteins known as Class I and II molecules. They are antigenic and involved in tissue typing for transplantation purposes.

Class I antigens are expressed on all cell types except erythrocytes and trophoblasts. They are 3 main loci, A, B and C.

Class II antigens are expressed on B cells, monocytes, dendritic cells and activated T cells. They are important in the presentation of antigen to subpopulations of T Cells.

Ref: Kumar & Clark. Clinical Medicine, 3rd Ed. W. B. Saunders. Ch. 2.

QUESTION 446

A. FALSE B. FALSE C. TRUE D. FALSE E. FALSE

An immune response is essential for survival after birth but not for normal growth and development in utero. IgM synthesis starts after 30 weeks gestation but the production of IgG is delayed until several weeks after birth. Premature infants have low levels of maternal antibody as active transport does not occur until the 3rd trimester. As there is little initial IgG production by the infant, levels of antibody fall after birth due to the loss of maternal IgG in the newborn period.

Ref: Kumar & Clark. Clinical Medicine, 3rd Ed. W. B. Saunders. Ch. 2.

QUESTION 447

A. FALSE B. FALSE C. TRUE D. TRUE E. TRUE

X-linked recessive disorders are transmitted by healthy females carrying one abnormal copy of the affected gene or affected males if they reach fertility. The disorders always present in males but may occur rarely in females homozygous for the affect gene. If the mother is the carrier and the father is normal, 50% of the girls born will be carriers of the abnormal gene and the other 50% will be normal. Of the boys, 50% will be affected and the other 50% normal as they inherit the normal X chromosome from the mother. If the father has the disease and the mother is normal, none of the male offspring will be affected but all of the female offspring will be carriers as they will inherit the affected X chromosome from the father. Random inactivation of the X chromosome may produce variably severe manifestations in women.

Ref: Kumar & Clark. Clinical Medicine, 3rd Ed. W. B. Saunders. Ch. 2.

QUESTION 448

A. TRUE B. TRUE C. TRUE D. FALSE E. TRUE

The common examples of X-linked recessive disorders include:

- Becker's and Duchenne muscular dystrophy
- Haemophilia A and B (Christmas disease)
- Colour blindness
- G-6-PDH deficiency
- Fabry's disease
- Fragile X syndrome
- Hunter's syndrome - mucopolysaccharidosis

- Nephrogenic diabetes insipidus
- Wiskott–Aldrich syndrome

Myotonic dystrophy is an example of a disease with autosomal dominant inheritance

Ref: Kumar & Clark. Clinical Medicine, 3rd Ed. W. B. Saunders. Ch. 2.

QUESTION 449

A. TRUE B. TRUE C. FALSE D. TRUE E. FALSE

Some of the common autosomal dominant disorders anaesthetists may encounter include:
- Acute intermittent porphyria
- C1 esterase inhibitor deficiency
- Adult polycystic kidney disease
- Hereditary angio-oedema
- Hereditary elliptocytosis and spherocytosis
- Huntingdon's chorea
- Marfan's syndrome
- Dystrophia myotonica
- Neurofibromatosis
- von Willebrand's disease

Beta thalassaemia and Friedreich's ataxia are examples of autosomal recessive disorders.

Ref: Kumar & Clark. Clinical Medicine, 3rd Ed. W. B. Saunders. Ch. 2.

QUESTION 450

A. FALSE B. TRUE C. TRUE D. TRUE E. FALSE

Autosomal recessive disorders only affect the individual with 2 abnormal copies of the gene. Parents are generally unaffected carriers and there is usually no family history. The offspring of an affected individual will be normal unless the partner is a carrier. If 2 carriers marry, 25% of the offspring will be normal, 25% will be affected with the condition and 50% will be carriers. Autosomal recessive conditions usually present early in life and are associated with a high mortality. Cystic fibrosis is the commonest recessive disease in Britain. Thalassaemia and sickle cell disease are very common world wide.

Vitamin D resistant rickets is the often quoted example of an X-linked dominant condition. G-6-PDH deficiency is X-linked recessive.

Ref: Kumar & Clark. Clinical Medicine, 3rd Ed. W. B. Saunders. Ch. 2.

QUESTION 451

A. TRUE B. TRUE C. FALSE D. TRUE E. TRUE

Plasmapheresis is indicated in conditions where there is hyperviscosity or where removal of serum antibodies is required. It is indicated in the early neurological stages of Guillain-Barré syndrome and non-oliguric Goodpasture's syndrome where there is an anti-GBM antibody. It may be used in Myasthenic crises or in the prethymectomy stage of the disease. It is not indicated in von Willebrand's disease which is due to deficiency or abnormality of factor VIII-vWF.

Ref: Kumar & Clark. Clinical Medicine, 3rd Ed. W. B. Saunders. Ch. 6.
Epstein RJ. Medicine for Examinations. 3rd Ed. Churchill Livingstone. Ch. 6.

QUESTION 452

A. TRUE B. TRUE C. FALSE D. TRUE E. TRUE

Selective IgA deficiency is the commonest immune defect in the UK with a prevalence of 1 in 700. Patients are often asymptomatic but some are prone to an increased risk of pyogenic infections (sinopulmonary). Many of these have an associated defect such as IgG2 deficiency. Patient's serum contains anti IgA antibodies that can trigger immune transfusion reactions and anaphylaxis in patients treated with gammaglobulin. Such patients should be treated with IgA deficient blood products. It is associated with other autoimmune disorders such as coeliac disease, rheumatoid arthritis and SLE.

Ref: Kumar & Clark. Clinical Medicine, 3rd Ed. W. B. Saunders. Ch. 6.
Epstein RJ. Medicine for Examinations. 3rd Ed. Churchill Livingstone. Ch. 6.

QUESTION 453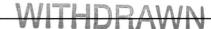

A. TRUE B. TRUE C. FALSE D. TRUE E. FALSE

Selective IgA deficiency is commonly sporadic and not inherited (incidence 1:700). Clinical features vary from asymptomatic (incidental finding) to recurrent chest infections and bronchiectasis and chronic diarrhoeal disease similar to coeliac disease. There is an increased incidence of other autoimmune disorders, e.g. SLE, chronic active hepatitis, RA, thyroiditis and pernicious anaemia. There may be an associated IgG subclass deficiency, but levels of IgG and IgM are usually normal. Intravenous immunoglobulin is not the preferred treatment as low quantities of IgA in the preparation may trigger an anaphylactic reaction. X-linked recessive immunodeficiency syndromes include Bruton's agammaglobulinaemia, Wiskott-Aldrich syndrome and chronic granulomatous disease.

Ref: Kumar & Clark. Clinical Medicine, 3rd Ed. W. B. Saunders. Ch. 6.
Epstein RJ. Medicine for Examinations. 3rd Ed. Churchill Livingstone. Ch. 6.

QUESTION 454

A. FALSE B. TRUE C. FALSE D. FALSE E. TRUE

Type I reactions (immediate) - IgE, IgG4, basophils and mast cells (e.g. atopic diseases - asthma, hayfever, anaphylaxis and drugs). There is associated oedema, vasodilatation and mast cell degranulation.
Type II reactions (cell-bound antigen) – membrane bound IgM/G causing cell lysis or

opsonisation (e.g. transfusion reactions, autoimmune haemolytic anaemias, ITP, Goodpasture's and Graves' disease, Myasthenia gravis).

Type III reactions (immune complex deposition) - caused by IgA/G immune complexes (e.g. Arthus reaction, serum sickness, SLE, Henoch-Schînlein and glomerulonephritis, low grade viral infections eg viral hepatitis). May be treated with plasmapheresis.

Type IV reactions (delayed type) - T-cell, macrophage mediated (e.g. graft rejection, tuberculin and graft versus host disease).

Grave's disease is sometimes referred to as Type V (stimulating). There exists a Type VI which is antibody-dependent cell-mediated cytotoxicity which is involved in autoimmune tumour rejection.

Ref: Kumar & Clark. Clinical Medicine, 3rd Ed. W. B. Saunders. Ch. 6.

QUESTION 455

A. TRUE B. FALSE C. TRUE D. TRUE E. FALSE

Hereditary angio-oedema is an autosomal dominant condition associated with C1 esterase inhibitor deficiency. This protein is responsible for the modulation of the intravascular activation of complement. Deficiency leads to angio-oedema due to the unregulated release of vasoactive mediators that increase vascular permeability. The classical picture is of oedema of the skin and mucous membranes. Severe airway obstruction may occur due to laryngeal oedema and lead to death. Diagnosis is on the basis of a family history, clinical manifestations and documentation of low or absent C1esterase inhibitor levels. About 15% of patients may have the disease in association with normal C1 esterase inhibitor levels. The functional activity of the protein is zero in these cases. An acquired form of the disease may be seen in patients with lymphoma. Fibrinolytics (tranexamic acid) and anabolic steroids (danazol, stanozolol) are used in long term prophylaxis. Short term treatment/prophylaxis includes the use of steroids, FFP and purified C1 esterase inhibitor. The key to management of anaesthesia is adequate preoperative prophylaxis.

Ref: Kumar & Clark. Clinical Medicine, 3rd Ed. W. B. Saunders. Ch. 20.
Stoelting & Dierdorf. Anaesthesia and Co-Existing Disease. 3rd Ed. Churchill Livingstone. Ch. 29.

QUESTION 456

A. TRUE B. FALSE C. FALSE D. TRUE E. TRUE

IL-1 is released by activated macrophages and antigen-presenting cells and leads to stimulation of helper (CD4^{+}) T cell proliferation and maturation. It also promotes B cell proliferation. IL-2 is produced by TH1 helper T cells (along with IL-1, gamma-IFN and TNF) and is mitogenic for T cells and NK cells. All these cytokines are pro-inflammatory and induce a catabolic state and fever. Only TNF has direct anti-tumour activity - the others enhance immune responses. IL-3 (also called multi-CSF) stimulates growth and differentiation of bone marrow stem cells and most haematopoietic cell lineages.

Ref: Kumar & Clark. Clinical Medicine, 3rd Ed. W. B. Saunders. Ch. 2.

QUESTION 457

A. FALSE B. TRUE C. TRUE D. TRUE E. FALSE

T lymphocytes are divided into subtypes on the basis of cell-surface markers as well as functional characteristics. All T cells express CD3 on their surface; this is in close relation to the T cell receptor and is involved in T cell activation. CD4-positive T cells are termed helper T cells and are further divided into TH1 and TH2 on functional characteristics.

TH1 cells primarily enhance immune responses and secrete IL-1, gamma-IFN, IL-12 and TNF. They promote T cell proliferation and macrophage activation. TH2 cells secrete IL-4, IL-5, IL-6, IL-10 and IL-13 and are involved primarily in enhancing humoral immune responses (B cell activation, Ig class switching, etc.). IL-15 has been shown to induce T cell activation and TNF production, especially in patients with rheumatoid arthritis. CD45RO is a cell-surface marker for memory T cells: these are the subgroup that circulates through the tissues screening for antigen. CD45RA is a marker for naive T cells.

QUESTION 458

A. FALSE B. FALSE C. TRUE D. TRUE E. TRUE

The MHC molecules are divided into class I and class II and both groups are encoded on the short arm of chromosome 6. HLA A, B and C (class I molecules) are single-chain polypeptides found on the surface of most nucleated cells (but not RBC or trophoblast cells). Their function is to present antigen to CD8+ T cells (cytotoxic) and they mediate graft rejection. On the cell surface they are closely associated with beta2-microglobulin. CD8 on the surface of T cells recognises non-polymorphic areas on the class I molecule and stabilises the interaction between the TCR and class I for antigen recognition. HLA DP, DQ and DR (class II molecules) are composed of two polypeptide chains and are found on the surface of antigen-presenting cells (macrophages, dendritic cells), activated T cells, B cells, sperm and epididymal cells. Their function is to present foreign antigen to helper T cells (CD4+). The class II molecules are the most important locus involved in graft rejection, and matching is essential for long-term survival. Siblings inherit one chromosome from each parent and so have a 1:4 chance of being identical (and 1:4 for being non-identical) in their HLA type. Identical twins are identical in their HLA type.

Ref: Kumar & Clark. Clinical Medicine, 3rd Ed. W. B. Saunders. Ch. 2.

QUESTION 459

A. TRUE B. FALSE C. FALSE D. TRUE E. FALSE

Estimation of the frequency of anaphylactic reactions associated with anaesthesia remains difficult. The incidence in France is estimated as 1 in 3,500-6,000. In Australia it is reported as 1 in 10,000-20,000. More reactions occur in females in particular for neuromuscular blocking drugs. A previous history of specific drug exposure is not necessary. For NMB there may be no history of previous drug exposure in as many as 80% of affected patients. Latex hypersensitivity typically occurs 30-60 minutes after the start of the procedure rather than at induction. There is a recognised cross-reactivity with bananas and avocados. Reaction to drugs is more common if they are given intravenously.

Ref : Association of Anaesthetists booklet: Suspected anaphylactic reactions associated with anaesthesia. 1995.

QUESTION 460

A. TRUE B. FALSE C. FALSE D. TRUE E. TRUE

Mast cell tryptase is the main protein in mast cell granules and is released with histamine and other amines. Release occurs in both IgE mediated anaphylactic reactions and non IgE mediated anaphylactoid reactions. Its concentration in plasma is raised between 1 and 6 hours after mast cell degranulation. It is not present if red cells or white cells. Plasma concentration is therefore not affected by haemolysis or neutrophil degranulation. Elevated concentrations may be detected for 12-14 hours even in the event of death. Concentrations of greater than 20 ng/ml may be seen after an anaphylactic reaction. It is both a specific and sensitive test for anaphylactic or anaphylactoid reactions. It is the most useful acute test available. Methyl histamine (main metabolite of histamine) levels in the urine are raised after reactions involving systemic histamine release. Levels need to be corrected for the urinary creatinine and this may cause some difficulty in interpretation.

The RAST test measures antigen-specific IgE antibodies in the serum. This is now only available for suxamethonium. The CAP test is a fluoro-immunoassay for the measurement of antigen-specific antibody which is more sensitive than RAST. It is useful in latex allergy.

Ref: Association of Anaesthetists booklet: Suspected anaphylactic reactions associated with anaesthesia. 1995.

QUESTION 461

A. TRUE B. TRUE C. FALSE D. TRUE E. FALSE

Treacher-Collins syndrome is the most common of the mandibular dysostoses. It is associated with micrognathia and early airway problems similar to patients with Pierre-Robin syndrome which is also associated with glossoptosis (posterior displacement of the tongue) and cleft palate. Choanal and not cloacal atresia is associated with breathing difficulty in the neonate. Eaton-Lambert is related to bronchogenic carcinomas and presents with a myasthenic like syndrome. It does not occur in neonates.

Ref: Stoelting & Dierdorf: Anaesthesia and Co-Existing Disease. 3rd Ed. Churchill Livingstone. Ch. 32.

QUESTION 462

A. TRUE B. FALSE C. TRUE D. TRUE E. FALSE

The common findings in pyloric stenosis are a hypokalaemic, hypochloraemic metabolic alkalosis due to the persistent vomiting of hydrogen ions with the consequent secretion of potassium in exchange for hydrogen by the kidneys to maintain a normal arterial pH. In addition to this the kidneys also excrete potassium and hydrogen in exchange for sodium as the infant becomes sodium deplete from vomiting. Hypoglycaemia may occur 2-3 hours after surgical correction of pyloric stenosis and there may be a period of postoperative depression of ventilation which may be related to CSF alkalosis.

Pyloric stenosis is more common in males and occurs in about 1 in 500 live births. It is as common in preterm neonates as it is in full term neonates.

Ref: Stoelting & Dierdorf: Anaesthesia and Co-Existing Disease. 3rd Ed. Churchill Livingstone. Ch. 32.

QUESTION 463

A. TRUE B. TRUE C. TRUE D. TRUE E. FALSE

All of the above may predispose to the development of RDS in the neonate except congenital heart disease which may be associated with RDS but is not strictly a predisposing factor for it.

QUESTION 464

A. FALSE B. TRUE C. TRUE D. TRUE E. TRUE

Kernicterus is a syndrome caused by the toxic effects of unconjugated bilirubin on the central nervous system. The immature blood-brain barrier of the neonate (preterm especially) allows bilirubin (which is not lipophilic) to enter the brain and cause cell damage. Hypoxaemia, acidosis and hypercapnoea may also facilitate this. Neonates with sepsis or RDS may have reduced bilirubin binding capacity and so be at increased risk. The clinical features of kernicterus include hypertonicity, opisthotonos and spasticity. Treatment includes phototherapy which converts bilirubin into water-soluble photobilirubin and exchange transfusions.

Ref: Stoelting & Dierdorf: Anaesthesia and Co-Existing Disease. 3rd Ed. Churchill Livingstone. Ch. 32.

QUESTION 465

A. TRUE B. FALSE C. TRUE D. FALSE E. FALSE

Tracheo-oesophageal fistulae has an incidence of 1 in about 3500 live births. 30-40% of patients are born preterm and are generally less than 1 week old at diagnosis. 20% of patients have an associated cardiac anomaly (VSD, Fallot's, coarctation or ASD). There is a recognised association with maternal polyhydramnios. The most common type (80%) is oesophageal atresia with a lower pouch fistula. 10% have oesophageal atresia with no fistula and only 2% have a tracheo-oesophageal fistula without oesophageal atresia.

Ref: Goldstone and Pollard. Handbook of Clinical Anesthesia. Churchill Livingstone.

QUESTION 466

A. FALSE B. FALSE C. TRUE D. TRUE E. FALSE

Omphalocele is associated with the external herniation of abdominal viscera through a defect at the base of the umbilical cord. Herniation through a defect lateral to the normally inserted umbilical cord occurs in gastroschisis. It occurs in about 1 in 5,000-10,000 live births and is more common in males. About one third of patients with this are born prematurely. However it is associated with a 75% incidence of other congenital defects including cardiac problems, Down's and Beckwith syndrome. Cardiac defects are the major cause of mortality.

Ref: Stoelting & Dierdorf: Anaesthesia and Co-Existing Disease. 3rd Ed. Churchill Livingstone. Ch. 32.

QUESTION 467

A. TRUE B. TRUE C. FALSE D. TRUE E. FALSE

Gastroschisis is more commonly associated with prematurity than omphalocele but is rarely associated with other congenital abnormalities. Unlike omphalocele the abdominal viscera are not covered with a hernia sac and the defect is through the anterior abdominal wall lateral to the umbilical cord. Fluid requirements are increased and the exposed bowel should be covered to reduce fluid and heat loss. The use of nitrous oxide is controversial. It may cause bowel distension and make returning the bowel to the abdomen more difficult. If it is not used, air should be used to dilute the oxygen due to the risk of retinopathy of prematurity.

Ref: Stoelting & Dierdorf: Anaesthesia and Co-existing Disease. 3rd Ed. Churchill Livingstone. Ch. 32.

QUESTION 468

A. TRUE B. FALSE C. TRUE D. TRUE E. TRUE

Reye syndrome is an acute encephalopathy associated with fatty infiltration of the viscera. Death is due to diffuse cerebral oedema which leads to brain infarction and herniation. It is usually found in children under 10 and follows a prodromal viral illness. There is a recognised association with the use of salicylates. The onset is heralded by protracted vomiting and signs of raised intracranial pressure. There is a tachycardia, mild fever and respiratory alkalosis. There may be a rapid deterioration in neurological state. Tendon reflexes are hyperactive. PT, TT, Liver enzymes and ammonia are all raised. Hypoglycaemia may occur. Patients have hepatomegaly and not splenomegaly. Injury to the brain and liver progresses for 3 to 6 days after which there is rapid resolution if death does not occur due to cerebral oedema. Treatment is supportive and aimed at maintaining cerebral perfusion.

Ref: Stoelting & Dierdorf: Anaesthesia and Co-Existing Disease. 3rd Ed. Churchill Livingstone. Ch. 32.

QUESTION 469

A. TRUE B. TRUE C. TRUE D. FALSE E. TRUE

Nephroblastoma occurs in 1 in 13,500 births and accounts for about 10% of solid tumours in children. It typically presents as an asymptomatic mass in the flank in a otherwise healthy child. Malaise, fever, vomiting, pain, haematuria, anaemia and urinary problems may occur later in the disease. Hypertension is particularly associated with bilateral tumours and may lead to encephalopathy and congestive cardiac failure. Hypokalaemia may occur due to secondary hyperaldosteronism due to renin release by the tumour. 75% of cases are diagnosed by the age of 4. It is an inherited cancer syndrome with the gene located at 11p13. Survival rates are excellent with a combination of nephrectomy, radiotherapy and chemotherapy even for those children with metastatic disease.

Ref: Stoelting & Dierdorf: Anaesthesia and Co-Existing Disease. 3rd Ed. Churchill Livingstone. Ch. 32.
Kumar & Clark. Clinical Medicine, 3rd Ed. W. B. Saunders. Ch. 9.

QUESTION 470

A. TRUE B. TRUE C. FALSE D. TRUE E. TRUE

The Apgar score assigns a value of 0, 1 or 2 to five vital signs observed at 1 minute and 5 minutes after delivery. Heart rate and respiratory effort are the most important criteria with colour being the least important. Significant hypoxaemia is generally signified by a heart rate below 100 which scores 1 point. Apgars correlate well with acid-base balance immediately after delivery but are not sensitive enough to detect or evaluate the subtle effects of obstetric anaesthetic technique on neonates.

SCORE

	0	1	2
Heart rate	Absent	<100	>100
Respiratory effort	Absent	Slow Irreg	Crying
Reflex irritability	No response	Grimace	Crying
Muscle tone	Limp	Flexion of extremities	Active
Colour	Pale, Cyanotic	Body pink extremities cyanotic	Pink

Ref: Stoelting & Dierdorf: Anaesthesia and Co-Existing Disease. 3rd Ed. Churchill Livingstone. Ch. 31.

QUESTION 471

A. FALSE B. TRUE C. TRUE D. FALSE E. TRUE

Infections due to Hib are an important cause of morbidity and mortality in young children. There are 6 encapsulated strains (a-f) that cause disease in man. Meningitis with bacteraemia is the most common presentation. 15% of cases present with epiglottitis and in 10% there is septicaemia without any other infection. Hib meningitis is associated with deafness, convulsions and intellectual impairment. The case fatality rate is about 4%. Hib occurred in about 1 in 600 children before their fifth birthday prior to vaccination programmes in the UK that commenced in 1992.

It is rare below the age of 3 months and the peak incidence occurs at the age of 10-11 months.

Ref: Immunisation against infective disease 1996. DoH. HMSO.

QUESTION 472

A. FALSE B. TRUE C. TRUE D. FALSE E. FALSE

The following are the commonly used live vaccines: Oral polio (Sabin), measles, mumps, rubella, yellow fever, BCG and Typhoid Ty 21a.

Haemophilus influenza type B is a non replicating bacterial capsular antigen vaccine. Menigococcal vaccine is a purified, heat stable lyophilised extract from the polysaccharide outer capsule of N meningitides. Tetanus vaccine is a toxoid.

Ref: Kumar & Clark. Clinical Medicine, 3rd Ed. W. B. Saunders. Ch. 1.

QUESTION 473

A. TRUE B. TRUE C. TRUE D. TRUE E. FALSE

The incubation period for rubella is between 14 and 21 days with infectivity from 1 week before to 4 days after the onset of the rash. Fetal damage occurs in up to 90% of cases of infection between 8 and 10 weeks gestation. Multiple defects are common and only perceptive deafness and pigmentary retinopathy occur alone. The risk of damage declines to 10-20% by week 16 and it is rare after that. Other defects include mental handicap, microcephaly, cataract, cardiac abnormalities (PDA and VSD), IUGR and inflammatory lesions of the brain, liver, lungs and bone marrow. Some patients may appear normal at birth.

Ref: Immunisation against infective disease. 1996. DoH. HMSO.

QUESTION 474

A. TRUE B. TRUE C. TRUE D. TRUE E. TRUE

NEC is a mainly a disease of preterm infants. Those less than 32 weeks gestation and 1500g are at greatest risk. Survivors often have long-term nutritional and developmental problems. The aetiology is multifactorial and all the above have been implicated. The common feature of the disease is mucosal and bowel ischaemia secondary to hypoperfusion of the GI tract. The clinical features include abdominal distension, bloody stool, hypovolaemic shock and metabolic acidosis. There is bleeding associated with thrombocytopenia.

Gas may be visible in the wall of the bowel. Treatment is supportive with surgery reserved for those in whom medical treatment has failed.

Ref: Stoelting & Dierdorf. Anaesthesia and Co-Existing Disease. 3rd Ed. Churchill Livingstone. Ch. 32.

QUESTION 475

A. TRUE B. TRUE C. TRUE D. TRUE E. TRUE

Intraosseus access was first described in the 1940s. It provides a safe and reliable method for rapidly administering most drugs and fluids into a non-collapsible marrow venous plexus. It is most useful for those under the age of 6. Onset of action and drug levels are comparable to iv administration. Fluids should be pressurised to overcome resistance of the emissary veins leading from the intramedullary cavity. Complications are minimal and occur in fewer than 1% but include fat and bone marrow emboli, compartment syndrome, skin necrosis, tibial fracture, and osteomyelitis.

Ref: Pediatric Advanced Life Support Manual. American Heart Association. 1997. Ch. 5.

QUESTION 476

A. TRUE B. FALSE C. FALSE D. TRUE E. TRUE

Intraosseus access is most useful for those under the age of 6. Onset of action and drug levels are comparable to iv administration. Fluids should be pressurised to overcome resistance of the emissary veins leading from the intramedullary cavity. Complications are minimal and occur in fewer than 1% but include fat and bone marrow emboli, compartment syndrome, skin necrosis, tibial fracture, and osteomyelitis. The flat anteromedial surface of the tibia 1-3cm below the tibial tuberosity is the preferred site (away from the growth plate).

Ref: Pediatric Advanced Life Support Manual. American Heart Association. 1997. Ch. 5.

QUESTION 477

A. FALSE B. FALSE C. TRUE D. TRUE E. TRUE

The following give rough approximations:

Body weight in kg = 2 × (Age in years + 4)
Defibrillation charge = 2 joules / kg
Correct endotracheal tube size (mm) = (Age in years / 4) + 4
Correct endotracheal length (in cm to the teeth) = (Age in years/2) + 12
5th centile systolic blood pressure = (Age in years × 2) + 70
Median systolic blood pressure is (Age in years × 2) + 90

Ref: Various & Pediatric Advanced Life Support Manual. American Heart Association. 1997. Ch. 2.

QUESTION 478

A. TRUE B. TRUE C. TRUE D. TRUE E. FALSE

Causes of neonatal jaundice include:

* Increased bilirubin production (haemolytic disease; extravasated blood; swallowed maternal blood; sepsis; polycythaemia; haemoglobinopathies; red-cell abnormalities).
* Increased enterohepatic circulation = unconjugated bilirubin (bowel obstruction; meconium plug; hypothyroidism).
* Decreased conjugation (breast milk jaundice; Crigler-Najjar syndrome).
* Impaired hepatocellular transport (Dubin-Johnson; Rotor's; congenital infection; TORCH; Galactosaemia; Tyrosinosis; alpha-1-antitrypsin deficiency; iv feeding).
* Biliary obstruction (atresia; coledochal cyst; bands).

Ref: A neonatal vade-mecum. Fleming & Spiedel. Lloyd-Luke. Ch. 17.

QUESTION 479

A. TRUE B. FALSE C. TRUE D. TRUE E. FALSE

Mean haematological values for the neonate include an Hb of 16.5-18.5 g/dl for the first week of life. This value falls over the next few months. Reticulocyte count at birth is normally 3-7% and this falls to zero by about day 7. Nucleated red cells are common at birth in cord blood (500/ml) but will be only 200/ml by day 1 and absent after day 3. Platelet count follows the normal adult range (150-400).

Ref: A neonatal vade-mecum. Fleming & Spiedel. Lloyd-Luke. Appendix.

QUESTION 480

A. FALSE B. TRUE C. FALSE D. TRUE E. TRUE

Blood gas values for pH and PCO_2 obtained from a capillary sample are generally close to those obtained from an arterial line if the baby is normotensive, well perfused and warm. Arterialized capillary samples are usually 0.65-1.3 kPa (5-10 mmHg) lower than arterial values for PaO_2 < 7.8 kPa (60mmHg). Above this value capillary PO_2 does not reflect arterial PO_2.

Normal arterial values at 24 hrs are: PO_2 = 7.8-10.4 kPa (60-80mmHg); PCO_2 = 3.9-5.2 kPa (30-40mmHg); pH = 7.30-7.35. 1 kPa = approximately 7.5 mmHg

Ref: A neonatal vade-mecum. Fleming & Spiedel. Lloyd-Luke. Appendix.

QUESTION 481

A. TRUE B. FALSE C. TRUE D. TRUE E. FALSE

Urinary pH is usually below 5.3; osmolality may range between 30 - 1400 mosmol/l depending on fluid and hormonal status. Urine normally contains under 150 mg of protein per 24 hrs. Various biochemical investigations can be used to help distinguish prerenal oliguria from acute renal failure; these include specific gravity (high in prerenal, low in renal failure), urine osmolality (high in prerenal, low in renal failure), urine sodium (low in prerenal, high in renal failure) and urine/plasma ratios for osmolality, urea and creatinine.

Ref: **Kumar & Clark. Clinical Medicine, 3rd Ed. W. B. Saunders. Ch. 9.**

QUESTION 482

A. TRUE B. TRUE C. FALSE D. TRUE E. FALSE

The vomiting in pyloric stenosis leads to a loss of hydrogen ions without loss of bicarbonate and it is this bicarbonate generated by gastric mucosal cells that increases plasma levels. Renal compensation initially increases bicarbonate excretion however, the degree of renal compensation may be limited by:

1. concurrent volume depletion leading to decreased glomerular filtration and;
2. loss of chloride ion in the vomitus leading to decreased iso-osmotic sodium reabsorption and ultimately increased hydrogen and potassium ion excretion in exchange for sodium.

The urine therefore becomes inappropriately acidic and stimulates inappropriate bicarbonate reabsorption. The further loss of potassium compounds the hypokalaemia due to vomiting and the associated alkalosis.

Ref: **Zilva JF, Pannall PR & Mayne PD. Clinical Chemistry in Diagnosis and Treatment.**

QUESTION 483

A. TRUE B. TRUE C. TRUE D. TRUE E. FALSE

A number of factors may influence biochemical tests and give erroneous results. Posture has an effect on plasma protein concentrations and hence substances bound to them. Levels tend to be lower in the supine patient. Hyperlipidaemia and hyperproteinaemia may both give rise to spuriously low sodium ion concentrations. Fluoride inhibits red cell glycolysis and thus enables an accurate glucose estimation to be made. Potassium is released from cells, especially platelets, during clotting which leads to over estimation of potassium in the clotted sample. Similarly estimation of calcium from a specimen collected into a tube containing EDTA (ethylenediamine tetra-acetate) will give a spuriously low result as the anticoagulant action of EDTA relies on the chelation / precipitation of calcium.

Ref: **Zilva JF, Pannall PR & Mayne PD. Clinical Chemistry in Diagnosis and Treatment.**

QUESTION 484

A. FALSE B. FALSE C. TRUE D. TRUE E. TRUE

Magnesium is a predominantly intracellular ion present mainly in bone and skeletal muscle. Approximately 35 % is protein bound within the plasma. Magnesium is required for protein and nucleic acid synthesis and is involved in the regulation of potassium and calcium homeostasis. Hypomagnesaemia is predominantly due to severe prolonged diarrhoea or intestinal fistulae. Some cytotoxic drugs e.g. cisplatin may cause hypomagnesaemia by impairing renal tubular reabsorption.

Ref: Zilva JF, Pannall PR & Mayne PD. Clinical Chemistry in Diagnosis and Treatment.

QUESTION 485

A. TRUE   B. TRUE   C. TRUE   D. TRUE   E. TRUE

Hyponatraemia may be associated with normal, decreased or increased extracellular volume and total body sodium content. The differential diagnosis depends on an assessment of the patients extracellular volume. It may rarely be due to hyperlipidaemia or hyperproteinaemia due to techniques of measurement of sodium in the aqueous phase but the expression of the concentration in relation to the total volume of plasma. Plasma osmolality is normal in this situation and the sodium is spuriously low and requires no treatment.

Normal ECF volume hyponatraemia
Abnormal ADH release - vagal neuropathy, Addison's, hypothyroidism, hypokalaemia
SIADH
Stress - surgery, nausea
Major psychiatric illness - psychogenic polydipsia
Increased sensitivity to ADH - chlorpropamide, tolbutamide
ADH like substances - oxytocin, DDAVP
Unmeasured osmotically active substances stimulating ADH release - glucose, alcohol, mannitol

Decreased ECF volume hyponatraemia
Gut loss due to vomiting, diarrhoea, haemorrhage
Renal losses - osmotic diuresis, excess diuretics, adrenocortical insufficiency, tubulo - interstitial renal disease, recovery phase ATN

Increased ECF volume hyponatraemia
Heart failure
Liver failure
Oliguric renal failure
Hypoalbuminaemia

Ref: Kumar & Clark. Clinical Medicine, W. B. Saunders. Ch. 10.

QUESTION 486

A. FALSE   B. FALSE   C. TRUE   D. TRUE   E. FALSE

Only about 0.1% of the total body iron circulates in the plasma , the vast majority (70%) circulates in erythrocyte haemoglobin. Iron is bound to transferrin in the ferric form. Plasma iron concentrations vary between the sexes, probably due to hormonal influences. Androgens tend to increase the level and oestrogens lower it. A rise in iron levels is seen in the first few weeks of pregnancy and with some oral contraceptives. Due to circadian rhythm there is an increase in levels in the morning.

Ref: Zilva JF, Pannall PR & Mayne PD. Clinical Chemistry in Diagnosis and Treatment.

QUESTION 487

A. TRUE B. FALSE C. TRUE D. FALSE E. FALSE

Electrophoresis separates proteins according to their electrical charge and may be performed by applying a small amount of serum to a strip of cellulose acetate and passing a charge across it. The strip is then stained. The proteins separate into five main groups- albumin, alpha 1, alpha 2, beta and gamma globulins. If plasma is used a sixth band - fibrinogen is detected. Total protein estimation is not a particularly useful tool. Acute changes in plasma protein concentration reflect changes in intravascular volume rather than changes in protein per se. Only significant changes in one of the major plasma protein groups e.g. albumin/immunoglobulins is likely to have a significant effect on the total protein estimation. Venous stasis will cause a rise in plasma protein concentration as the combined effect of raised venous pressure and vessel wall hypoxia will cause the leak of water and small molecules out of the vessel increasing the protein concentration.

Ref: Zilva JF, Pannall PR & Mayne PD. Clinical Chemistry in Diagnosis and Treatment.

QUESTION 488

A. TRUE B. TRUE C. FALSE D. FALSE E. TRUE

Albumin, with a molecular weight of 65,000 Da and a plasma half life of 20 days is synthesised in the liver. Approximately 60% of albumin in the extracellular compartment is in the interstitial compartment though the concentration in the plasma compartment is very much higher. Albumin levels vary by as much as 5-10g/litre in the recumbent patient due to fluid redistribution. Analbuminaemia is a rare condition in which despite the complete lack of albumin there is only minimal ankle oedema following prolonged standing

Ref: Zilva JF, Pannall PR & Mayne PD. Clinical Chemistry in Diagnosis and Treatment.

QUESTION 489

A. FALSE B. FALSE C. FALSE D. FALSE E. FALSE

Assessment of free T4 is the first and most useful test of thyroid function. T3 changes tend to mirror those of T4 in most instances. In addition T3 levels are affected by a variety of non thyroid factors. Both T3 and T4 are highly protein bound (> 99%), predominantly to thyroxine binding globulin (TBG), an alpha globulin. TBG levels may be altered by a range of conditions. It is increased by pregnancy, OCP, oestrogens, acute intermittent porphyria, myxoedema and reduced by androgens, danazol, acromegaly and thyrotoxicosis. Thyroid hormones demonstrate only very minor circadian variation and tests may be performed at any time. TRH test is not a first line test and is used only in difficult cases.

Ref: Zilva JF, Pannall PR & Mayne PD. Clinical Chemistry in Diagnosis and Treatment.
Oxford Textbook of Medicine, 3rd Ed. Oxford University Press.

QUESTION 490

A. TRUE B. TRUE C. FALSE D. TRUE E. FALSE

Hypernatraemia is defined as a plasma Na greater than 145 mmol/l. It may be caused by:

Sodium excess e.g. Cushing's syndrome, hyperaldosteronism and following Na bicarbonate therapy due to the sodium load
Free water loss either through renal system e.g. diabetes insipidus or through insensible losses
Sodium loss with excess water loss e.g. osmotic diuresis (mannitol), diabetes mellitus, vomiting and diarrhoea
Inadequate water intake
Drugs - steroids, liquorice and oral contraceptives

Ref: Zilva JF, Pannall PR & Mayne PD. Clinical Chemistry in Diagnosis and Treatment.

QUESTION 491

A. TRUE B. TRUE C. FALSE D. TRUE E. TRUE

Urate is the end product of purine metabolism. Hyperuricaemia may result from a number of mechanisms:

1. Increased urate formation secondary to increased purine synthesis, increased purine intake or increased nucleic acid turnover
2. Decreased excretion

Psoriasis and starvation lead to an increase in nucleic acid turnover and may thus lead to hyperuricaemia. Acidosis reduces renal excretion as do thiazide and loop diuretics. Glucose -6-phosphatase deficiency increases uric acid levels through two mechanisms. Increased purine synthesis due to increased activity in the pentose phosphate pathway and by causing an acidosis which reduces renal urate excretion.

Ref: Zilva JF, Pannall PR & Mayne PD. Clinical Chemistry in Diagnosis and Treatment.

QUESTION 492

A. TRUE B. TRUE C. FALSE D. TRUE E. FALSE

The Carcinoid syndrome results from tumours of argentaffin cells which, under normal circumstances synthesise 5 hydroxytryptamine (serotonin) from the amine precursor tryptophan. 5-HT is metabolised to 5-hydroxyindole acetic acid (5-HIAA) which is excreted in the urine and thus provides a useful tool in the diagnosis of the syndrome. Symptoms of carcinoid, which tend to occur only after the tumour has metastasised include flushing, bronchospasm and profuse diarrhoea which may well be severe enough to cause fluid and electrolyte disturbances. Nicotinamide metabolism may affected by the diversion of tryptophan from nicotinamide synthesis to 5-HT and may result in a pellagra type syndrome.

Carcinoid tumours may also be associated with increased plasma concentrations of gastrin, insulin, ACTH and parathyroid hormone.

Ref: Zilva JF, Pannall PR & Mayne PD. Clinical Chemistry in Diagnosis and Treatment. Oxford Textbook of Medicine, 3rd Ed. Oxford University Press.

QUESTION 493

A. TRUE B. TRUE C. TRUE D. FALSE E. TRUE

The main clinically important causes of hypophosphataemia include:

- Hyperparathyroidism
- Insulin treatment of diabetic ketoacidosis
- Alcoholic withdrawal supported by dextrose infusions
- Proximal renal tubule dysfunction
- Starvation
- Severe burns
- Hypovitaminosis D (rickets, osteomalacia)
- Iatrogenic causes -Hyperalimenation with inadequate phosphate repletion, phosphate binding antacids, anticonvulsants, prolonged use of thiazides and paracetamol due to increased renal losses

Other associations include malabsorption, GH deficiency, diarrhoea, vomiting, severe hypercalcaemia of any cause, gout, pregnancy and hypothyroidism.

Ref: Epstein RJ. Medicine for Examinations. 3rd Ed. Churchill Livingstone. Ch. 8.

QUESTION 494

A. TRUE B. TRUE C. FALSE D. TRUE E. TRUE

Potassium is predominantly an intracellular ion. Hypokalaemia i.e. plasma potassium less than 3.5 mmol/l is caused by:

1. Reduced intake
2. Excessive loss e.g. renal or from GI tract
3. Redistribution i.e. movement into cells under influence of insulin

Cushing's syndrome causes hypokalaemia through a mineralocorticoid action on the distal convoluted tubule. Crush injury tends to cause hyperkalaemia due to potassium release into the plasma from damaged cells.

Ref: Zilva JF, Pannall PR & Mayne PD. Clinical Chemistry in Diagnosis and Treatment.

QUESTION   495

A. TRUE B. FALSE C. TRUE D. TRUE E. TRUE

Addison's disease (primary hypoadrenalism) is a condition in which there is destruction of the entire adrenal cortex and absent or reduced excretion of glucocorticoids, mineralocorticoids and sex hormones. The classic biochemical picture is one of hyponatraemia, hyperkalaemia and increased urea as a consequence of reduced mineralocorticoid action and resultant water depletion. Hypoglycaemia and hypercalcaemia may also occur.

Ref: Zilva JF, Pannall PR & Mayne PD. Clinical Chemistry in Diagnosis and Treatment.

QUESTION   496

A. TRUE B. TRUE C. FALSE D. FALSE E. FALSE

Alkaline phosphatases are a group of enzymes that hydrolyse phosphates at high pH. Though present in most tissues, concentrations are high in the hepatobiliary tree, osteoblasts, intestinal wall, renal tubules and the placenta. Increased levels may be physiological or secondary to bone and liver disease or in malignant involvement of the liver/bone. Low levels are associated with arrested bone growth and hypophosphatasia.

Myeloma in general does not cause increased alkaline phosphatase levels unless there is liver involvement. Acute hepatitis is associated with only modest increases in ALP levels.

Ref: Zilva JF, Pannall PR & Mayne PD. Clinical Chemistry in Diagnosis and Treatment.

QUESTION   497

A. TRUE B. TRUE C. TRUE D. TRUE E. TRUE

Amylase is predominantly present in pancreatic secretions and saliva although may be extracted from a variety of tissues e.g. gonads. It has a relatively low molecular weight and is therefore excreted via the kidneys. Levels may be increased 1-2 times the upper limit of normal in renal failure without significance. In such cases urine amylase levels are low. Spasm of the sphincter of Oddi following morphine administration may also lead to increased plasma levels as do a variety of acute abdominal conditions e.g. ruptured ectopic. Levels tend to be low in the infant under 1 year and patients with cystic fibrosis or pancreatic insufficiency. High levels in alcoholics, pregnancy and diabetic ketoacidosis are of salivary rather than pancreatic origin.

Ref: Zilva JF, Pannall PR & Mayne PD. Clinical Chemistry in Diagnosis and Treatment.

QUESTION   498

A. TRUE B. FALSE C. FALSE D. TRUE E. TRUE

Cushing's syndrome describes the clinical situation in which there is an increased level of circulating cortisol. The resulting biochemical profile is a result of both the glucocorticoid and mineralocorticoid activity of cortisol. Glucose tolerance is impaired leading to hyperglycaemia and glycosuria. The mineralocorticoid action results in the retention of sodium and water which lead to hypertension. Potassium is lost in the urine leading to hypokalaemia which may contribute to the muscle weakness seen in this condition. Increased triglycerides are a common finding in patients with Cushing's even if they are not overtly diabetic. Increased skeletal turnover accounts for the hypercalciuria which may result in urinary tract stones in about 10% of cases.

Ref: Zilva JF, Pannall PR & Mayne PD. Clinical Chemistry in Diagnosis and Treatment.

QUESTION   499

A. TRUE B. TRUE C. FALSE D. FALSE E. FALSE

Creatine kinase (CK) is an enzyme that is abundant in heart and skeletal muscle. It consists of two protein subunits which combine to give 3 isoenzymes enabling the determination of the source tissue. Plasma CK levels are elevated in the muscular dystrophies but do not increase in neurogenic muscular disorders such as multiple sclerosis. Plasma levels may be elevated in hypothyroidism due to decreased breakdown of the enzyme.

Ref: Zilva JF, Pannall PR & Mayne PD. Clinical Chemistry in Diagnosis and Treatment.

QUESTION   500

A. TRUE B. TRUE C. FALSE D. FALSE E. TRUE

Hyperparathyroidism and malignant disease (myeloma, SCC lung and renal cell carcinoma) are the commonest causes of hypercalcaemia. Other endocrine causes include hyperthyroidism (as a direct calcium releasing action of thyroid hormones) and Addison's disease. Paget's disease, milk-alkali syndrome, vitamin D excess and sarcoidosis are also associated with hypercalcaemia. Thiazide diuretics are a rare cause of hypercalcaemia. They increase renal tubular resorption of calcium.

Ref: Zilva JF, Pannall PR & Mayne PD. Clinical Chemistry in Diagnosis and Treatment.

QUESTION   501

A. TRUE B. TRUE C. TRUE D. TRUE E. FALSE

Initiation of insulin treatment may cause oedema as may feeding following malnutrition; the mechanisms for this are complex. Non-steroidal anti-inflammatory drugs may produce oedema where the renin angiotensin system is activated e.g. heart failure, liver cirrhosis. Oestrogen has a mild aldosterone effect; nifedipine, with other calcium channel blockers, may alter capillary pressure by relaxation of pre-capillary arterioles and result in oedema. Metolazone is a powerful thiazide diuretic used in the treatment of heart failure.

Ref: Kumar & Clark. Clinical Medicine, 3rd Ed. W. B. Saunders. Ch. 10.

QUESTION 502

A. FALSE B. FALSE C. TRUE D. TRUE E. FALSE

In hypothyroidism and sick cell syndrome, hyponatraemia with normal extracellular volume occurs. Hypoalbuminaemia secondary to nephrotic syndrome results in hyponatraemia with increased extracellular volume. Causes of hyponatraemia with decreased extracellular volume include gastro-intestinal fluid loss, osmotic diuresis (due to e.g. hyperglycaemia, mannitol), excessive diuretic use and unilateral renal artery stenosis.

Ref: Kumar & Clark. Clinical Medicine, 3rd Ed. W. B. Saunders. Ch. 10.

QUESTION 503

A. TRUE B. TRUE C. TRUE D. FALSE E. TRUE

Excessive use of 0.9% or hypertonic saline, 8.4% sodium bicarbonate or high sodium content drugs (such as piperacillin) may all result in hypernatraemia, as may osmotic diuresis. Desmopressin is a vasopressin analogue which is used in the treatment of diabetes insipidus and haemophilia.

Ref: Kumar & Clark. Clinical Medicine, 3rd Ed. W. B. Saunders. Ch. 10.

QUESTION 504

A. FALSE B. FALSE C. FALSE D. FALSE E. TRUE

Hypomagnesaemia, metabolic alkalosis and increased aldosterone secretion are all associated with hypokalaemia. A 'sine wave' pattern on electrocardiogram is a feature of hyperkalaemia and is a sign of imminent cardiac arrest. Bartter's syndrome comprises hypokalaemia, alkalosis, normal blood pressure and elevated plasma renin and aldosterone; there are many causes of this.

Ref: Kumar & clark. Clinical Medicine, 3rd Ed. W. B. Saunders. Ch. 10.

QUESTION 505

A. TRUE B. TRUE C. TRUE D. TRUE E. TRUE

Hypomagnesaemia occurs when there is diminished intake or absorption and/or increased loss from either the kidney or gastrointestinal tract. If severe (less than 0.7 mmol/l) it results in neurological symptoms, such as hyperreflexia, confusion, hallucinations, convulsions and electrocardiogram changes (e.g. prolonged QT interval, broad flat T waves).

Ref: Kumar & Clark. Clinical Medicine, 3rd Ed. W. B. Saunders. Ch. 10.

QUESTION 506

A. TRUE B. FALSE C. TRUE D. FALSE E. TRUE

Metabolic acidosis with a normal anion gap occurs when either HCl is being retained or $NaHCO_3$ is being lost e.g. in type 4 renal tubular acidosis (aldosterone deficiency) and hyperparathyroidism. If the anion gap is increased there is an excessive amount of an unmeasured anion e.g. lactate, ketones, salicylate.

Ref: Kumar & Clark. Clinical Medicine, 3rd Ed. W. B. Saunders. Ch. 10.

QUESTION 507

A. FALSE B. FALSE C. TRUE D. FALSE E. TRUE

Hypophosphataemia (serum phosphate less than 0.8 mmol/l) may be caused by hyperparathyroidism, carbohydrate administration after fasting, acute alkalosis, ketoacidosis, hypomagnesaemia and chronic alcoholism. It results in muscle weakness, myocardial depression, irritability, convulsions, coma and haematological abnormalities (haemolysis, platelet and leucocyte dysfunction). The oxyhaemoglobin dissociation curve may shift to the left because of reduced 2, 3-diphosphoglycerate. Overtreatment and resultant hyperphosphataemia may cause hypocalcaemia and hypomagnesaemia. Hyperphosphataemia is common in patients with chronic renal failure.

Ref: Kumar & Clark. Clinical Medicine, 3rd Ed. W. B. Saunders. Ch. 10.

QUESTION 508

A. FALSE B. TRUE C. TRUE D. TRUE E. TRUE

Nephrotic syndrome causes a dilutional hyponatraemia. Hypopituitarism produces adrenal failure and so sodium depletion (low sodium with raised potassium and urea).

Causes of hyponatraemia may be divided into pseudo- and true-hyponatraemia:

1. Pseudo-hyponatraemia: The presence of other agents in the plasma causes an apparent reduction in sodium, but the actual plasma sodium in the 'plasma-water' compartment remains normal, e.g. hypertriglyceridaemia, raised gammaglobulins (e.g. myeloma), hyperglycaemia or another osmotic agent (mannitol, ethanol, etc.).

2. True-hyponatraemia: This may be due to sodium depletion or water excess. Sodium depletion may result from renal losses (e.g. diuretic excess, osmotic diuresis in hyperglycaemia, Addison's disease, intrinsic renal disease - nephrocalcinosis, medullary cystic disease), GI losses (e.g. diarrhoea, fistula losses, villous adenoma of colon, bowel obstruction) or skin losses (e.g. heat exposure with inadequate salt replacement). Water excess and dilutional hyponatraemia may be iatrogenic (over-replacement with 5% dextrose without saline) or due to cardiac failure, cirrhosis of the liver, nephrotic syndrome, hypothyroidism and SIADH (syndrome of inappropriate ADH secretion).

Causes of SIADH: Malignancy (small cell lung cancer, pancreas, prostate, adrenal, lymphoma, leukaemia, etc.); intra-cranial causes (malignancy - primary or secondary, CVA, head injury, meningoencephalitis, abscess, intracranial haemorrhage, vasculitis, etc.); chest (pneumonia, TB, abscess, aspergillosis, etc.); drug-induced (e.g. chlorpropamide, opiates, phenothiazines, carbamazepine); and metabolic diseases (e.g. porphyria).

QUESTION 509

A. FALSE B. TRUE C. TRUE D. TRUE E. FALSE

Other causes of hypocalcaemia include chronic renal failure, phosphate therapy, hypomagnesaemia (alcoholism, diabetes, diuretics, amphotericin, aminoglycosides, cyclosporin, cisplatinum, malabsorption, diarrhoea, Conn's syndrome), massive blood transfusion, vitamin D deficiency or resistance. Di George syndrome is congenital parathormone deficiency and is associated with mental retardation, cataracts, calcified basal ganglia and organ-specific AI disease.

Primary hypoparathyroidism is a failure of the parathyroid glands. It may be autoimmune and is associated with other autoimmune diseases such as hypothyroidism, pernicious anaemia, hypogonadism and Addison's disease. Pseudohypoparathyroidism is an end-organ unresponsiveness to PTH. It is associated with short metacarpals and metatarsals and round face and biochemically the patients are similar to those with primary hypoparathyroidism (low calcium, normal or raised phosphate) but with normal or raised alkaline phosphatase and PTH. Patients with pseudo-pseudohypoparathyroidism have the morphological features of pseudohypoparathyroidism but normal calcium.

Ref: Kumar & Clark. Clinical Medicine, 3rd Ed. W. B. Saunders. Ch. 8.

QUESTION 510

A. FALSE B. TRUE C. TRUE D. FALSE E. FALSE

All forms of metabolic alkalosis have a low serum chloride level. Urinary chloride is low when alkalosis is associated with hypovolaemia. Hypovolaemia stimulates ADH secretion and both sodium and chloride are conserved by the kidney. Urine chloride is normal or increased in primary hyperaldosteronism, Bartter's syndrome and Cushing's syndrome.

QUESTION 511

A. FALSE B. TRUE C. FALSE D. TRUE E. TRUE

The anion gap is calculated by $Na - Cl - HCO_3$ (not phosphate); the normal range is 8-12 mEq/l. High anion-gap metabolic acidosis is seen with uraemia, ketoacidosis, lactic acidosis and overdose with aspirin, methanol, ethylene glycol and paraldehyde. A low anion gap is seen with hypoalbuminaemia, paraproteinaemia, hypercalcaemia, hypermagnesaemia and lithium intoxication. Acidosis in the presence of a normal anion gap (bicarbonate loss, hyperchloraemic) is seen in renal tubular acidosis, GI losses (diarrhoea, pancreatic/biliary fistula). Bicarbonate loss through the GI tract and urine (RTA) is increased with acetazolamide.

QUESTION 512

A. TRUE B. TRUE C. FALSE D. FALSE E. FALSE

Causes of hypophosphataemia include insulin treatment of DKA, alcohol withdrawal syndrome treated with IV dextrose, renal tubular acidosis (proximal), osteomalacia (unless accompanied by renal failure), starvation, severe burns, paracetamol overdose (by increased renal excretion) and hyperalimentation, etc. Clinical features include confusion, ataxia and seizures (reduced 2, 6-DPG and tissue hypoxia), bleeding (platelet dysfunction), haemolysis, rhabdomyolysis, renal failure and cardiomyopathy.

QUESTION 513

A. TRUE B. FALSE C. TRUE D. FALSE E. FALSE

The abnormalities are low sodium (severe), low potassium, low serum osmolarity and an inappropriately concentrated urine. The diagnosis is SIADH (syndrome of inappropriate ADH release). In primary adrenal failure (Addison's disease), there is renal loss of sodium with hyponatraemia, but with hypovolaemia, raised potassium and urea. Nephrotic syndrome results in dilutional hyponatraemia and the urine osmolarity is usually lower.

Antidiuretic hormone, ADH (= vasopressin) is synthesised by the paraventricular and supraoptic regions of the hypothalamus. Release is usually controlled by the serum osmolarity (normal range 282-292 mOsm). Inappropriate release is seen in a variety of conditions: malignancy (small cell lung cancer, pancreas, prostate, adrenal, lymphoma, leukaemia, carcinoid, etc.); intracranial causes (malignancy - primary or secondary, CVA, head injury, meningoencephalitis, abscess, intracranial haemorrhage, vasculitis, etc.; chest (pneumonia, TB, abscess, aspergillosis, etc.); drug-induced (e.g. chlorpropamide, opiates, phenothiazines, carbamazepine); and metabolic (e.g. severe pain, porphyria).

Treatment: fluid restriction, demeclocycline, hypertonic saline (very cautiously) and occasionally glucocorticoids. Too-rapid correction of the hyponatraemia may result in central pontine myelinolysis. Search for and try to treat the underlying cause of SIADH (and in elderly patients always exclude hypothyroidism and pneumonia).

QUESTION 514

A. TRUE B. TRUE C. FALSE D. TRUE E. TRUE

Patients with primary polydipsia most commonly present with fitting due to severe hyponatraemia. Up to 80% have underlying schizophrenia. Generally associated with a low plasma osmolality (~275 mOsm/kg c.f. nephrogenic diabetes insipidus where the plasma osmolality rarely falls below 295 mOsm/kg). Diagnosis is by water deprivation test: the normal response is to concentrate the urine (urine osmolality > 800 mOsm/kg); in patients with psychogenic polydipsia the urine osmolality may rise slightly but unless they are contained and prevented access to water scrupulously, the rise is less than normal. In diabetes insipidus the urine remains abnormally dilute (urine osmolality < 400 mOsm/kg).

Persistent hypokalaemia can damage the renal tubules and results in polyuria due to nephrogenic diabetes insipidus. Other causes of this include hypercalcaemia, lithium, demeclocycline and intrinsic renal disease..

QUESTION 515

A. TRUE B. TRUE C. TRUE D. TRUE E. TRUE

Urine specific gravity compares the mass of a solution to an equal volume of water. It is therefore related to but not an exact measure of the number of particles. Urinometer readings should be corrected for temperature, protein and glucose in the urine.

Specific gravity is increased by all the above as well as dextran and radiographic contrast media.

Ref: Wallach. Interpretation of diagnostic test. 5th Ed. Little Brown.

QUESTION 516

A. FALSE B. FALSE C. FALSE D. TRUE E. FALSE

Flecainide is a Type Ic antiarrhythmic drug and binds to activated sodium channel with a long half-life and so demonstrates use-dependence. In the CAST study (Cardiac Arrhythmia Suppression Trial) patients with >6 ventricular premature complexes per hour received flecainide iv; the drug increased mortality in this group of patients. It is very effective (70-80%) in cardioverting patients in acute AF back into sinus rhythm: use with caution in patients with impaired left ventricular function as it is negatively inotropic. In WPW it acts by slowing conduction through the accessory pathway rather than the AV node.

QUESTION 517

A. TRUE B. FALSE C. FALSE D. TRUE E. TRUE

Some drugs are metabolised by enzymes susceptible to polymorphisms which affect their activity. This is the basis of fast and slow acetylation (e.g. hydralazine) and slow and poor metabolism (e.g. debrisoquine). The prevalence of these polymorphisms shows considerable variation between racial groups.

Genetic polymorphisms are determined by abnormalities of gene expression and are not dependent on the pharmacological actions of the drug. However, the consequences of poor metabolism of a particular drug are clearly dependent on its pharmacological actions: drugs with a steep dose-response curve or a low therapeutic index may well produce toxic effects in poor metabolisers.

QUESTION 518

A. TRUE B. FALSE C. TRUE D. FALSE E. TRUE

Angiotensin-converting enzyme inhibitors (ACE inhibitors) have been shown to reduce mortality in congestive cardiac failure and following myocardial infarction. ACE inhibitors inhibit the conversion of angiotensin-I to angiotensin-II, a potent vasoconstrictor. They also result in inhibition of the feedback mechanisms which suppress plasma renin levels - thus plasma renin levels are greatly elevated in patients receiving ACE inhibitors.

One form of secondary hypertension is glucocorticoid suppressible. In these patients the 5'-regulatory region of 11-beta-hydroxylase is linked to aldosterone synthase. Suppression of ACTH by dexamethasone inhibits aldosterone synthesis and reduces blood pressure in these patients.

Renal artery stenosis reduces the blood flow to the kidney and stimulates renin secretion. This in turn leads to high levels of angiotensin-II which drives the hypertension. Inhibition of angiotensin-II production using an ACE inhibitor will reduce blood pressure.

QUESTION 519

A. FALSE B. TRUE C. TRUE D. FALSE E. FALSE

Standard heparin is a mixture of sulphated glycosaminoglycans with a range of molecular weights from 3,000 to 40,000. Low molecular weight heparin is produced from this and has a molecular weight range of 3,000-8,000. These compounds bind antithrombin-III but not thrombin. They are less prone to non-specific effects such as promoting platelet aggregation but are as effective as standard heparin in anticoagulating the patient.

Hirudin is the most potent naturally occurring (in leeches) inhibitor of thrombin. Recombinant hirudin is now available and is being investigated in the treatment of unstable angina and myocardial infarction.

GP IIb/IIIa receptors on platelets are critical for platelet aggregation. Fab fragments of mon-oclonal antibodies against this protein inhibit aggregation and are being investigated in the treatment of unstable angina, prevention of restenosis following angioplasty and a number of other clinical situations.

Alteplase is a recombinant tissue-type plasminogen activator based on the human sequence; unlike streptokinase it is not antigenic. It may be used in patients with antibodies to streptokinase.

Aspirin combined with thrombolytic agents has been shown to reduce mortality in the early period post myocardial infarction.

QUESTION 520

A. TRUE B. FALSE C. TRUE D. TRUE E. TRUE

Originally marketed as an anti-anginal drug, amiodarone is a widely used antiarrhythmic drug with Class III activity. Other side effects of amiodarone include rash, headache, tremor, sleep disturbance, corneal deposits (do not usually interfere with vision), nausea, constipation, peripheral neuropathy and pulmonary fibrosis. It contains high amounts of iodine and can affect thyroid function causing hypothyroidism more frequently than hyperthyroidism. It has a very long half life and accumulates in the liver and thyroid (increasing the density of the liver on CT). Intravenous amiodarone can precipitate profound hypotension and bradycardia and should be used with caution.

QUESTION 521

A. FALSE B. TRUE C. FALSE D. TRUE E. FALSE

The calcium antagonists inhibit calcium INFLUX not efflux. Diltiazem is a benzothiazepine that is a potent coronary vasodilator but less potent on other vascular beds. Its effect on the AV node is to increase the refractory period and slow the heart rate, which makes it useful for treating SVTs. Nifedipine is not licensed for use in pregnancy. There are some reports of teratogenicity in animals but not humans. Other causes of gum hypertrophy include cyclosporin, chronic myelomonocytic leukaemia and phenytoin. Phenytoin is the drug of choice for arrhythmias from digoxin toxicity.

QUESTION 522

A. FALSE B. TRUE C. TRUE D. TRUE E. FALSE

Quinidine is a class Ia antiarrhythmic with good oral bioavailability. 80% is protein bound causing the resulting drug reactions (displacing warfarin and digoxin, etc.). The main indication for use is atrial arrhythmias. It has a slight vagolytic effect and may accelerate the ventricular rate in AF unless digoxin is given concomitantly.
Disopyramide has both class Ia and III activity and an anticholinergic effect. For similar reasons to quinidine it should not be used for AF alone.

QUESTION 523

A. TRUE B. FALSE C. TRUE D. FALSE E. FALSE

Digoxin toxicity may be precipitated by:

*   *Metabolic imbalance* – hypokalaemia, hypomagnesaemia, hypercalcaemia, hypoxia, hypothyroidism.
*   *Drug interactions* – either displacement from protein binding (e.g. quinidine, amiodarone, etc.) or by inhibiting tubular secretion of digoxin (calcium channel blockers, nifedipine, verapamil).
*   *Other predisposing factors* – old age, renal failure, cardiac amyloid, pre-existing cardiac disease.

Toxicity may cause pulsus bigeminus, bradycardias, AV block, SVTs and ventricular arrhythmias. Patients notice nausea, vomiting, abdominal pain, xanthopsia (yellow vision), confusion and blurred vision. Treatment: stop digoxin and correct electrolyte abnormalities. Phenytoin for tachyarrhythmias and atropine or pacing for bradyarrhythmias. Antidigoxin antibodies or dialysis may be required.

QUESTION 524

A. TRUE B. TRUE C. FALSE D. TRUE E. FALSE

Enoximone is a selective phosphodiesterase inhibitor and exerts most of its effects on the myocardium. It reduces afterload and increases cardiac contractility and cardiac output.

Adrenaline acts on both alpha and beta receptors. At low doses, beta effects predominate (tachycardia, increased cardiac output, lower SVR) but at higher doses alpha effects take over with peripheral vasoconstriction. Noradrenaline is mainly an alpha-agonist and increases the SVR. Isoprenaline is a beta-agonist and produces a tachycardia, increasing myocardial consumption. Dobutamine increases cardiac output and vasodilates by acting on beta-adrenergic receptors.

QUESTION 525

A. TRUE B. FALSE C. TRUE D. TRUE E. TRUE

Digoxin toxicity may be precipitated by either displacement from protein binding (e.g. quinidine, amiodarone, etc.) or by inhibiting tubular secretion of digoxin (calcium channel blockers, nifedipine, verapamil). Metabolic imbalance (such as hypokalaemia, hypomagnesaemia, hypercalcaemia, hypoxia or hypothyroidism) can also trigger toxicity. Amphotericin can produce severe hypokalaemia and hypomagnesaemia and thus precipitate digoxin toxicity.

QUESTION 526

A. FALSE B. FALSE C. FALSE D. FALSE E. TRUE

The volume of distribution (Vd) of the drug determines how effective dialysis will be in removing the drug from the body. Drugs for which haemodialysis is effective include salicylates, phenobarbitone, methanol, ethylene glycol and lithium. Digoxin, opiates, tricyclics and lipid-soluble beta-blockers have a very large Vd. More effective supportive measures are antidigoxin antibody/atropine/correction of hypokalaemia for digoxin; naloxone for pethidine; beta-blockers for arrhythmias from tricyclics, pacing/glucagon/isoprenaline for propranolol.

Haemoperfusion is effective for short and medium acting barbiturates, chloral hydrate, meprobamate and theophylline.

Activated charcoal should be given for aspirin, carbamazepine, dapsone, phenobarbitone, quinine and theophylline.

QUESTION 527

A. TRUE B. FALSE C. TRUE D. FALSE E. TRUE

In first-order kinetics, the rate of elimination of a drug is dependent on the concentration of the drug and this applies to the majority of drugs in clinical use (the concentration of the drug in plasma falls in an exponential manner). Zero-order (or saturation kinetics) refers to the situation where the rate of elimination is independent of concentration and the drug levels fall at a constant rate. Examples of this are ethanol and salicylate. Phenytoin elimination is first-order at low concentrations and then zero-order.

One consequence of zero-order metabolism is that the duration of action of the drug is more dependent on the dose and another is that once the maximum rate of elimination is reached, in theory the concentration of the drug in the body can increase indefinitely with no steady-state level being achieved.

QUESTION 528

A. FALSE B. FALSE C. TRUE D. TRUE E. TRUE

The most common adverse drug reactions are gastrointestinal (nausea) and dermatological (rashes). Approximately 3% of hospital admissions are directly related to adverse drug interactions.

QUESTION 529

A. TRUE B. FALSE C. FALSE D. TRUE E. FALSE

Theophylline poisoning produces vomiting, restlessness and agitation, tachycardia, dilated pupils, haematemesis and tachyarrhythmias. Hypokalaemia and hyperglycaemia may be found. Elimination may be enhanced by activated charcoal. Correction of hypokalaemia is effective in reducing the risk of tachyarrhythmias. Other drugs effectively cleared by charcoal include aspirin, carbamazepine, dapsone, phenobarbitone and quinine.

Haemodialysis is effective in removing salicylates, phenobarbitone, methanol, ethylene glycol and lithium. Forced alkaline diuresis is no longer recommended for salicylates and bicarbonate infusion is as effective.

Tricyclics delay gastric emptying time and thus gastric lavage should still be attempted.

QUESTION 530

A. FALSE B. FALSE C. FALSE D. TRUE E. TRUE

Drugs can harm the fetus by altering organ development in the first trimester of pregnancy or inhibiting organ function later in gestation. ACE inhibitors impair fetal renal function and are associated with oligohydramnios and neonatal anuria. Methyldopa is the safest drug for the treatment of blood pressure in pregnancy. Low-dose aspirin is used in patients with pre-eclampsia. Warfarin can cause fetal intracranial haemorrhage and is associated with chondrodysplasia punctata. Carbamazepine and phenytoin can both cause early neonatal haemorrhage (vitamin K deficiency related) and are teratogenic (carbamazepine - CNS, limb and cardiac; phenytoin - craniofacial, limb; valproate - neural tube).

QUESTION 531

A. TRUE B. TRUE C. TRUE D. TRUE E. TRUE

Stevens-Johnson syndrome is most commonly precipitated by a drug (sulphonamides, penicillin, some sedatives) but also occurs with viral infections (cf. Herpes simplex), and some malignancies. Characterised by fever, arthralgia, myalgia, pneumonitis, uveitis, vesicles on the oro-genital mucosa and conjunctiva, with 'target' lesions on the skin. Treatment: topical calamine, steroids (topical and systemic in severe cases).

QUESTION 532

A. TRUE B. TRUE C. TRUE D. FALSE E. FALSE

Diazepam is metabolised to nordiazepam which is further metabolised to oxazepam, both of which are still active benzodiazepines. Amitryptilline is metabolised to nortryptilline which is still an active tricyclic antidepressant. Zidovudine is an inactive pro-drug and is metabolised to zidovudine triphosphate which is the active drug. Other drugs with active metabolites include heroin and codeine (to morphine), propranolol (to 4-hydroxy propranolol), imipramine (to desmethylimipramine). Pro-drugs that require activation include cortisone (to hydrocortisone), prednisone (to prednisolone), cyclophosphamide (to phosphoramide mustard), azathioprine (to mercaptopurine) and enalapril (to enalaprilat).

QUESTION 533

A. TRUE B. TRUE C. FALSE D. TRUE E. TRUE

For beta-blocker overdose, try atropine, glucagon infusion and temporary pacing. Tricyclic overdose may require iv neostigmine to counteract the anticholinergic effects and a beta-blocker for treatment of SVTs. Phenytoin is useful for convulsions and VT in TCA poisoning. Other antidotes include desferrioxamine for iron, calcium EDTA and/or dimecaprol for lead poisoning, dimecaprol for heavy metal poisoning, ethanol for ethylene glycol, dicobalt edetate for cyanide, digoxin-specific antibody for digoxin, naloxone for opiates, N-acetylcysteine for paracetamol, Fuller's earth for paraquat, vitamin K for warfarin.

QUESTION 534

A. TRUE B. TRUE C. TRUE D. FALSE E. FALSE

Chlorpropamide, carbamazepine, thiazides and ethacrynic acid all increase sensitivity of tubules to ADH. Chlorpropamide is ineffective for nephrogenic diabetes insipidus but is effective in incomplete central diabetes insipidus. Lithium (along with demeclocycline and amphotericin B) are recognised causes of nephrogenic diabetes insipidus.

QUESTION 535

A. TRUE B. TRUE C. TRUE D. FALSE E. FALSE

Drugs that undergo extensive pre-systemic elimination (first-pass metabolism) include aspirin, chlormethiazole, chlorpromazine, dextropropoxyphene, GTN, imipramine, isosorbide dinitrate, levodopa, lignocaine, metoprolol, morphine, nortryptilline, pethidine, propranolol, salbutamol, verapamil. Gentamicin is not absorbed orally. Ciprofloxacin has excellent oral bioavailability.

QUESTION 536

A. TRUE B. FALSE C. TRUE D. FALSE E. TRUE

Other drugs that cause pulmonary fibrosis include busulphan, chloramphenicol, bleomycin, nitrofurantoin, melphlan and paraquat. Lung fibrosis is also a feature of tuberculosis, Aspergillus infection, Klebsiella pneumoniae, silicosis, radiation, chronic extrinsic allergic alveolitis, coal workers pneumoconiosis (all mainly upper lobes). Lower zone lung fibrosis is a feature of bronchiectasis, asbestosis, rheumatoid arthritis, scleroderma, radiation, cryptogenic fibrosing alveolitis, sarcoidosis, tuberose sclerosis and neurofibromatosis.

QUESTION 537

A. TRUE B. TRUE C. TRUE D. FALSE E. FALSE

The list of drugs unsafe for patients with acute intermittent porphyria is vast. Drugs which are safe are easier to remember and include aspirin and pethidine (analgesia for acute attacks), chlorpromazine and diazepam (sedation for agitation, psychosis, etc.), penicillin (for infections), beta-blockers, thiazides (for hypertension), bumetanide and amiloride (for fluid retention), glipizide (for NIDDM), certrizine, chlorpheniramine and steroids (for allergic reactions).

QUESTION 538

A. TRUE B. TRUE C. TRUE D. FALSE E. TRUE

Nicorandil is a powerful coronary vasodilator due to its effect as a potassium channel opener and is used in the treatment of angina. The side-effect profile is similar to nitrates.

Losartan (and valsartan) are specific angiotensin II receptor antagonists (at the AT1 receptor) used in the treatment of hypertension. They have similar properties to ACE inhibitors but unlike the latter do not inhibit the breakdown of bradykinin and so cough is not a common side effect.

Nitroprusside is an arteriolar vasodilator that releases nitric oxide, a potent vasodilator.

Gabapentin potentiates GABA responses and blocks sodium channels and is used as an antiepileptic.
Lanzoprazole (like omeprazole) is a proton pump inhibitor used in the treatment of peptic ulcer disease.

QUESTION 539

A. TRUE B. TRUE C. FALSE D. FALSE E. FALSE

There are at least two kinds of alpha adrenergic receptor: the alpha1 receptors are found on vascular smooth muscle cell membranes and stimulation produces vasoconstriction; alpha2 receptors are found on the presynaptic nerve terminals and arterioles of human skin together with alpha1 receptors. On the presynaptic terminals, activation reduces neurotransmitter release. The effects of alpha stimulation (e.g. with noradrenaline) results in vasoconstriction and hypertension, decreased insulin secretion in response to a glucose load and axillary sweating. Lipolysis is beta adrenergic receptor mediated.

QUESTION 540

A. TRUE B. FALSE C. TRUE D. TRUE E. TRUE

The endothelins are a family of vasoactive peptides. Three members have been identified: endothelin-I is the most potent vasoconstrictor identified to date. It stimulates growth in a number of cell types including vascular smooth muscle cells.

The endothelins are generated from precursor molecules by endothelin–converting enzyme (like angiotensin II by ACE). The enzymes degrading endothelins have not yet been characterised but include endopeptidase-24.11.

Nitric oxide (also known as EDRF-endothelium derived relaxant factor) is cleaved from L-arginine by nitric oxide synthetase. NO is produced continuously by the vascular endothelium and maintains the vasculature in a state of active vasodilatation; thus antagonists (e.g. L-NMMA or L-NAME) produce vasoconstriction in normal human volunteers. NO stimulates soluble guanylate cyclase to produce cyclic GMP which mediates its actions. Inhibition of cGMP breakdown will potentiate NO activity.

QUESTION 541

A. TRUE B. FALSE C. TRUE D. TRUE E. TRUE

Felty's syndrome is Rheumatoid arthritis associated with splenomegaly and neutropenia, whilst Caplan's syndrome is a nodular pulmonary fibrosis in patients with Rheumatoid that have been exposed to various industrial dusts. Effusions are the commonest lung problem, whilst nodules may be mistaken for carcinoma. The fibrosing alveolitis found in Rheumatoid is indistinguishable from the cryptogenic form.

Ref: Kumar & Clark. Clinical Medicine, 3rd Ed. W. B. Saunders. Ch. 8.

QUESTION 542

A. TRUE B. FALSE C. FALSE D. FALSE E. FALSE

Calcium pyrophosphate crystals are brick-shaped and positively birefringent, whilst uric acid crystals of gout are needle-shaped and negatively birefringent. Renal stones due to uric acid deposition and tophi only occur in gout. Allopurinol is the treatment of choice in gout.

Ref: Kumar & Clark. Clinical Medicine, 3rd Ed. W. B. Saunders. Ch. 8.

QUESTION 543

A. TRUE B. FALSE C. TRUE D. TRUE E. FALSE

Anti-ds DNA antibodies are associated with Systemic lupus erythematosis (SLE), while the anti-cardiolipin antibody is associated with both SLE and cardiolipin syndrome/antiphospholipid syndrome (a connective tissue disease originally thought to be a variant of SLE but now considered a condition in it's own right). CREST syndrome is calcinosis (C), Raynaud's phenomenon (R), oesophageal involvement (E), sclerodactyly (S) and telangiectasia (T).

Ref: Kumar & Clark. Clinical Medicine, 3rd Ed. W. B. Saunders. Ch. 8.

QUESTION 544

A. FALSE   B. FALSE   C. TRUE   D. FALSE   E. TRUE

Rheumatoid arthritis is a symmetrical polyarticular arthritis i.e. more than four joints are involved and although rheumatoid factor is present in 80% of cases, it is not essential to the diagnosis. Neutrophils are present in the synovial fluid under several circumstances and therefore, the presence of bacteria is the only true way to differentiate.

Ref: Kumar & Clark. Clinical Medicine, 3rd Ed. W. B. Saunders. Ch. 8.

QUESTION 545

A. TRUE   B. TRUE   C. FALSE   D. FALSE   E. FALSE

The Boutonniere and Swan neck deformities are classically found in the fingers of patients with Rheumatoid arthritis. Osler's nodes are hand lesions found in patients with infective endocarditis.

Ref: Kumar & Clark. Clinical Medicine, 3rd Ed. W. B. Saunders. Ch. 8.

QUESTION 546

A. FALSE   B. TRUE   C. FALSE   D. TRUE   E. TRUE

Immune-complex mediated glomerulonephritis is a penicillamine induced condition which limits the use of penicillamine in the treatment of some patients with Rheumatoid arthritis. Although both retro-peritoneal fibrosis and renal cell carcinoma can occur in any circumstance, they are not specifically associated with Rheumatoid arthritis.

Ref: Kumar & Clark. Clinical Medicine, 3rd Ed. W. B. Saunders. Ch. 8.

QUESTION 547

A. TRUE   B. TRUE   C. TRUE   D. TRUE   E. TRUE

The following are all accepted complications of Systemic lupus erythematosis (SLE): glomerulonephritis; cerebellar ataxia; pericarditis; aseptic necrosis of the hip; restrictive lung defect.

Ref: Kumar & Clark. Clinical Medicine, 3rd Ed. W. B. Saunders. Ch. 8.

QUESTION 548

A. TRUE B. TRUE C. TRUE D. FALSE E. TRUE

Although antinuclear antibodies occur frequently in systemic sclerosis, they can occur in other conditions such as systemic lupus erythematosis.

Ref: Kumar & Clark. Clinical Medicine, 3rd Ed. W. B. Saunders. Ch. 8.

QUESTION 549

A. FALSE B. TRUE C. TRUE D. FALSE E. FALSE

Polyarteritis nodosa is more common in men than women. Churg-Strauss syndrome is a condition associated to Polyarteritis nodosa with allergic angiitis, granuloma formation and asthma. The cause of the granulomas in Wegener's is unknown but is not due to immune complex deposition. Polymyalgia rheumatica is a relatively benign condition treated with corticosteroids, but rarely there may be an associated temporal arteritis which could lead to permanent visual defects and neurological defects unless treated quickly.

Ref: Kumar & Clark. Clinical Medicine, 3rd Ed. W. B. Saunders. Ch. 8.

QUESTION 550

A. TRUE B. FALSE C. TRUE D. FALSE E. TRUE

Keratoconjunctivitis sicca is part of the sicca syndrome that occurs in Sjögren's syndrome as well as other rheumatological disorders, whilst Keratoderma blenorrhagica is a skin condition seen in Reiter's syndrome. Although senile cataracts may occur in rheumatological diseases they are not a specific complication. Vitreal haemorrhages may be associated with Systemic lupus erythematosis.

Ref: Kumar & Clark. Clinical Medicine, 3rd Ed. W. B. Saunders. Ch. 8.

QUESTION 551

A. FALSE B. TRUE C. TRUE D. TRUE E. TRUE

Patients with polymyalgia are typically >50 years and present with proximal muscle tenderness and weakness; shoulder and pelvic muscle stiffness are worse in the mornings. Other features include anorexia, weight loss and low-grade fevers. Investigations: ESR > 50 mm/h; elevated alkaline phosphatase and gamma-GT; normal creatinine kinase, EMG and muscle biopsy. The condition responds to low-dose steroids. 50% of patients with temporal arteritis have symptoms of polymyalgia and 50% of patients with polymyalgia have temporal arteritis on biopsy.

QUESTION 552

A. TRUE B. TRUE C. TRUE D. TRUE E. TRUE

Ankylosing spondylitis is a disease of the insertions of tendons into bone (i.e. an enthesitis). This produces heel pain (plantar fasciitis), achilles tendonitis, quadriceps tendonitis, iliac crest pain, etc. In addition, other organ systems may be involved. Chest pains are common and may be due to pericarditis, costochondral disease or dilatation of the aortic root and aortic incompetence (aortic valve involvement is accompanied by first-degree heart block). Other features include urethritis and chronic prostatitis, anterior uveitis, apical pulmonary fibrosis, cauda equina syndrome and amyloidosis.

QUESTION 553

A. TRUE B. TRUE C. TRUE D. TRUE E. TRUE

Pulmonary involvement in rheumatoid arthritis may precede the onset of arthritis. Commonly it produces pleural adhesions and effusions (typically the effusion has low glucose). Obliterative bronchiolitis is a rare but recognised complication and may respond to steroid therapy. Stridor is due to involvement of the cricoaryetenoid joints and may be accompanied by dyspnoea and occasionally obstruction necessitating tracheostomy. Rheumatoid nodules, single or multiple, may occur in the lungs and frequently cavitate. Caplan's syndrome occurs in patients exposed to coal or other inorganic dusts. There is massive pulmonary fibrosis and nodule formation. Pulmonary fibrosis is less common but occurs with chronic disease.

QUESTION 554

A. TRUE B. TRUE C. FALSE D. FALSE E. TRUE

Other infective agents that have been associated with a reactive arthritis include *Salmonella*, and *Yersenia*. Arthralgia (but no arthritis) may occur following infections with influenza virus, Coxsackie virus, EBV, mumps, *Mycoplasma pneumoniae* and *Brucella*. Clinically there is usually knee or joint pain and swelling which settles over 3 months. 50% will have a recurrence of the disease.

QUESTION 555

A. TRUE B. TRUE C. FALSE D. FALSE E. FALSE

An acute attack may be treated with NSAIDs and/or colchicine. A short course of corticosteroids (oral or injected into the inflamed joint - once infection is excluded) produces symptomatic relief.

Allopurinol should not be given in the acute stages as it increases the pain and inflammation.

Paracetamol is usually inadequate in the early stages. Probenecid increases renal excretion of urate and may be used for long-term prophylaxis but exacerbates symptoms in an acute attack. Other drugs to avoid in gouty patients (i.e. drugs that inhibit urate excretion) are thiazides, ethambutol, low-dose salicylates and cyclosporin A.

NOTES

NOTES

NOTES

QBase Anaesthesia: 3
on CD-ROM

SYSTEM REQUIREMENTS

An IBM compatible PC with a minimum 80386 processor and 4Mb of RAM VGA Monitor set up to display at least 256 colours.

CD-ROM drive

Windows 3.1 or higher with Microsoft compatible mouse

The display setting of your computer must be set to display "SMALL FONTS".

See Windows manuals for furthe instructions on how to do this.

INSTALLATION INSTRUCTIONS

The program will install the appropriate files onto your hard drive. It requires the QBase CD-ROM to be installed in the D:\drive.

In order to run to run QBase the CD-ROM must be in the drive.

Print Readme.txt and Helpfile.txt on the CD-ROM for fuller instructions and user manual

WINDOWS 95

1. Insert the QBase CD-ROM into drive **D:**
2. From the **Start Menu,** select the RUN **option**
3. Type **D:\setup.exe and press enter or return**
4. **Follow the Full Installation** option and accept the default directory for installation of QBase.
   The installation program creates a folder called **QBase** containing the program icon and another called **Exams** into which you can save previous exam attempts.
5. To run QBase double click the **QBase** icon in the QBase folder. From windows Explorer double click the **QBase.exe** file in the QBase folder.

WINDOWS 3.1/WINDOWS FOR WORKGROUPS 3.11

1. Insert the QBase CD-ROM into the drive D:
2. From the **File Menu,** select the **RUN option**
3. Type **D:\setup.exe and press enter or return**
4. Follow the instructions given by the installation program. Select the **Full Installation** option and accept the default directory for installation of QBase

   The Installation program creates a program window and directory called **QBase** containing the program icon. It also creates a directory called **Exams** into which you can save previous attempts.
5. To run QBase double click on the **QBase** icon in the QBase program. From File Manager double click the **QBase.exe** file in the QBase directory.